HANDBOOK OF

Home Health Standards

Quality, Documentation, and Reimbursement

FIFTH EDITION

Tina M. Marrelli
MSN, MA, RN
Health Care Consultant
Editor, *Home Healthcare Nurse*

With assistance from

Patrice D. Artress
PhD, RN
Health Care Consultant

MOSBY
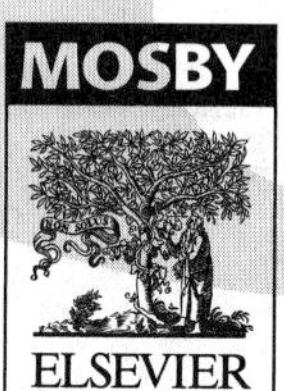
ELSEVIER

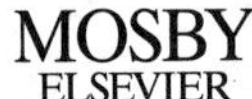

11830 Westline Industrial Drive
St. Louis, Missouri 63146

HANDBOOK OF HOME HEALTH STANDARDS:
QUALITY, DOCUMENTATION,
AND REIMBURSEMENT, FIFTH EDITION ISBN 978-0-323-05224-5

Notice

Neither the Publisher nor the Author assumes any responsibility for any loss or injury and/or damage to persons or property arising out of or related to any use of the material contained in this book. It is the responsibility of the treating practitioner, relying on independent expertise and knowledge of the patient, to determine the best treatment and method of application for the patient.

The Publisher

Library of Congress Cataloging-in-Publication Data
Marrelli, T. M.
Handbook of home health standards : quality, documentation, and reimbursement / Tina M. Marrelli ; with assistance from Patrice D. Artress. -- 5th ed.
p. ; cm.
Rev. ed. of: Handbook of home health standards & documentation guidelines for reimbursement. 4th ed. c2001.
Includes bibliographical references and index.
ISBN 978-0-323-05224-5 (pbk. : alk. paper) 1. Home care services--Standards--United States--Handbooks, manuals, etc. 2. Home care services--United States--Medical records--Handbooks, manuals, etc. 3. Insurance, Health--United States--Handbooks, manuals, etc. 4. Medicare--Handbooks, manuals, etc. I. Artress, Patrice D. II. Marrelli, T. M. Handbook of home health standards & documentation guidelines for reimbursement. III. Title.
[DNLM: 1. Home Care Services--standards--United States--Handbooks. 2. Insurance, Health, Reimbursement--United States--Handbooks. 3. Reimbursement Mechanisms--United States--Handbooks. WY 49 M358hb 2009]
RA645.35.M37 2009
362.1'4021873--dc22
2008016005

Acquisitions Editor: Linda Thomas
Developmental Editor: Carlie Irwin
Book Production Manager: Gayle May
Project Manager: Tracey Schriefer
Designer: Paula Catalano

Printed in the United States of America

Last digit is the print number: 9 8 7 6 5 4 3 2 1

REVIEWERS

Ida Blevins, RHIA
Supervisor, Reimbursement and Information Management
St. John's Hospital Home Health Services
Springfield, Illinois

Beki Burtscher, RN, BSN
Chief Executive Officer
Live Longer at Home Health Care Services, Inc.
Arcadia, Florida

Barbara Campbell, RN, MS, CNS
Home Care/Hospice Consultant
Good Samaritan Home Health Care
Sioux Falls, South Dakota

Arlene J. Chabanuk, MSN, RN, CDE, HCS-D
Project Coordinator
Quality Insights of Pennsylvania
Wayne, Pennsylvania

Cindy Farris, MPH, BSN, RN
Medical Assistant, Program Faculty Member
South College
Knoxville, Tennessee

Blake Godfrey, MS, CCC-SLP
Director of Rehabilitation Services,
Speech Language Pathologist
Caring Nurses, Inc.
Las Vegas, Nevada

Claire Gold, MSPT, MBA, CPHQ, COS-C
National Manager, Therapy Practice
Gentiva Health Services
Melville, New York

Margery Harvey-Griffith, MS, RN
Vice President Operations
Boca Home Care, Inc.
Boca Raton, Florida

Nancy H. Kendrick, RN, MS
Clinical and Operations Consultant
Hammonds and Consociates, Inc.
Atlanta, Georgia

Diana L. Kornetti, MA, PT, HCS-D, COS-C
Administrator/Co-Owner
Integrity Home Health Care, Inc.
Ocala, Florida

Cindy Krafft, PT, MS, COS-C
Assistant Director Operational Consulting—Rehabilitation
Fazzi Associates, Inc.
Northampton, Massachusetts

Mary Curry Narayan, MSN, APRN, BC, CTN
Home Health Nursing Clinical Specialist, Transcultural Nurse Specialist, Nursing Education Consultant
Visiting Nurse Service Network
Vienna, Virginia

Janet Puglisi, RN, BSN
Director
Professional Home Health Care, Inc.
Denver, Colorado

Jeanne Ryan, MA, OTR, CHCE, COS-C
Executive Director
VNA and Hospice of Cooley Dickinson, Inc.
Northampton, Massachusetts

Rebecca B. Smarr, PT, COS-C
Physical Therapist and Home Health Consultant
Kingwood, Texas

Joanne Steemer, RN, BSN, CLNC, HCS-D, CCP
Administrator
Medical Legal Connection
Duncanville, Texas

Martha A. Tice, MS, RN, ACHPN
Clinical Educator
Capital Hospice
Falls Church, Virginia

Deanna Whitlatch, RN, BS
Manager, Provider Outreach and Education
Cahaba GBA
Des Moines, Iowa

Sandra Whittier, RN, BC, MSN, COS-C
Admission Nurse/Educator
Northeast Senior Health
Beverly, Massachusetts

Rhonda M. Will, RN, BS, COS-C, HCS-D
Assistant Director, Home Care Quality Institute
Fazzi Associates, Inc.
Northampton, Massachusetts

PREFACE

Some years ago, this book started out as a very slim, small, pocket-sized red book. It was written for a great team of home care and hospice clinicians in the 1980s. In the ensuing years, home care has faced many challenges, including the interim payment system, the prospective payment system (PPS), and most recently the "refinement" of the PPS.

The changes have been so significant that in this revised fifth edition even the title has changed; quality, reimbursement, and documentation will be the drivers for health care into the future. Those of you who knew the first four editions as the "little red book" can still refer to this text with the knowledge that by following these guidelines you are assisting your organizations, your patients, and their families by providing quality care. Like previous editions, this handbook provides both new and experienced nurses, therapists, social workers, and other clinicians the tools to support coverage and medical necessity through documentation while providing skillful home health care to patients and their families.

Even if your clinical documentation is totally automated, this book is a needed review; for this reason, thousands of clinicians carry them in their visit bags. The care planning and other information in this handbook assists in individualizing patient care because there is no way in the complexity of home health care that we can know and remember it all!

GUIDELINES FOR USE

Home health care has changed in ways that were unimagined when this book was first published over 20 years ago. The fifth edition represents a major revision of this widely used handbook, and the purpose remains the same: to provide information and resources to enhance the quality of care, to emphasize the importance of clinical documentation, and to assist in appropriate reimbursement of services provided to patients and families in their homes. Home care has changed radically over the years; so too has this totally rewritten fifth edition.

This handbook contains 26 care guidelines: A Template for Quality Care of the Older Adult, The Hospice and Palliative Care Guideline, 12 Adult "Medical Surgical" Care Guidelines, and 12 "Maternal Child" Care Guidelines. Like the fourth edition, the adult clinical care and maternal child guidelines are arranged alphabetically and in order of body systems (e.g., cardiovascular, integumentary, musculoskeletal).

These care guidelines provide new and experienced home care clinicians examples of interventions and other considerations to assist in assessment, care planning, reimbursement, and other processes. The emphasis on the importance of teaching interventions is emphasized and reiterated throughout this fifth edition. The systems-based model continues; home health care organizations and clinicians think in groups of similar or "like" patients, such as patients with heart failure or other aggregate populations. In fact, the PPS is based on a number of home health resource groups (HHRGs), which is one way to categorize patients into a specialized case mix with similar characteristics, with the rationale that the resource utilization for this group of patients is usually comparable.

Certain assumptions have been made regarding home health care services; the main assumption is that provided services meet recognized organizational and payer standards and are therefore justified and appropriate for reimbursement.

Part One: Home Care: A Unique Specialty presents information about home care and addresses fundamentals for effective practice and operations that new and experienced clinicians will find helpful. Also included is an overview of documentation and the many roles documentation plays in assessment, care planning, coordination, coverage, and reimbursement of home care services. Because coding plays an increasing role of importance in compliance and reimbursement, this edition also specifies coding standards.

Part Two: Clinical Practice in Home Care presents an overview and provides practical insights for effective home care practice; describes the basic requirements for the Outcome and Assessment Information Set (OASIS), details a patient example and the corresponding comprehensive assessment with the OASIS, Plan of Care (POC), and HHRG worksheet; and discusses home health quality initiatives including Home Health Compare, Outcome-Based Quality Monitoring, Outcome-Based Quality Improvement, and others.

Part Three: Adult Clinical Guidelines: A Systems Approach for Assessment, Care Planning, and Documentation

1. **General Considerations**—This section contains general considerations such as statistics and aspects of care that impact the health of the home care population.

2. **Potential Diagnoses and Codes**—This section lists some of the most commonly seen conditions in home care related to the system and lists the International Classification of Diseases, Ninth Revision, Clinical Modification (ICD-9-CM) codes. The source for all the codes was the current edition of the ICD-9-CM. The codes are listed alphabetically to assist in easy identification.

Because coding is important in health care, the ICD-9-CM system contains more than 10,000 diagnosis code categories and more than 40,000 cross-referenced diagnosis terms; there are more codes than could be listed in this handbook. *This book is not intended to be used as a stand-alone coding book; when additional information or codes are needed, readers should refer to official coding books and a qualified, credentialed coder.*

3. **OASIS Considerations**—This section highlights certain OASIS data elements and emphasizes the complete, accurate, and timely completion of the data elements as an integral part of comprehensive assessment and the primary basis for determining the patient's HHRG in the PPS model.

4. **Associated Nursing Diagnoses**—This section refers readers to Part Seven for a listing of the most recent approved nursing diagnoses. In the interest of keeping this text a handbook, in the fifth edition, the list is located in one place in its entirety for easy review and retrieval of needed information. The identified nursing diagnoses are approved by the North American Nursing Diagnosis Association-International (NANDA-I) and may be used as the focus for intervention by nurses in home care practice.

5. **Supportive Factors for the Determination and Documentation of Homebound Status**—In this section, specific examples of patients by system illustrate homebound status. Please keep in mind that these are examples only. Patients' reasons for homebound status will vary and must be documented in terms of functional limitations and other health-related reasons; the documentation must show that the patient has a "normal inability to leave home," if they leave home it is with "considerable and taxing effort," and those absences meet the listed, definitional requirements. Readers are referred to the *Medicare Home Health Agency Manual* and Part Six for actual language related to homebound status.

Homebound is an admission and qualifying criteria for Medicare home care. It is imperative that the documentation for homebound patients supports the Medicare definition of homebound. Readers are encouraged to memorize and/or review the Medicare definition of homebound. There are examples of homebound in the *Medicare Home Health Agency Manual*. In addition, the OASIS data elements must be congruent and "paint the picture" that the patient is homebound. Questions about homebound status should be referred to your manager.

6. **Potential Interdisciplinary Goals and Outcomes—** Patient-centered goals/outcomes are a required component of the POC and help the clinician project what will be achieved as a result of care and interventions with the patient and family/caregiver. Goals or outcomes often begin with the statement "By the end of the projected episode of care, the patient and/or caregiver will…." Like all components of care planning, these will be individualized to your patients and families and determined to be appropriate for your patient.

7. **Skills/Interventions/Services and Management—** Home care clinicians must exercise acute and effective clinical thinking, observation, technical, teaching, and evaluation skills while performing clinical assessments, interventions, and management of home care patients. This section lists the home care team members and some of their specialized functions or interventions based on the patients' problems and unique circumstances. The skills and services identified in this section include those of nursing, home health aide, physical therapy, occupational therapy, speech-language pathology, medical social services, nutritional and dietary counseling, and pharmacy services. (Hospice and Palliative Care is in Part Four and has additional team members and services for patients and families.) Nursing is listed as the first service because it is the most frequently used. Because of the multifaceted interventions and complex coordination of activities that must occur with home care, the nursing section is subdivided into seven areas: (1) Critical Thinking/ Assessment Components, (2) Teaching, (3) Medication Therapeutic Regimens, (4) Nutrition/Hydration/Elimination,

(5) Safety, (6) Care Coordination/Case Management/Discharge Planning, and (7) Other Considerations. This specificity should assist care planning in the identification and prioritization of patient/family care interventions. Interventions for all services often use verbs in the description of care to support effective documentation. These services may also be used, when appropriate, as orders for the POC. It is important to note that care must be individualized, and there must be physician orders.

The information is provided as a list to assist in the easy identification of needed home care services and to assist all team members by providing an understanding of the range of available services based on the specialized team member's education and professional scope of practice. A handbook such as this one that is used by each/all team member(s) assists in the standardization of care and care processes across an organization and disciplines because everyone is truly "on the same page."

8. **Tips to Support Medical Necessity, Quality, and Reimbursement**—This section contains tips for Medicare coverage and documentation requirements specific to patient problem(s). Regardless of payer, the documentation must demonstrate and support the provided care and the patient's response to that care. Readers are also referred to Part Two for an "Overview of Documentation."

9. **Evidence-Based and Other Resources for Practice and Education**—This section provides useful, often free, patient education or professional resources. These resources were chosen specifically to support the educational needs of patients and clinicians. Readers are encouraged to contact the author via email with suggestions for additional resources they believe should be included in a subsequent edition at news@marrelli.com.

Part Four: Hospice and Palliative Care: Clinical Guidelines for Assessment, Care Planning, and Documentation contains tips for practicing skillful and compassionate hospice and end-of-life care for patients and families. In addition to the descriptions of team members in Part Four, this specialized section contains interventions for Emotional/Spiritual Considerations, Volunteer Support, Spiritual Counseling, Bereavement Counseling, and Music, Art, and Other Therapies and Services.

Part Five: Maternal/Child Care: Clinical Guidelines for Assessment, Care Planning, and Documentation provides 12 Maternal/Child Care Guidelines that have been significantly updated, and because pediatric home care continues to grow, numerous codes have been added.

Part Six: Medicare Home Care Guidelines for Coverage of Services contains parts of the *Medicare Manual* for easy reference. Readers are encouraged to review the Coverage of Services section, particularly the homebound section and the six covered services with examples.

Part Seven: NANDA-I–Approved Nursing Diagnoses lists the NANDA-I–Approved Nursing Diagnoses.

Part Eight: Home Care Definitions and Abbreviations provides a glossary and abbreviations that are useful to clinicians and managers in home care.

Part Nine: Guidelines for Home Medical Equipment and Supply Considerations details the scope of services to home health patients to facilitate greater independence, function, and a higher quality of life.

Part Ten: Directory of Evidence-Based and Other Resources

Appendix A: Home Care Orientation: Important Foundation for Success

Appendix B: Sample Case-Mix Grouper Worksheet

Appendix C: Non-Routine Supplies (NRS) Case-Mix Adjustment Variables and Scores

Appendix D: Home Health Prospective Payment System Final Rule (from the Federal Register 2007)

Appendix E: Draft of OASIS C

ACKNOWLEDGMENT

This book is dedicated to all the clinicians and managers who make home care "work" in their communities daily. Home care and hospice operations demand a commitment and attention to detail rarely found in other businesses or work settings. This book is for the nurses, physical therapists, occupational therapists, aides, social workers, dietitians, pharmacists, and others who provide hands-on skilled care while meeting often difficult and multilevel regulations. This also includes everyone in the office—the schedulers, on-call teams, secretaries, administrative staff, QI team members, HR team members, educators, billers, CFOs, and CEOs—those who strive for "business as usual" whether there is an ice storm, a hurricane pending, a power outage, or any of numerous other events that impact home care and hospice operations.

Our hope is that this book will streamline the time spent performing required documentation activities while assisting in individualizing care planning for patients. As always, thanks to the many people who offered guidance throughout this 5th edition.

As this book went to press, we had a limited time with documenting the Medicare PPS "refinements." Our lasting hope is that policy makers and politicians will do the right thing in the years to come by creating a working system that allows people to stay in the lowest health care setting of their choice—usually their own home. Such a model will only emerge if home care "experts"—and if you are using this book you are included here—take policy makers, such as your elected officials (both state and national), on home care visits. Only in this way will they "get" the vision of professional, competent, and compassionate care in the safest setting.

The rhetoric of "aging in place" and "doing the right thing" need to come together. It is through all of our collective efforts that such a vision may be visualized… and our hope is that we are all a part of that new home care effort.

Thanks to you all and for what you contribute to the profession everyday!

ABOUT THE AUTHOR

Tina M. Marrelli, MSN, MA, RN

Tina M. Marrelli, MSN, MA, RN, is President of Marrelli and Associates, Inc., a health care consulting and publishing firm, and the editor of the peer-reviewed journal *Home Healthcare Nurse*. Ms. Marrelli is the author of numerous books including the *Nurse Manager's Survival Guide* (Mosby), the *Nursing Documentation Handbook* (Mosby), *The Hospice and Palliative Care Handbook* (Mosby), and *Mosby's Home Care & Hospice Drug Handbook* (Mosby). She is also the author of *Home Health Aide: Guidelines for Care* (Marrelli, 2008) and *Home Health Aide: Guidelines for Care Instructor Manual* (Marrelli, 2008).

Ms. Marrelli received a Bachelor's degree in Nursing from Duke University School of Nursing, a Master of Arts in Management and Supervision, Health Care Administration, and a Master's in Nursing. She has directed various home care programs and has extensive experience in home care, hospice, and hospital settings. Ms. Marrelli worked at the central office of the Health Care Financing Administration, now the Centers for Medicare and Medicaid Services, for four years in home care and hospice policy and operations, and she received the Bureau Director's Citation.

Marrelli and Associates, Inc. provides consultative services to universities, insurers, hospitals, home health agencies, and hospice programs in management, compliance, case management, other quality initiatives, daily operations, and documentation projects.

Correspondence, including feedback, recommendations, or suggestions about this book may be directed to Tina Marrelli by e-mail at news@marrelli.com.

Patrice D. Artress, PhD, RN

Patrice D. Artress, PhD, RN, is a gerontologist and health care consultant working with health care organizations in the areas of quality, outcome management and research, and clinical trials. Dr. Artress has extensive experience with the older adult population, especially in home care settings, and has worked in various capacities in development of clinical resources, research, and education.

Dr. Artress received a Bachelor's degree in nursing from Andrews University, a Master of Science in community health nursing, and a Doctorate in nursing and gerontology from the University of Michigan.

CONTENTS

PART ONE **Home Care: A Unique Specialty, 1**

PART TWO **Clinical Practice in Home Care, 75**

PART THREE **Adult Clinical Guidelines: A Systems Approach for Assessment, Care Planning, and Documentation, 127**

1

PART ONE

HOME CARE: A UNIQUE SPECIALTY

A UNIQUE SPECIALTY

Home care is very different from other types of healthcare. First and foremost, the home care clinician is a guest in someone's home; no one dictates visiting hours, the required age of visitors, what to wear, when to go to bed, what to eat, and the myriad of other details that historically have been a standard part of most healthcare facilities. The home care clinician may be the only healthcare provider seeing the patient on a particular day or week and therefore must feel comfortable working independently, yet recognize they are part of a larger team of service providers.

Home Care: A Working Definition

Home care has many and varying definitions. As the government and other insurers shift from an intervention cost-based focus to a preventive-prospective payment model, a definition that incorporates prevention is imperative. The U.S. Public Health Service defines home care as "that component of a continuum of comprehensive healthcare whereby health services are provided to individuals and families in their places of residence for the purpose of promoting, maintaining, or restoring health, or maximizing the level of independence, while minimizing the effects of disability and illness, including terminal illness. Services appropriate to the needs of the individual patient and family are planned, coordinated, and made available by providers organized for the delivery of home care." [1]

This classic definition provides a good framework for two reasons: it is not prescriptive as to the services provided, does not limit services, and refers to "individuals and families." It acknowledges that in home care, patients are cared for in the context of the family whose members, when capable, able, and willing to provide care, can make a lot of difference. The definition uses the words *promotion* and *restoring*. In *promotion*, health is a lifestyle choice with certain preventive components that are under the individual's control and that empower healthcare. Historically, Medicare did not pay for or cover preventive care. Medicare now covers some preventive care services, such as certain vaccines, mammography, Pap smears, and other prevention-focused interventions. Because most home care patients are older adults, *restoring* refers to efforts directed toward the restoration or maintenance of safe, independent functioning.

This definition is comprehensive because it addresses numerous aspects of care, especially when referring to the inclusion of terminal illness. The care of patients at the end of life is a large part of home care practice. Cancer is the second leading cause of death in the United States (after cardiovascular disease) and is a common diagnosis in home care. In fact, cancer is the diagnosis in 80% of all patients in hospice. (It is estimated that 29% of hospices are home healthcare agency-based or affiliated.)

The emphasis in the definition on the "individual patient and family" demonstrates the return to community-based care in which the patient and family (and their environment) may be valued as predictors and supports to achieving (or not achieving) predetermined health goals. Finally, the services are "planned and coordinated" which refers to care coordination and communication among all parties involved in the provision of care. This definition summarizes the best components of home healthcare delivery.

The term *home care* is used in the broadest sense throughout this book and includes all kinds of in-home services: home health agencies (HHAs), hospices that provide care in the patient's home, public health or other municipality-coordinated services, private duty care, various community programs, and other services that provide health or supportive care to patients in their homes. Whatever the specific definition of home care or the services your organization provides, one main tenet remains; we strive to provide patients and their families with quality, patient-centered care. This means that care is customer-service oriented, that the patient, family and care provider decide upon and agree on the goals, and that the care processes and interventions are based on clinically-sound, evidence-based data and research. The best models of home care operations today promote patient-centered care and ongoing staff education and evaluation to be successful.

Home Care: The Big Picture

As noted above, home care is complex and varied but can be viewed as having four distinct areas or components: (1) Reimbursement/Payer Processes; (2) Quality and Customer Service Imperatives; (3) Home: the Environment of Care (thus, the unique nature of home care!); and (4) Patient Care Planning and Related Processes (Figure 1-1).

The home care clinician must have a working knowledge of all four components to be successful in this specialty area and to positively impact patient outcomes. The following sections address the home care clinician's role in meeting the myriad requirements of home care, often simultaneously. The information is organized so that it moves from the larger external environment to the actual care processes in home care that support quality, evidence-based patient care from a holistic, interdisciplinary perspective— the main focus of this text.

Component One: Reimbursement/Payer Processes

Medicare has set many of the standards for home care. Because of this, all home care clinicians need a working knowledge of Medicare: how patients qualify for coverage, rules related to specific services, and other information that can assist the clinician when addressing Medicare issues.

All Medicare-certified home care programs are structured by the Medicare Conditions of Participation (COPs). To participate in the Medicare program, as addressed in the Medicare COPs, HHAs and hospices must meet specific regulations. From a home care clinician's perspective, effective patient care and daily home health activities should support the intent of the COPs. Box 1-1 lists

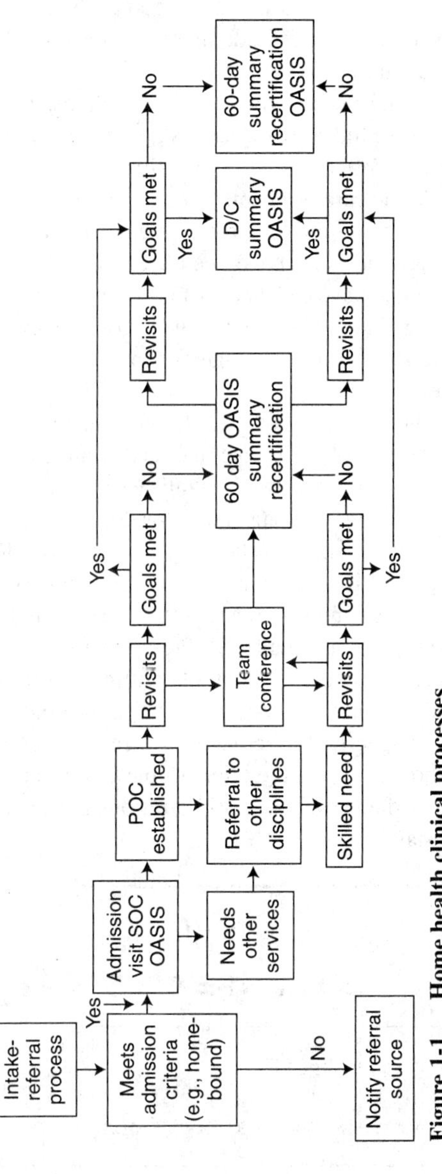

Figure 1-1 Home health clinical processes.

the COPs with the standards that support each one. References to the Code of Federal Regulations (CFR) refer to the citation in the law. Medicare-certified home care organizations must comply with these standards. The COPs can be viewed online at www.access.gpo.gov/nara/cfr/waisidx_99/42cfr484_99.html or obtained through your state or national home care or hospice organization.

State rules in relation to home care agencies and practice vary widely. Some states have licensure requirements for home care, some have certificate of need processes or related regulatory legislation that many believe controls growth and the number of provider organizations, and other states have neither.

In addition to the Medicare COPs and Medicare certification, and applicable state rules and regulations, policies and procedures that have been established by individual home care organizations must be followed. There are other certifying agencies such as The Joint Commission (JC), the Community Health Accreditation Program (CHAP), and the Accreditation Commission for Health Care (ACHC). Surveyors may cite an agency for failure to adhere to its own policies, as well as failure to comply with federal or state regulations, and claims can be denied. From a home care clinician's perspective, effective patient care and daily HHA activities should support the intent of the COPs, and Medicare-certified home care organizations must comply with these standards.

BOX 1-1

MEDICARE COPS

1. Patient rights (42 CFR 484.10)
    a. Notice of rights
    b. Exercise of rights and respect for property and person

c. Right to be informed and to participate in planning care and treatment
d. Confidentiality of medical records
e. Patient liability for payment
f. Home health hotline

2. Release of patient identifiable OASIS information (CFR 484.11)
3. Compliance with federal, state, and local laws, disclosure and ownership information, and compliance with accepted professional standards and principles (42 CFR 484.12)
   g. Compliance with laws and regulations
   h. Disclosure of ownership and management information
   i. Compliance with accepted professional standards and principles
4. Organization, services, and administration (42 CFR 484.14)
   a. Services furnished
   b. Governing body
   c. Administrator, supervising physician, or registered nurse
   d. Personnel policies
   e. Personnel contracts
   f. Coordination of patient services
   g. Services under arrangements
   h. Institutional planning-capital expenditure plan
   i. Preparation and annual review of plan and budget
   j. Laboratory services
5. Group of professional personnel (42 CFR 484.16)
   a. Advisory and evaluation function
6. Acceptance of patients, plan of care, and medical supervision (42 CFR 484.18)
   a. Plan of care
   b. Periodic review of plan of care
   c. Conformance with physician orders
7. Reporting OASIS information (42 CFR 484.20)

Continued

BOX 1-1

MEDICARE COPS—cont'd

8. Skilled nursing services (42 CFR 484.30)
   a. Duties of the registered nurse
   b. Duties of the licensed practical nurse
9. Therapy services (CFR 484.32)
   a. Supervision of physical therapy assistant and occupational therapy assistant
   b. Supervision of speech therapy services
10. Medical social service (42 CFR 484.34)
11. Home health aide services (42 CFR 484.36)
    a. Home health aide training
    b. Competency evaluation and in-service training
    c. Assignment and duties of the home health aide
    d. Supervision of home health aides
12. Qualifying to furnish outpatient physical therapy or speech-language pathology services (42 CFR 484.38)
13. Clinical records (42 CFR 484.48)
    a. Retention of records
    b. Protection of records
14. Evaluation of the agency's program (42 CFR 484.52)
    a. Policy and administrative review
    b. Clinical record review
15. Comprehensive assessment of patients (42 CFR 484.55)

Medicare Update

The Centers for Medicare and Medicaid Services (CMS, formerly known as the Healthcare Financing Administration or HCFA) manage the Medicare and Medicaid programs. Medicare is the largest medical insurance program in the world, and is the national medical health insurance program for Medicare beneficiaries. These beneficiaries consist primarily of three groups: (1) persons over 65 years of age (the largest group of beneficiaries); (2) the disabled population (regardless of age); and (3) persons with end-stage renal disease and amyotrophic lateral sclerosis (Lou Gehrig's disease). When Medicare began July 1966, approximately 19 million people enrolled; Medicare now covers approximately 44 million older and disabled individuals.

Medicare traditionally consisted of two parts: Hospital Insurance, also known as Part A, and Supplementary Medical Insurance, also known as Part B. The Medicare+Choice program, sometimes known as Part C, was established by the Balanced Budget Act of 1997 (Public Law 105-33) and expanded beneficiaries' options for participation in private-sector healthcare plans. More recent legislation has established Part D, the prescription drug benefit.

Home care spending is difficult to estimate; however, the total spending for home care in 2006 was estimated to be $52.7 billion. According to the CMS, Medicare benefit payments totaled $295 billion for 2004, 4% of which was spent on home health ($11.8 billion). The largest percentage of Medicare dollars went to inpatient care, followed by outpatient care, and the smallest percentage was spent on nursing home care.

Government Contractors

Regional Home Health Intermediaries (RHHIs) or Medicare Administrative Contractors (MACs) are the insurance companies who contract with CMS to process claims and make payment determinations on home care and hospice claims from across the country. Each contractor is allowed to implement local coverage determinations, and the reader is strongly encouraged to review applicable local coverage determinations for the particular contractor. Local coverage determinations are an administrative and educational tool that specify under what clinical circumstances a service is reasonable and necessary (www.cms.hhs.gov/MedicalReviewProcess/04_ncds.asp). The up-to-date toll-free number and website for each state's RHHI or MAC is found at the CMS Home Care website (www.cms.hhs.gov/center/hha.asp).

CMS instructs the contractors about administering the Medicare home health and hospice programs. An in-depth discussion of documentation follows later in this section, but it is important to note that the contractors look at clinical documentation to assist in supporting covered care, such as the patient's homebound status and the need for skilled care. *The contractors can pay only for care under Medicare provisions that are covered by law. The clinical documentation in the patient's health/clinical record contains the essential information either to support or not support Medicare coverage and payment for services.*

Prospective Payment System: The Big Picture

A prospective payment system (PPS) is a third-party payment system, such as Medicare, that establishes certain payment rates for services or categories of patients, regardless of the actual costs of that care. The Medicare diagnostic-related group (DRG) system for acute inpatient care is the most widely used example of this type of payment.

Clinicians and managers may remember when hospitals implemented their PPS mechanism based on DRGs in the early 1980s pursuant to the passage of the Tax Equity and Fiscal Responsibility Act of 1982. Hospices have been paid prospectively based on four levels of care since Medicare started the Medicare Hospice Benefit in the 1980s. Skilled nursing facilities are reimbursed prospectively according to the Minimum Data Set collected on the patient at set time points, similar to home care Outcome and Assessment Information Set (OASIS) data collection.

Home care was one of the last provider types to move to a PPS reimbursement system based on the patient's condition, not the actual costs of the services/care provided.

Implemented October 1, 2000, as mandated by Congress, *this became the biggest change in Medicare home care since the inception of the program, and changed, or realigned, incentives from overutilization to underutilization.* With PPS, Medicare beneficiaries receive services for an unlimited number of 60-day episodes of care if they meet home health eligibility and coverage requirements, such as homebound and skilled care. (See specific Medicare coverage and eligibility as addressed in Part Six of this text). The initial and each subsequent 60-day episode period correspond with the Plan of Care (POC) based on continuing needs identified by the clinician(s) and ordered by the physician.

Home care has its own mechanism or unit of payment, similar to DRGs, on which the PPS is based, and is paid per episode of care. The home care PPS assigns a Home Health Resource Group (HHRG) score based on the OASIS documentation that uses a case-mix classification system reflecting the severity of the patient's condition in three domains: clinical, functional, and service utilization. The standardized 60-day base rate is determined annually (e.g., $2339 for 2007) and is adjusted by the area wage index.

There are a finite number of possible combinations of patient severity or case-mix groups. In 2008, the number of case-mix groups increased from 80 to 153. Each HHRG has a different dollar amount attributed or assigned based on its "weight," which reflects the average level of resources used to provide home health services to patients, and is updated annually or as needed. This amount includes all the service disciplines, an OASIS adjustment, non-routine medical supplies, an outpatient therapy adjustment, and a standardization factor for wage index (other adjustments may be included). This standardized payment is then specifically adjusted for each HHA based on geographic locations and the specific case-mix adjusted category for the patients served. The payment covers one individual for 60 days of care (the unit of reimbursement is the 60-day episode) regardless of the number of days or of actual care services rendered within the episode. The episode begins on the first billable visit and generally ends on day 60 or at discharge, with a few exceptions.

The HHRG assignment is driven by the OASIS data items based on the severity of the patient's condition in terms of clinical factors and functional status, and adjusted by episode number and number of therapy visits. It provides the weighting or multiplier for the standard PPS rate, designed to reflect varying patient care costs. The severity calculations are determined by the clinician when scoring the OASIS items based on the comprehensive assessment. Because of these defined HHRGs, organizations are reimbursed the same amounts for similar patients, with adjustments for different regions of the country. An example of a sample case-mix grouper worksheet is provided in Appendix B of this text.

Organizations must continue to focus their efforts in terms of patient populations and cohorts of "like" patients; clinicians must begin assessing patients from a body systems or functional perspective, such as musculoskeletal or endocrine rather than relying solely on a diagnostic category (e.g., arthritis, diabetes mellitus). In this way, trends in care, variances, and outcomes may be more easily reviewed and identified, and changes for quality and efficiency may be implemented for a category or a given patient population. For this reason, the care guidelines presented later in this book are primarily systems-based.

Other PPS design features include adjustments and exceptions to the usual 60-day episode. These occur when the basic episode of care is interrupted and the payment is prorated accordingly. These are as follows:

1. The Low Utilization Payment Adjustment (LUPA) occurs when a patient is seen or provided with a certain number of visits in a given episode. When PPS was initially implemented, the LUPA was four or fewer visits in an episode. In these LUPA instances, the agency is not reimbursed the full episode amount, but provided a dollar

amount per visit determined by Medicare that is specific to the service area. The specific medical review aspects of PPS are identified in the following section, "Documentation: An Overview."

A low number of visits may be appropriate for some patients (e.g., catheters, B-12 injections). However, if there is a concern about underutilization (the patient is not getting an appropriate number of visits based on clinical condition), the quality of the care, or possible inappropriate (under)utilization, this may be the focus of a medical review of the documentation by the RHHI or Medicare contractor. Organizations that have a trend of five to six visits per episode must be prepared to support the level of care for these individual patients through documentation.

2. Partial episode payment (PEP) occurs when a patient changes HHAs during an episode of care or when the patient is discharged with all goals met and is later readmitted to the same agency within the original 60-day period, and is the mechanism that determines how the payment will be allocated or prorated between agencies.
3. "Outliers" are a small group of unusual patient cases that are not adequately accounted for in the national payment rate structure and have high cost resource needs. Like the hospital DRG system, HHAs are reimbursed more for these patients, although the costs often exceed the outlier revenue. Because of specific Congressional mandates for PPS to remain "budget neutral," the outlier reimbursement is based on a "shared loss" concept with Medicare sharing the loss with HHAs through a complex formula of outlier reimbursement of costs.
4. Clinicians must be cognizant of the costs of medical supplies and thrifty in their planning and use of supplies necessary for the patient's care. Reimbursement of non-routine supplies is determined by the interaction of select diagnoses with specific OASIS data item responses when the supply appears on the claim. Readers are

referred to Appendix C for Table 10A and Appendix D for Table 10B.

Home care can learn much from other PPS-reimbursed providers. The good news is that many hospitals are still in business and their lengths of stays continue to decrease even though they have had this reimbursement mechanism for almost three decades. Like the hospitals, home care has seen the emergence of clinical paths, more interdisciplinary collaboration, the change to case management models and roles, an increased interest in and use of telehealth, the standardization of care and care processes, and many other changes to manage closely the care and services and support the timely achievement of patient outcomes.

The OASIS and PPS: Critical Interface for Success and Survival

The move to PPS brought its own glossary of terms and demanded an immediate change in the mindset and behavior of clinicians and managers to be successful (read: *survive*) in home care. Successful home care organizations moved from reimbursement-focused thinking to practice-based thinking, and from patient dependence to patient independence—and became facilitators for patients to achieve outcomes. This has been effectively accomplished with visits and other non-traditional patient contacts (e.g., phone calls, telemonitoring), and other innovative delivery models that closely manage clinical care and promote evidence-based practice.

PPS success depends on the clinician's skills, understanding, and accurate completion of the comprehensive assessment, including the OASIS, and its integral role in the interface with PPS. The OASIS, the set of mandated data elements, must be understood as a significant part of the patient's assessment, and also the structure that underlies the determination for the PPS case-mix payment. The OASIS is a significant driver to identify the patient's care needs and services. An analogy is that the scoring of data elements from OASIS provides the fuel that determines the trajectory for the PPS rocket.

The OASIS is administered at specified time intervals: admission, discharge, transfer, resumption of care, recertification, and when there is a significant change in the patient's condition that was not anticipated. OASIS is used to measure three major outcomes for specific patient status attributes—improvement, stabilization, and deterioration. The OASIS data, which are transmitted to the state, are the basis for Outcome-Based Quality Monitoring (OBQM), Outcome-Based Quality Improvement (OBQI), and Home Health Compare reports. These reports are benchmarking tools that identify the organization's status as determined by specified clinical, functional, and service utilization indicators. These reports must be reviewed by agencies and are used for quality improvement purposes. The data analysis and findings also informs and suggests future adjustments and refinement of the OASIS and PPS to the CMS.

Clinicians must understand and be competent in the comprehensive patient assessment, including the OASIS data elements. All patients must be assessed accurately on each data element, and each piece of the assessment needs to correlate and be consistent with other parts of the assessment. This is best accomplished by a thorough orientation to OASIS, training followed by testing, and verification of OASIS skills, consistency, and similar assessment findings (e.g., interrater reliability).

PPS reimbursement continues to be weighted towards therapy services, and it is reasonable to assume that significant medical review of the documentation of therapy services will continue because it is a utilization parameter controlled by the home care agency. Therapy team members are usually involved in performing OASIS assessments, care coordination/case management, and interdisciplinary care planning. Therefore, therapy team members play a significant role in determining the amount of therapy visits needed for patients to reach goals.

When both nursing and therapy care are ordered at the time of the initial referral, the COPs state that the nurse must perform the initial assessment and gather the OASIS data. Although dependent on state law and practice acts, a therapist, most often a physical therapist (PT), performs the start of care (SOC) comprehensive assessment, including the OASIS, when therapy is the *only* skilled service required by, or initially ordered for, the patient. This visit then becomes one visit counted toward the therapy visit threshold. A registered nurse (RN), physical therapist (PT), occupational therapist (OT), or speech-language pathologist (SLP) may complete the assessment at other time points according to agency policy.

Clinicians are referred to the *HHA Manual* in Part Six, in which the coverage section for all skilled services is reprinted in its entirety.

Compliance: Everyone's Role

No discussion of Medicare would be complete without addressing compliance issues. Compliance and quality go hand-in-hand; in fact, they can be seen as two sides of the same coin (quality is discussed in more depth in the next section). All Medicare providers have an obligation to conform and "comply" with the rules and requirements of the Medicare program. Stated simply, all team members must have a working knowledge of the Medicare program and comply with the rules related to the law, coverage, and payment determination. Unfortunately, stories about unscrupulous providers and evidence of fraud sometimes make newspaper and headline news. However, there are some fundamental steps that can assist organizations in their quest for compliance and quality.

Strategies for Ensuring Ongoing Compliance

- **Make sure that staff know the "rules" related to Medicare.** This includes the *HHA Manual* Coverage of Services section—the definition of homebound status, covered nursing, therapy, and aide services; accurate completion of the plan of care (POC) and the comprehensive assessment, including the OASIS; compliance related to physician orders (e.g., state licensure and other requirements); and general and specific documentation requirements used by individual organizations related to accuracy, completeness, and timelines for submission.

- **Perform comprehensive audits that encompass the span of care activities from admission through discharge.** Typical review questions include: Does the patient meet Medicare and the organization's admission policies and criteria? Are physician orders timely? Are all business practices and billing processes in compliance with Medicare and other requirements?
- **Standardize care and operational processes.** Strive to decrease the risk caused by varying or different systems, methods, practices, and operations whenever possible.
- **Provide patient education handouts and tools.** This assists in identifying that the patient meets Medicare criteria (e.g., homebound, skilled care) and in establishing mutually agreed-upon goals with projected timelines for achievement.
- **Verify and document that there are physician orders prior to the provision of care.** Physician orders not only include medical treatment orders but also orders for services and the projected frequency and duration of visits during the certification period (episode of care).
- **Validate that the physician orders are signed and dated by the physician prior to billing for the provided care.**
- **Use checklists for clinical record reviews.** This and other methods will assist in monitoring compliance and quality on an ongoing basis.
- **Develop mechanisms to verify that patients are provided care as ordered.** This includes that the written documentation and related components of care planning (e.g., how verbal orders are obtained, evidence of care coordination, conformance with the ordered care) support Medicare and other requirements.
- **Perform unannounced or random supervisory visits.** This is a way to support compliance—a kind of ongoing mini "mock survey" related to the most important kinds of compliance.
- **Promote awareness among agency staff that the federal government has made controlling healthcare fraud and**

abuse a high priority. It is critical that home care clinicians know and adhere to the rules—this is the basis for everyone's important role in ongoing compliance.

Medicare Requirements for Home Care

All home care team members must know and understand Medicare coverage. Other regulations governing care include the Medicare COPs, the hospice COPs, the state operations manual, and the Intermediary Manual. The hospice Manual lists the rules related to hospice and the four levels of care. Part Six of this handbook has the full text of the coverage section of the *HHA Manuals*.

A Medicare beneficiary must meet all of the following "qualifying" criteria to be covered under the Medicare home health benefit:

1. Is eligible for Medicare;
2. Is provided services by a Medicare-certified home health agency;
3. Is homebound as defined by Medicare;
4. Is provided services as defined in the *HHA Manual* and meets the specific coverage rules related to the six services (nursing, physical therapy [PT], occupational therapy [OT], speech/language pathology [SLP], medical social services [MSS], home health aide [HHA]);
5. Is provided medically reasonable and necessary services; and
6. Receives physician certification and oversight of the patient's POC.

If all of these conditions are met, Medicare will pay for part-time or intermittent skilled nursing, physical, occupational, and speech therapy; medical social services; and home health aide visits. Beneficiaries are not liable for any co-insurance or deductibles for these services and may receive an unlimited number of visits, provided the coverage criteria are met.

Homebound: A Major Qualifying Criteria

Homebound status is an essential qualifying requirement or criteria that must be met for Medicare coverage. The patient is either homebound and the POC is initiated, or the patient is identified as not being homebound or confined to the home as defined by Medicare and therefore cannot be admitted to the organization's home care program under the Medicare benefit. Thus, when performing the initial assessment, the clinician must identify the functional criteria that support the homebound status. Box 1-2 is the definition of homebound as found in the *HHA Manual*.

BOX 1-2

HHA MANUAL DEFINITION OF HOMEBOUND

204.1 F(Cont.) COVERAGE OF SERVICES 07-02

A. *Patient Confined to The Home*—In order for a patient to be eligible to receive covered home health services under both Part A and Part B, the law requires that a physician certify in all cases that the patient is confined to his/her home. (See §240.I.) An individual does not have to be bedridden to be considered as confined to the home. However, the condition of these patients should be such that there exists a normal inability to leave home and, consequently, leaving home would require a considerable and taxing effort. If the patient does in fact leave the home, the patient may nevertheless be considered homebound if the absences from the home are infrequent or for periods of relatively short duration, or are attributable to the need to receive healthcare treatment. Absences attributable to the need to receive healthcare treatment include, but are not limited to, attendance at adult day centers to receive medical care, ongoing receipt of outpatient kidney dialysis, and the receipt of outpatient chemotherapy or radiation therapy. Any absence of an individual from the home attributable to the need to receive healthcare treatment, including regular absences for the purpose of participating in therapeutic, psychosocial, or medical treatment in an adult day-care program that is licensed or certified by a State, or accredited, to furnish

Continued

BOX 1-2

HHA MANUAL DEFINITION OF HOMEBOUND—cont'd

adult day-care services in a State shall not disqualify an individual from being considered to be confined to his home. Any other absence of an individual from the home shall not so disqualify an individual if the absence is of an infrequent or of relatively short duration. For purposes of the preceding sentence, any absence for the purpose of attending a religious service shall be deemed to be an absence of infrequent or short duration. It is expected that in most instances, absences from the home that occur will be for the purpose of receiving healthcare treatment. However, occasional absences from the home for non-medical purposes, e.g., an occasional trip to the barber, a walk around the block, a drive, attendance at a family reunion, funeral, graduation, or other infrequent or unique event would not necessitate a finding that the patient is not homebound if the absences are undertaken on an infrequent basis or are of relatively short duration and do not indicate that the patient has the capacity to obtain the healthcare provided outside rather than in the home. The examples provided above are not all-inclusive and are meant to be illustrative of the kinds of infrequent or unique events a patient may attend.

Generally speaking, a patient will be considered to be homebound if he/she has a condition due to an illness or injury that restricts his/her ability to leave his/her place of residence except with the aid of supportive devices such as crutches, canes, wheelchairs, and walkers, the use of special transportation, or the assistance of another person or if leaving home is medically contraindicated. Some examples of homebound patients that illustrate the factors used to determine whether a homebound condition exists would be: (1) a patient paralyzed from a stroke who is confined to a wheelchair or requires the aid of crutches in order to walk; (2) a patient who is blind or senile and requires the assistance of another person to leave his/her residence; (3) a patient who has lost the use of his/her upper extremities and, therefore, is unable to open doors, use handrails on stairways, etc., and requires the assistance of another individual to leave his/her residence; (4) a patient who has just returned from a hospital stay involving surgery suffering from resultant weakness and pain and, therefore, his/her actions may be restricted by his/her physician to certain specified and limited activities such as getting out of bed only for a specified period of time, walking stairs only once a day, etc.; (5) a patient with arteriosclerotic heart disease of such severity that he/she must avoid all stress and physical activity; (6) a patient with a psychiatric problem if the illness is manifested in part by a refusal to leave home or is of such a nature that it would not be considered safe to leave home unattended, even if he/she has no physical limitations; and (7) a patient in the late stages of ALS or neurodegenerative disabilities.

In determining whether the patient has the general inability to leave the home and leaves the home only infrequently or for periods of short duration, it is necessary (as is the case in determining whether skilled nursing services are intermittent) to look at the patient's condition over a period of time rather than for short periods within the home health stay. For example, a patient may leave the home (under the conditions described above, e.g., with severe and taxing effort, with the assistance of others) more frequently during a short period when, for example, the presence of visiting relatives provides a unique opportunity for such absences, than is normally the case. So long as the patient's overall condition and experience is such that he or she meets these qualifications, he or she should be considered confined to the home.

14 Rev. 302

07-02 COVERAGE OF SERVICES 204.1 (Cont.)

The aged person who does not often travel from home because of feebleness and insecurity brought on by advanced age would not be considered confined to the home for purposes of receiving home health services unless he/she meets one of the above conditions. A patient who

Continued

BOX 1-2

HHA MANUAL DEFINITION OF HOMEBOUND—cont'd

requires skilled care must also be determined to be confined to the home in order for home health services to be covered.

Although a patient must be confined to the home to be eligible for covered home health services, some services cannot be provided at the patient's residence because equipment is required that cannot be made available there. If the services required by a patient involve the use of such equipment, the HHA may make arrangements or contract with a hospital, skilled nursing facility, or a rehabilitation center to provide these services on an outpatient basis. (See §§200.2 and 206.5.) However, even in these situations, for the services to be covered as home health services, the patient must be considered confined to his/her home; and to receive such outpatient services a homebound patient will generally require the use of supportive devices, special transportation, or the assistance of another person to travel to the appropriate facility.

If a question is raised as to whether a patient is confined to the home, the HHA will be asked to furnish the intermediary with the information necessary to establish that the patient is homebound as defined above.

Daily Care

Medicare defines daily care as care delivered seven days a week. Patients who receive daily care must have a realistic projected end date. *This means that the home care nurse needs a projected endpoint for daily visits. Patients who need daily nursing care for an unspecified amount of time or indefinitely do not receive coverage under Medicare.* The *only* exception to an endpoint for daily care is insulin injections and only under certain circumstances.

When admitting a patient who needs daily (7 days a week) wound care or other daily care such as Calcimar injection administration, the documentation needs to support medical necessity and ensure the meeting of intermittent requirements. Specify the projected endpoint on the POC. It must be specific, not "when the wound is healed." This finite and estimated endpoint must be stated as a specific date. For example, "Daily RN visits until physician re-evaluates patient for further wound surgery on 2/22/08." Another example is "Daily for 3 months, 02/01/08 to 05/01/08."

Project the date daily visits will no longer be necessary (end date) by considering specific clinical progress or patient/caregiver behavior that will occur in order to reduce visits less often than daily. Critically think/ask yourself the following:

When will care (e.g., wound care) be less complex?
When can patient/caregiver be taught procedure?
What are the barriers to reducing care from daily to less often than daily?
When/where can a willing and able caregiver be found?

When determining the projected date, it should be realistic based on the patient's unique medical condition—and that date is usually *not* the end of the episode. For example, if the patient has had a wound for 2 years and is referred to your HHA, it may not be realistic that the wound will now heal. In this case the patient may not be appropriate for home care because this patient may need a level of care (full time) that the Medicare program does not cover. Such cases need to be discussed with your manager.

If the initial orders were three-times-per-week skilled wound care and the physician increases these to daily, be sure to discuss and obtain a supplemental or telephone order with a projected endpoint in either a date format or a specific number of days or weeks. Be certain to include this updated order in the clinical record. Remember that it is only for daily visits that a finite, projected endpoint is needed.

Document progress or lack of progress and the specific clinical findings related to the wound and other problems having an impact on the care provided. For wound care patients, this includes accurate size, drainage, amount, character, presence of odor, etc.

Insulin administration is the only exception to daily intermittent care that requires a specific endpoint. For unusual circumstances in which the patient is physically or mentally unable to self-inject and there is no available able and willing caregiver, the HHA can provide daily visits, while trying to locate a caregiver. This is the only type of daily visits that usually do not need a projected ending date, although it is still prudent to project one. Of note, with the right equipment and circumstances, even blind persons with diabetes can be taught to give themselves insulin injections.

Management and Evaluation of the POC

Management and evaluation (M&E) of the POC is a covered Medicare service for homebound patients requiring complex intervention and care coordination and is called various things, including skilled management, skilled planning and assessment, skilled management and planning, case management, and M&E.

Before this was a covered service by Medicare, clinicians practicing in home health had limited exposure to this level of care. Many times patients were kept on the service by HHAs with no reimbursement because the patient had an extensive medical history of multifaceted problems, no caregivers, safety problems, or multiple needs that the caregiver could not safely and effectively meet. However, these patients were frequently readmitted to home care after rehospitalization (e.g., fell and refractured hip, acute exacerbation of heart failure [HF] or chronic obstructive pulmonary disease [COPD]).

The following are typical issues that need to be addressed to determine that the patient is appropriate for M&E. Evaluation of need and subsequent documentation may support M&E services: (1) the patient's medical history; (2) the caregiver's support system; (3) current or highly probable medical concerns based on past history;

(4) multiple medications listed on the POC indicating complex management issues; (5) functional limitations that affect care; (6) safety or other high-risk factors identified; (7) unusual home and/or other environment; (8) ordered disciplines and interventions; (9) diagnoses and underlying pathologies that affect the POC; (10) patient's and/or caregiver's mental status; and (11) history of frequent hospitalizations. The clinician needs to assess and document why the skills of an RN or therapist are needed to promote the patient's stabilization and/or (document evidence of movement toward patient goals) and ensure medical safety.

In discussing M&E as a skilled service, the Medicare manual states: "Skilled nursing … where underlying conditions or complications require that only a RN can ensure that essential nonskilled care is achieving its purpose.... The complexity of the necessary unskilled services which are a necessary part of the medical treatment must require the involvement of skilled nursing personnel to promote the patient's recovery and medical safety in view of the beneficiary's overall condition." Also, "management and evaluation of a patient care plan … constitute skilled therapy services when...those activities require the involvement of a skilled therapist to meet the patient's needs, promote recovery, and ensure medical safety." Please refer to this section in Part Six for further clarification and examples of the kinds of patients that may be appropriate for M&E.

Documentation to Support Covered Care

The RHHI or MAC is responsible only for paying for care that is covered under the Medicare home care program guidelines. The contractors make these decisions or adjudicate the claims and make payment determinations based on a careful review of the patient's clinical record. This section addresses the major components of required documentation for Medicare and other third-party payers.

Because Medicare is a medical insurance program, there must be justification in the clinical notes supporting medical necessity for the care and for the level of intensity (frequency and duration) of the care. *It is the responsibility of all clinicians to provide the clinical documentation that identifies their role in all components of the provision of home care, including assessment information, care planning, interventions, communications and care coordination, and evaluation.* Thus the burden is on the clinician to document the care, provide the rationale for care, report the patient's response and progress, and support covered care throughout the patient's stay in home care.

Documentation: An Overview

Documentation in the clinical record plays a critical role in home care. Home care practice is described every day to surveyors, peers, managers, and any third-party payer through the review of clinical home care records. Home care clinicians must integrate knowledge of regulatory criteria, care coordination, and practice into effective documentation that supports coverage and demonstrates quality. The increased specialization of practice, the complexity of patients' problems, and advanced technologies have contributed to providing more services to patients in their homes. The clinical record is the only source of written communication, and sometimes the only source of *any* communication, for the team members involved in the patient's care. The team members not only contribute their unique assessments, interventions, and outcomes, but may also actually base their subsequent actions on events documented by another team member.

Documentation is effective when it:

1. Demonstrates the standard of care provided to a patient;
2. Provides the basis for coverage and reimbursement;
3. Protects the clinician and the organization from alleged malpractice or fraud complaints;
4. Provides the organization with information for data collection and benchmarking;

5. Supports the tenets of quality care, and recognizes that quality is in the details (e.g., completion, accuracy, adherence to organizational timelines, and other standards);
6. Provides the primary written source for reference and communication among members of the home care team;
7. Validates the standardization of care and care practices;
8. Provides the basis for staff education; and
9. Acts as the basis for reviews related to quality of care, reimbursement, and documentation for the organization's licensing (where applicable), accreditation, and state surveys.

The clinical HHA record is the only document that chronicles a patient's stay from the SOC through discharge. For greatest accuracy, documentation should be completed at the time the care is provided—ideally in the home—or as soon as possible thereafter and ***ALWAYS*** before the next visit. Home health documentation includes the POC, the comprehensive assessment which includes the OASIS, the daily visit record or clinical notes, and other required forms. A change in the patient's POC and any discussion with the patient and/or other team members must be recorded as evidence of care coordination. Important facets of the documentation also include the patient's condition, the environment of care, a description of the specific care provided, any communication with the physician, and the observed or verbal patient responses to completed interventions.

When admitting the patient, verify that the particular insurance requirements are met. For example, for Medicare, the patient must meet the homebound and other qualifying criteria. How the patient specifically meets the homebound criteria must be reflected in the clinical documentation on admission and also be documented every visit on your visit note. Documentation should be objectively reviewed after it is completed. The reviewer should ask, "Does this POC, OASIS comprehensive assessment, or visit note reflect why the patient is homebound and how and why the skills of the home care clinician are needed?"

Box 1-3 lists documentation essentials, and Box 1-4 is a checklist for effective documentation to ensure that quality and reimbursement requirements are met. Effective documentation is a learned skill, and as with any skill, improvement comes *only with practice and effort.*

BOX 1-3

DOCUMENTATION ESSENTIALS

DO

- If handwritten, write legibly or print neatly. The record must be readable.
- Use permanent, black ink.
- Identify the time and date for every entry, sign the entry, and include your title.
- Describe care or interventions provided and patient's response or mark appropriate box on flow sheet.
- Write objectively when describing findings (e.g., behaviors).
- Document in consecutive and chronologic order with no skipped areas.
- Document or enter information either at the patient's home (if safe and appropriate) or as soon as possible after care is provided.
- Be factual and specific.
- Use the patient's name (e.g., "Mr. Smith") or ask what they prefer to be called.
- Use patient, family, or caregiver quotes that are in response to instruction or any other care intervention.
- Document patient complaints or needs and their resolutions. (Also remember to discuss complaints with your manager, who may document them in the complaint log and note the resolution or follow-up actions taken and any trends.)

- Make sure the patient's complete name is listed correctly on the visit record, daily note, and other forms.
- Be accurate, complete, and thorough.
- Avoid non-standard abbreviations—some abbreviations are not allowed if JC-accredited (see Part Eight of this text)—and refer to your agency's approved list of abbreviations.
- Chart only the care that you provided.
- Promptly document any change in the patient's condition and the actions taken based on that change.
- Document the patient's, family's, or caregiver's response to all teaching and other care interventions.
- To correct an error: draw a line through the erroneous entry and add your signature and the date and time. Check your organizational policy related to errors.
- When using electronic documentation on a Point-of-Service device: balance responses from drop-down boxes and checklists with narrative comments to describe unique nature of patient; and read output for clarity before uploading data.

DO NOT

- Rely on memory.
- Use liquid eraser or erase entries—this may appear to be an attempt to cover up incriminating entries and is illegal.
- Cross out words beyond recognition.
- Make assumptions, draw conclusions, or blame.
- Leave blank lines between entries and your signature.
- Wait too long to record entries.
- Leave gaps or blank lines in documentation.
- Use abbreviations unless they are clear and appear on the organization's list of approved abbreviations.

Adapted with permission, *Home Care and Hospice Update*, Vol. 7, No. 3, March 2000.

BOX 1-4

CHECKLIST FOR EFFECTIVE DOCUMENTATION

- Recognize that at the first visit the nurse or therapist initiates the process of claims payment (or denial) with completion of the initial comprehensive assessment, including OASIS items, and the POC.
- Read your documentation objectively. Ask yourself if the comprehensive assessment, including OASIS items, the POC, and daily visit records reflect why the patient is homebound (if the patient has Medicare or another insurance that requires that criteria), and how the skills of a nurse or therapist are needed. (Many HHAs have a peer review process that significantly helps home care clinicians objectively review documentation.)
- Emphasize (1) why the care was initiated, (2) what the skilled interventions are, (3) what the intended outcomes/goals of the patient's POC are, and (4) what the plans are for discharge (rehabilitation potential).
- Complete your patient documentation as soon as possible. Document all care and related activities in the patients' home unless your safety is a concern. This includes the initial comprehensive assessment, including OASIS items, daily visit notes, updating the medication sheet, care coordination, scheduling, and physician calls. Make this a norm! It is not correct to write after other visits or at the end of the day from a risk management perspective. Relying on memory or rough notes after seeing multiple patients at the end of a day can be difficult and is an unsafe practice. Explain to your patients that the last few moments of every visit are for completing the documentation required by Medicare or other payer. Patients and their families understand. In fact, during this time the patients may think of questions to ask you and thereby reduce the number of calls after you leave. This is particularly important when working with new admissions because

of all the forms that the patients must sign, the information you need for the completion of the comprehensive assessment, the OASIS items, the POC, and the initial and daily visit notes.

- The comprehensive assessment, including OASIS items, and the POC are the most important components of the home care clinical record—they must be complete, accurate, and the content should clearly describe the patient. All other information flows from the services and needs identified and ordered on the POC.
- Make sure your patient meets the organization's and insurance program's admission criteria. This is important from both risk management and reimbursement perspectives. The need for skilled, covered services should be clearly evident.
- Focus on the patient's problems in your documentation. They are the reason home care is being provided, and the payers must see evidence of such to validate the coverage criteria.
- Demonstrate through your documentation that the care provided is patient-centered. For example, make your patient goals measurable and your outcomes realistic and specific to the patient's unique problems and needs.
- Remember that anyone who looks at your patient's clinical record does not have the depth of knowledge that you have gained from providing services to the patient in the home setting. Because of this, document information that is objective and clearly "paints a picture" of the patient, the relevant problems and needs, and how the care is directed toward goal achievement and discharge.
- Remember that effective documentation does not have to be wordy. However, the contents should convey to any reader, such as your manager or a state surveyor, the status of your patient, adherence to the ordered POC, and consistent progress toward predetermined patient-centered goals.

Continued

BOX 1-4

CHECKLIST FOR EFFECTIVE DOCUMENTATION—cont'd

- Check that the information in the clinical record flows well and that a reader can understand, through objective evidence, what is happening with the patient. This includes the problems and the skilled services that are needed, again based on the clear picture presented in the documentation.
- Use the OASIS items to effectively "paint a picture" of the patient congruent with all other documentation. This may require adding comments in addition to merely marking the selected OASIS item response box.
- Document homebound status at the time of admission to the agency—this information verifies the patient's eligibility for the Medicare home care benefit—and at each subsequent visit.
- Remember that entries on the clinical record need to be legible, neat, and consistently organized. How the clinical record looks may be seen as an indicator of care and the quality of the organization.
- If using electronic records, entries need to be organized and information regarding the patient easy to retrieve and review.
- Look at the documentation objectively. Does it tell the story of the patient's progress (or lack of progress) and the interventions implemented based on the initial assessment, OASIS information, and the POC?
- Make sure telephone calls and other communications with physicians, community agencies, and other team members are documented. Include interdisciplinary team conferences and discussions. Does the documentation explain what occurred with the patient; what actions were ordered, modified, and implemented; and what the patient's response was to these interventions?

- Explain a significant decline or improvement in the patient's condition, and document findings in an updated OASIS assessment.
- Each visit by a nurse or therapist should include the elements of assessment, care planning, interventions and actions, progress toward patient-centered goals, assessment of the patient's response, and continued evaluation.
- Document goal achievement and/or progress toward goals and outcomes. Are the goals realistic, quantifiable, and patient centered?
- Remember that care and services need to be directed toward needs identified by the OASIS. This supports the level of care (HHRG reimbursement) the HHA provided (e.g., the documented care must be consistent with the case-mix grouper score used to bill Medicare).
- If progress has not occurred as planned, explain the reasons in the documentation. If a patient is too ill for a rehabilitation service or refuses the service, is there written communication with the doctor about this included in the record? Has an order been received and documented to place the service on hold or to discharge the patient from that service?
- Documentation should include family/caregiver education and their responses to, and demonstration of, the specific education and objective results of the education.
- Document the patient's response to care interventions and other activities.
- Modify interventions based on the patient's response, when appropriate.
- Document evidence of interdisciplinary team conferences and discussions.
- Show continuity of care planning goals and consistent movement toward outcomes/goal achievement by all members of the team on the chart.
- Generally, the record should tell the story of the patient's care, needs, and progress while receiving home care services and reflect the plan of care.

Continued

BOX 1-4

CHECKLIST FOR EFFECTIVE DOCUMENTATION—cont'd

- The entries and overall information need to reflect the level of care expected by today's healthcare consumers and their families.
- The clinical documentation should demonstrate compliance with regulatory, licensure, and quality standards.

Adapted with permission, *Home Care and Hospice Update,* Vol. 7, No. 3, March 2000.

Documentation Problems: Common Reasons for Payment Denials

Denials are always a traumatic experience for the home care clinician who provided the care, the patient who receives the denial notice, and the home care organization that must follow-up with a labor-intensive, time-consuming, and costly process to recover the cost of visits and care they thought was covered. Home care services are under an intense level of scrutiny due to suspected fraud and abuse. Some of the "focused" or other reviews are triggered by high or low utilization patterns, such as excessive therapy visits that result in higher reimbursement to the agency. The payer determines whether the frequency and duration of the services provided were medically reasonable and necessary. Because the determination will be based on review of the clinical record, it is imperative that clinicians provide documentation that supports the medical necessity of each visit.

Some reviews are random and others are based on screening for outliers or patterns of aberrancy as compared with other home care or similar organizations. As you see in Box 1-5, most review issues are problems related to the need

BOX 1-5

TRIGGERS FOR DENIALS

- Incomplete or no physician orders for service, treatment, or visit frequency
- Skilled services (e.g., nursing, PT, OT, SLP) not reasonable and necessary
- Missing/incorrect documentation of orders or care provided
- No valid certification or recertification of the POC
- Poor assessment, prior level of patient function not addressed
- Lack of documented objective goals with functional measurements
- Use of "check box" forms without enough unique patient information
- Record does not support the need for the specialized skills of the nurse, therapist, etc. (i.e., functional score)
- Frequency and duration does not appear to be appropriate or correlated with the documented functional needs
- Repetitive and unclear notes of routine services that do not support medical necessity and need for the clinician
- Documentation does not support Medicare coverage criteria (e.g., homebound, covered services, etc.)

for the documentation to be timely, clear, and support why the skills of the clinician are needed based on the patient's unique medical problems. Keep these in mind as you comprehensively document your patient's care. Strive to document correctly and thoroughly for every visit and ask yourself the following:

Do these notes support Medicare coverage?
Do I have orders for all services rendered?
Would I pay for this visit if I were a reviewer?

Medical Review Considerations

Because of the high volume of claims, the payer cannot examine each home care or hospice claim individually. Because of this, medical review efforts are directed toward areas and claims with the greatest risk of/for inappropriate payment. This process is called Progressive Corrective Action (PCA), and home care and hospice claims are subject to PCA based on the payer's initiatives and findings identified in claims processing, the survey process, and other sources of data collection. PCA entails the screening of claims with the greatest risk of overutilization of program payment.

The designated contractors or payers also have responsibilities related to timeliness of payments, fraud, and abuse initiatives; improving or assuring the quality of care provided to beneficiaries; and the ongoing education of providers. The largest impact of all contractors or payers from an organizational perspective is the specific medical review component. All contractors or payers are under pressure from the CMS to decrease claims that are not covered or not appropriate for Medicare and simultaneously avoid inconveniencing providers who do things right (bill correctly and adhere to coverage and other requirements). This is a big job, although sometimes it is only associated with additional documentation or development requests (called ADRs or 488s) received in the office. ADRs must be addressed promptly (within the required time frame; less than 30 days). All the requested documentation (such as specific visit information, physician orders to cover the entire period, etc.) should be contained in the clinical information within the record and correlate *exactly* with the requested bill(s).

The extent and depth of the review can vary, but it results in the claim being either paid or denied. Ineligibility continues to be problematic, whether due to lack of knowledge of coverage or other reasons. Surprisingly, "no physician orders obtained for the services billed," "the physician orders were not timely," "skilled nursing visit(s) not documented," "supplies not documented," "more visits provided than ordered," and "no physician certification obtained" continue to be among the top reasons for denials of home care claims.

Denials of any kind, including those just listed, can identify a trend to the payer, resulting in the review of even more claims. This has been called the "cascade effect" because the review goes deeper. For example, the contractor requests 20 clinical records (charts). During the review it is noted that the charts are missing visit notes, there are no verbal orders to continue the care, and supplies are not listed on the POC or mentioned elsewhere. The specific denials are identified, and the agency manager is notified. As a result, the organization is asked to submit more charts, and the cycle continues. Organizations or programs experiencing these reviews find the process costly and time-consuming because it is difficult to keep up with daily operations and effectively care for patients while also addressing these concerns. Prevention of medical review problems is the best solution. Always document treatment and services and have physician orders for all care anticipated and provided. The goal is that documentation is reviewed and no problems or irregularities are found. Periodic reviews and quality improvement processes will help to identify and address problem areas early and lower the risk for your agency.

PCA: An Overview

PCA is defined as a process for identifying and targeting limited medical review dollars on claims for which the greatest risk of inappropriate payment exists (see http://www.cms.hhs.gov/Transmittals/Downloads/R66PI.pdf for the full text in the *Medicare Program Integrity Manual*, Pub 100-08, Transmittal 66). Stated simply, the RHHIs find problems and focus efforts where there may be the most reward for their activities. This may be identifying a provider who clearly does not know coverage or collecting data for a fraud investigation or other program integrity (PI) initiative. They are then appropriately directed by CMS to target organizations and providers that do not adhere to the Medicare program requirements.

Providers frequently ask "Why me?" when chosen for a medical review or other kind of audit process. Providers and claims may be identified during statistical analysis (norms, outliers, thresholds, standards) or the number of visits billed. Agencies may be on review for a certain diagnosis, such as diabetes mellitus, or for any other selected parameters.

The Interface of Medical Review and PPS: Old and New

The more claims that are reviewed, the higher the likelihood of identifying problems. With this in mind, organizations should make coverage and associated documentation requirements an area for ongoing education and evaluation. These important skills should also be a component of the performance evaluation.

PPS brings additional topics for medical review because certain areas may involve heightened risk for financial loss or compromised quality of care. Questions that immediately come to mind regarding PPS and medical review:

- Is the case mix correct and congruent with the documented patient condition?
- Are all therapy visits necessary and is progress toward goals documented every visit?
- Do we have many episodes containing just five to six visits (which may suggest that you are avoiding LUPA episodes or trying to maximize revenues without a focus on medical necessity and quality)?
- Is OASIS seen as the basis for accurate payment?
- Do the POC, visit notes and documentation support the OASIS findings?
- Is the total number of visits provided consistent with patient care needs?

These and other important questions must be reviewed frequently. The government has allocated resources for review efforts to detect unnecessary episodes and flag underutilization within episodes of care on an ongoing basis.

Overall, efforts are directed toward ensuring that patient classification and billing data are accurate and that the payments made are appropriate.

Specific Areas for Medical Review

Therapy services continue as a focus of medical review because therapy services continue to weight the HHRG score, and agencies determine who receives/needs therapy services. LUPAs are another opportunity for medical review because of the nature of the threshold; making one or two additional visits (not based on patient need) results in the entire episode payment instead of payment per visit (a much reduced amount) based on three or four visits. For example, if an agency provides just enough visits to qualify for the full episode payment rather than the LUPA payment, that agency may have more than a cursory review, and be closely monitored and reviewed. Overall, CMS and its contractors are looking for significant patterns or changes in provider behavior that may be reimbursement-driven.

Diagnosis and Coding: Increasing Importance in Home Care

Like hospitals in the early 1980s with the inception of their PPS based on DRGs, determining the most appropriate diagnosis and codes for the episode is critical for appropriate reimbursement for home care. Determination of the primary and secondary diagnoses are the responsibility of the assessing clinician in collaboration with the physician. Poorly coded claims and claims that are questioned or further reviewed for lack of medical necessity are a concern for all administrators and financial officers. From a coding perspective, this diagnosis criterion is a significant factor because assignment of the ICD-9-CM code is intricately tied to reimbursement. Following up-to-date coding and other references and materials is important to remain compliant and to be apprised of changes in codes and regulations. Readers are referred to the American Health Information

Management Association (www.ahima.org) for further information regarding professional coding and coding standards of conduct.

The Health Insurance Portability and Accountability Act (HIPAA) of 1996 highlights the federal government's seriousness in uncovering and preventing Medicare fraud relative to the incorrect coding of Medicare patient records. In addition, the Office of the Inspector General (OIG), in its published compliance plan guidelines, lists specific areas of risk in health information and coding protocols. Historically the HIPAA and the OIG's focus has been on inpatient and outpatient settings; however, home care is now under continued, intense review as PPS is, in part, based on diagnostic coding.

Although PPS makes coding very important in numerous ways, as outcome studies become the norm in home care, diagnostic coding is also paramount in the determination of accurate and appropriate resource utilization for certain conditions. Managers and team members increasingly need accurate, timely patient care resource data for effective care planning and budgeting purposes that can be aggregated to the most appropriate category. That category will probably be a medical diagnosis or a group of similar medical diagnoses. In addition, OASIS patient information provides critical outcome data related to medical diagnosis(es) for calculations of recent (January 2008) and future refinements of the home care reimbursement rates. Coding is discussed further in the OASIS documentation section.

Back To The Future

Those of us who were (first) public health nurses remember having just a few visits after hospitalization to teach a family caregiver what he or she needed to know to function and who to call in an emergency. In fact, many believe that Medicare is trying to change from a high-tech intervention-focused model (in a patient population that generally needs medications assessed and ongoing case management) to that of a prevention-focused model.

There is Medicare coverage for care that is preventive in nature. Examples include immunizations, calcitonin (Calcimar) for osteoporosis, mammograms, colon cancer screening, and diabetes care and supplies. Some believe that the Balanced Budget Act, which passed some of these preventive initiatives set the stage for future Medicare reform. Changes to the law are beginning to build the framework of a grander plan for the Medicare program and make the change from administrator/ payer to purchaser with all the attendant implications of value, cost, and effective resource management. The Medicare Drug Benefit (Part D), however confusing, has proven to help ease the burden of prescription drug costs.

Whatever Medicare looks like in the future, older adults and other Medicare beneficiaries will not make hospitals their first choice for healthcare. Increasing inpatient costs, exposure to sometimes untreatable and increasing numbers of superinfections, the emphasis on patient rights and choice, and numerous safety and risk concerns all make home the setting of choice. Home care has survived the new landscape for practice-PPS. We must continue to improve practice, assist patients in their quest for self-care, and serve our communities. This is something home care has done for hundreds of years. In-home services will continue to expand in the coming years; but it will look very different from our historical perspectives of "how it used to be." The future of home care may well be better than how we remember it (see Box 1-6).

BOX 1-6

TIPS FOR SUCCESS

Changing Our Thinking

- Think episodes of care, not visits.
- Think maximizing patient self-care abilities and function to reduce emergent care visits and rehospitalizations.

Continued

BOX 1-6

TIPS FOR SUCCESS—cont'd

- Examine different case management models to determine which is best for your agency's practice and patient population.
- Study the OASIS data elements that determine the HHRGs—what the patients "look like" clinically.
- Remember that discharge planning begins at the initial SOC visit.
- "Front-load" visits at the beginning of the episode with intense interventions, particularly with therapy and home health aides, to prevent rehospitalization and hasten rehabilitation.
- Identify early in the episode if therapy, social work, or other services are needed to get patients to earlier optimal functioning and discharge.
- Practice patient education skills with each patient/family; learn what works for difficult or non-compliant patients. Involve social work early for these types of patients.
- Sign up for a patient assessment class to better hone physical and other assessment skills.
- Get physician orders signed as quickly as possible.
- Consult with/use wound care specialists (WOCNS and others) for wound care patients, cardiac clinical specialists for challenging heart failure patients, and certified diabetes educators for patients with diabetes.
- Remember the saying, "If we always do what we've always done, we'll always get what we've always gotten"—we cannot afford *not* to change.
- Know that PPS can be better—we know the parameters.
- Be a leader and embrace change—it will continue.
- Know that the PPS reimbursement model values critical thinking (our cognitive skills—teaching, training, managing services) rather than hands-on psychomotor activities!
- Develop and use clinical paths or protocols (the paths may have corresponding patient education paths or patient contract components).

- Treat your patients as essential partners in education and outcome achievement—they must be!
- Implement computer-based (clinical automation) charting systems to enhance and expedite charting.
- Embrace the clinical automation system if your organization already has one. Information "at your fingertips," needed to closely manage and evaluate care, is more important than ever.
- Teach a new team member or peer about PPS—the more you say it, practice it, and learn the glossary, the greater your comfort level.
- Subscribe to publications and read everything you can about evidence-based, innovative practices. Although it may be hard to try new things in such a regulated environment, we must—the incentives have been realigned for us to assess, treat, teach, and discharge.
- Sign up for telehealth education programs and learn that new glossary—it will become a common part of home care.
- Think in terms of groupings of patients (e.g., cardiovascular, neurologic) to identify trends and opportunities for improvement and increased efficiency across patient populations.
- Collaborate with clinical and non-clinical team members—the financial and clinical sides must be fully integrated.
- Educate physicians regarding changes—they must be our partners in patient care.
- Determine the specific plan and interventions for each visit at SOC.
- Involve the patient *and* the family/caregiver in care, beginning with the first visit.
- Identify any on-site visits that can be supplemented with telehealth protocols.
- Increase exponentially the speed of patient and family/caregiver education.
- Start with "What can I do to help you be independent (again)?" If that is not an option; what can you do to facilitate community and other caregiver supports for this patient?

Continued

BOX 1-6

TIPS FOR SUCCESS—cont'd

- Help with the development of standardized patient education tools at your organization.
- Know that now is the time to begin practicing evidence-based care.
- Communicate to your manager when a patient's status changes and intervene early.
- Use supplies and medical equipment judiciously; this may include treatments, dressings that are not changed as often, and intravenous pumps that are multidosage.
- Remember that Medicare home care fundamentals remain—homebound and other criteria—but there is generally a focus on underutilization.
- Attend in-services and other educational programs that provide up-to-date evidence-based care practices.
- Implement disease management programs to assist in helping clinicians improve patient outcomes.
- Remember that we are here to provide quality home care; the mission has not changed—but the methods may!

Component Two: Quality and Customer Service Imperatives

Three major problems have continued to plague the United States healthcare "system": access, cost, and quality. The continuing problem of access (lack of) and cost escalation of healthcare services is frequently cited in the newspapers and television news and provides grist for the political mill. It is no secret that the United States spends more than any other country in the world on healthcare, and yet, our morbidity and mortality rates remain higher for certain health problems than other countries. Consumers of healthcare want value for their healthcare, regardless of who pays for it. We have numerous external factors that demand quality, safety, and mandate measurable outcomes related to the provision of healthcare. Some of these factors include accreditation bodies such as The Joint Commission (JC, www.jointcommission.org), Community Health Accreditation Program (www.chapinc.org), Accreditation Commission for Health Care (ACHC), and others; utilization review entities; case management firms; and others. All these factors demonstrate that the cost/quality equation is becoming harder to balance for everyone concerned: patients, clinicians, home care organizations, and insurance payers.

Quality: An Overview

Quality emerged as a buzzword almost three decades ago, but is a critical concept that is here to stay in healthcare, and has become a cornerstone for successful organizations and their staff members. The basic premise of quality in home care is that the right clinicians provide the right interventions for the right patient at the right time. This means "doing it right the first time." Having the "right clinicians" starts with hiring skilled clinicians, with defined performance expectations clearly specified in the job or position descriptions. Competence or competency assessment is a long-term, ongoing, quality process that includes initially assessing the knowledge and skills of the clinical team members with on-going assessment, reassessing that the knowledge and skills are up-to-date, evidence-based, and appropriate for the patients being treated. In this way patients and their families are assured that competent clinicians knowledgeable in their area of expertise will contribute to the achievement of patient outcomes in a safe and standardized manner. This process of continually reviewing clinical team members' knowledge and skills is key to the provision of the best home care. Cross training, interdisciplinary orientation, and ongoing education also contribute to improved team work, standardized care, and effective operations.

The best organizations "walk the talk" of quality. These are organizations where "questioning why" is seen as a good thing, where the culture is that "no one is as smart as all of us," and there is true team work in which staff members work with each other as part of a cohesive team that revolves around patient needs. Quality improvement is the hallmark of the quality imperative and is key to survival in the health vision of the future. There is a saying, "If you cannot measure it, you cannot manage it." With this in mind, organizations set quality expectations and evaluate quality based on collected data.

Evaluating Quality: Focus on Data Management and Analysis

Organizations must effectively manage and analyze their data to evaluate the quality of the care they provide. The OASIS has brought home care up-to-date with other health entities such as hospitals which must track results of their care. The Home Health Compare website (www.medicare.gov/HHCompare) is sponsored by CMS and provides updates on home health quality measures from the OASIS information collected by Medicare and Medicaid-certified HHAs. These quality measures provide information about patients' physical health, whether their ability to perform basic daily activities improved, and whether emergent and/or hospital services were required to manage acute instabilities. Even if a patient's health condition (such as heart failure or diabetes) is not expected to get better, patients can usually improve how they manage and live with their illness. OBQM and OBQI reports are also based on the OASIS data, and contain outcome measures that are used for quality improvement. Home Health Compare, as well as OBQM and OBQI, are discussed in more depth in Part Two.

In addition to the above, many home care organizations track other statistics and trends, including: (1) average visits and length of stay by diagnoses or major diagnostic category; (2) average visits and length of stay or service by payer (such as Medicare, private insurance); (3) average visit and length of time spent per visit by discipline; (4) percentage of patients admitted to home care from an inpatient setting; and (5) rehospitalization rates. Other measures of quality include customer service and satisfaction survey feedback from patients, family, and referral sources; infection control information; incident reports; turn-around times for physician signatures for POCs and other physician orders; safety-related data such as falls; outcome reports that demonstrate appropriate care and visit patterns; and other resource utilization information. Some of this data can then be used as marketing materials to referral sources and consumers, especially when displayed in graph format.

Whatever the information collected, the data must be systematically aggregated and analyzed, summarized, and activities planned to further improve the quality of that process. Organizations and clinicians continually seek new ways to think about how to provide quality services and seek opportunities to streamline or redesign activities to support the best work of any home care organization. The goal is for patients to have achieved agreed-upon predetermined outcomes attributable to clinician interventions provided in an equal partnership with the patient. Only through this mechanism can the value of home care continue to be successfully demonstrated. Clinicians and organizations should ask, "What is/was the impact of my care/intervention/management on this particular patient?" The other hallmark that supports quality and survival in this competitive and changing environment is customer service.

Customer Service

Excellence in customer service is the cornerstone of quality. The external environment, including increased competition and regulatory entities, has brought the concept of customer service to a new and important level. In some cases, organizations may lose sight that home care is essentially a *service industry*. Customer service is a skill that too often has not been stressed and valued enough in the healthcare environment. Unfortunately, in some instances, it has been completely neglected. In the past, many customers or consumers of healthcare accepted less than perfect or merely adequate customer service, attributing it to the way the healthcare industry has "always" operated. Clinicians may sometimes think of customer service only in relation to the patient and family satisfaction survey or a form that may be sent out after discharge or at other times, depending on the organization. It is most important to think of quality far beyond the confines of patient satisfaction. Regular customer service in-services are needed to reinforce this quality indicator.

There are many "customers" in any home care or hospice organization. There are the external customers—patients, their families, and companies connected with patients, such as hospital referral sources, referring physicians, managed care company nurses, and others. Equally important are the internal customers—the home care team members, including clinical, managerial and administrative, billing, and others who work together to create an effective team. How positively and collaboratively the whole team works together and communicates is a measure of customer service. In fact, many organizations value and heavily weigh customer service from a performance evaluation perspective. In larger organizations, in which there are multiple office locations or local offices and corporate headquarters, these entities and the team members are also customers of the organization. Members of alliances, networks, systems, and other relationships of which the organization is a part are also customers.

Another measure of customer service attributes is the use of customer service satisfaction evaluation tools or survey forms. The patient's perception of care or satisfaction has emerged as a necessary monitor in this world of increased competition. All clinicians know that "bedside" manners are very important to patients and their families. In the past, good bedside manners were thought to be "enough" to define customer service. However, the home as a healthcare setting has introduced a whole new aspect to the traditional meaning of bedside manners.

With home care's direct patient and family contact, one of the most important ingredients for success is the human element. All team members should treat every phone or in-person encounter positively, always keeping in mind that the person is a customer. Of course, tasks need to be prioritized, but from a customer service perspective, some activities are to be valued more than others. For example, because home care services rely heavily on phone calls, this may be an opportunity for improved customer service. Remember if you answer a call from a referral source or family member, *you* are the first impression of home care. Numerous studies have shown how important first impressions are—after an assessment has been made by the customer or consumer, it is difficult to change.

One way to learn how your organization is perceived is to call your organization as a customer. Is the name of the organization and the person answering clearly stated? How does the person sound? Phones should always be answered timely and per agency policy to meet customer service goals. For example, many organizations have a standard of three rings maximum prior to answering; others may have a policy that calls are always returned within a certain period of time (e.g., within one hour) when following up on phone mail messages. In-services on phone etiquette are helpful for all staff.

The level of customer service that an organization provides on a daily basis can make *the* difference in its reputation and long-term survival. The goal of the organization and its team members is to meet the specific home healthcare needs of the public. Being on-time for scheduled appointments, calling if you are running late or early, and communicating changes support positive customer service feelings and are valued by many patients. Be aware of the crucial role that you have in facilitating the achievement of your organization's customer service goals.

Summary

Quality, customer service, and respect for patient rights go hand-in-hand in organizations that seek to provide excellent care for their patients. Quality must be a hallmark of every home care and hospice organization. Data is collected and analyzed, results are distributed and studied, specific areas are chosen for improvement, and educational and other efforts are directed toward ongoing improvement. This cycle is the force that drives the achievement of both quality and customer service imperatives.

Component Three: Home: The Environment of Care

Providing care in the patient's home and environment is why home care is so different from other care settings. Home care clinicians are guests in the patient and family's personal space, the opposite of the relationship in the hospital or other outpatient settings. In the patient's home, the clinician is immediately exposed to relevant data related to the patient's environment.

The home care clinician's observational and assessment/evaluation skills are key to early identification of potential safety problems or hazards in the patient's home environment. A home safety assessment is a part of the mandated comprehensive assessment in home care. Some of the more common safety hazards include ferocious or unusual pets (or unsanitary pet care), uneven steps or sidewalks, lack of maintenance on floor boards or porches, throw rugs, and space heaters. Rugs may slide and rug edges can pose a safety threat and contribute to falls. Other hazards include hallways that are cluttered, long, loose telephone cords or oxygen tubing, excessive noise such as from blaring televisions, inadequate lighting, and excessive smoke.

Environmental Safety Considerations: Identifying At-Risk Patients

Patients may have one or more environmental factors contributing to their inability to achieve established goals.

Although each factor, by itself, may not trigger the need for intervention by other team members, the clinician may see multiple factors that indicate a trend that needs to be evaluated to ensure the patient's long-term safety. Factors that may be high-risk indicators relative to the patient's home safety status are shown in Box 1-7.

BOX 1-7

HOME SAFETY RISK FACTORS

- Older age, frailty
- Living alone
- Caregiver's age and ability, capability, and willingness to care for the patient
- Patient (or caregiver) not answering the phone or door
- Incontinence problems or complaints (including odors)
- Impaired ability or inability to perform ADLs
- Lack of basic requirements or inadequate requirements for safety and health (e.g., food or refrigeration availability/capability, safe municipal or other water for drinking and hygiene needs, heat, air conditioning, protection from the natural elements)
- Environments in which either the patient or caregiver is abusive/abused
- Problematic social interactions (e.g., no or poor relations with others, loner, hermit-like, geographically or socially isolated, history of "firing" aides or others, refuses family help)
- Lack of appropriate equipment and limited adaptability to such equipment (e.g., bathtub upstairs with no railing on stairs)
- Physical structure of the home is of concern (e.g., wood stove is used for heat in winter and patient on oxygen therapy)
- Financial resource limitations

Continued

BOX 1-7

HOME SAFETY RISK FACTORS—cont'd

- Poor understanding, confusion, sundowning, inappropriate affect, paranoia, perceptual or judgment impairment, cognitive problems, behavioral problems, other psychological problems
- Patient/caregiver not following safety precautions
- Depression or grief symptomatology (e.g., tearful, crying, sad, history of loss)
- Poor appetite or impaired nutritional status
- Poor quantity/quality of sleep
- Multiple pathologies or co-morbidities (e.g., HF, COPD, cancer)
- Non-compliant with recommended therapeutic regimens
- Hygiene concerns from pets, pests or infestations such as roaches, fleas, lice, worms, or inappropriate defecation
- Language barriers or difficulty in accessing assistance
- Multiple/habitual emergency room visits and/or hospitalization/rehospitalizations in lieu of primary care
- History of falls or fractures (e.g., hip, wrist) due to falls
- Physical or geographical location (e.g., patient lives where there are few or no community resources)
- Substance abuse (patient or caregiver)
- Inability to perform IADLs (such as banking, shopping, acquiring prescriptions, laundry, cleaning house, preparing meals)
- Other factors

Home environmental problems as listed above should lead the clinician to two important questions: "What impact are the environmental problems having on the patient's health status?" and "Does this patient need a medical social worker or other interdisciplinary referral, such as occupational therapy or physical therapy?" Safety considerations may determine the need or trigger the mechanism for an evaluation by another member of the interdisciplinary team, discussed more fully in the next section, Component Four: Patient Care Planning and Related Processes.

Summary

The patient's home environment, when looked at holistically, often makes the difference between a patient being able to remain at home while receiving healthcare services or having to find an alternate setting, such as an assisted living or skilled nursing facility. The home care interdisciplinary team must use creative skills to develop a net for these at-risk patients, particularly older adults who want to remain in their own homes. Problems with safety issues could trigger problems in OBQM and OBQI data. The assessment information gathered by all team members and referrals made to other team members can often enable patients to remain safely in their home environments.

Component Four: Patient Care Planning and Related Processes

The formation of the POC is the essential component that creates the route or road map for the interdisciplinary team and patient to follow to achieve desired outcomes. Once the assessment has been done, thoughtful analysis of the data occurs, the goals are identified, and the patient's POC is established with direction from the physician and input from the patient/caregivers and other team members.

Because care planning and patient and family needs are directed from the assessed and reassessed findings, the services are based on the patient's specific pathology that requires intervention and other problems specific to their needs. It is this vision of where the patient can/will be upon discharge that creates the path to meeting the goals that all team members, most importantly the patient, support. See *Part Two: Clinical Practice in Home Care,* for a more detailed discussion of care planning and related processes.

Home care is delivered by an interdisciplinary team of clinicians with differing scopes of practice, standards, and clinical guidelines that contribute to improved care for patients and to the standardization of care and processes from an organizational perspective. Care is being reframed as advanced technology, specialized knowledge, and evidence-based practices of each discipline are implemented in the home care environment. It is essential that home care team members who can best meet the needs of the patient and family be consulted as early as possible after the need is identified and that the care be coordinated by the case manager. It should also be noted that Medicare, Medicaid, and other insurance payers may pay for only certain disciplines and services so it is always important to check and verify coverage.

Home care team members may include the following:

- Home health nurse, hospice nurse
- Other specialty, advanced practice nurses including psychiatric nurse, wound, ostomy, continence nurse specialist, certified diabetes educator (CDE)
- Physical therapist
- Occupational therapist
- Speech-language pathologist
- Medical social worker
- Home health aide
- Respiratory therapist
- Homemaker
- Dietitian
- Pharmacist
- Spiritual counselor, chaplain
- Physician
- Volunteers

HOME HEALTH, HOSPICE NURSE, PSYCHIATRIC NURSE, WOUND SPECIALIST, CERTIFIED DIABETES EDUCATOR: With some exceptions, home health and hospice nurses generally act as the case manager while a patient is receiving services. This care must always be provided within a medically-approved POC—physician orders are needed for all care and changes to the POC. Clinicians must possess excellent communication, assessment, planning, intervention, and teaching skills, and be able to work independently and in collaboration with other disciplines efficiently and effectively. Additionally, those clinicians who work with hospice or hospice-type patients should be experienced in the art and science of pain and symptom management.

The role of the psychiatric nurse in home care has been expanding as more care is provided in the community setting. The specific coverage of services related to psychiatric evaluation and therapy are found in Part Six of this book. The kinds of problems seen in home care by psychiatric nurses include depression and therapy, bipolar disorder, evaluation of medication therapeutic levels and effectiveness, and many geriatric-affective disorders.

The psychiatric nurse is primarily needed for the skills of medication evaluation, observation and assessment, and evaluation and therapy; the social worker may also be involved in counseling. Sometimes it may be appropriate for cases to be shared. The psychiatric nurse visit, which is a skilled nursing visit, may be covered for that expertise. For example, the patient with medical-surgical problems and depression or manipulative behavior may be seen by the psychiatric nurse, the same way that the primary nurse may arrange for a wound care specialist to see a patient with complex wound problems. The psychiatric nurse would set up the POC in conjunction with the primary nurse and other team members to establish a behavioral plan for the team. The documentation needs to focus on the psychiatric needs as documented by the psychiatric data base, such as a mental status exam and other interventions.

Some HHAs have a wound care specialist available as a consultant and clinical specialist. This role is particularly important in the HHA and in hospice settings with a high volume of patients with ostomies and complex wounds.

The certified diabetes educator (CDE) is important in diabetes case management, program development, and patient and clinician education.

Some agencies have other clinical specialists, such as heart failure or cardiac clinical specialists or infusion care, to assist with case management, program management, and patient and clinician education.

PHYSICAL THERAPIST: Physical therapists (PTs) have an important role as members of the rehabilitation team. The PT assists home care patients to attain the maximum level of safety and independence in physical function. This is accomplished by addressing strength, range of motion, pain, balance, and neuromotor deficits. Cardiopulmonary re-conditioning, transfer and gait training, and wound care are other physical therapy interventions that may be provided at home. The PT must possess excellent communication, assessment, planning, and intervention skills, and serve as the case manager with patients who require therapy services only. The PT, like other team members, provides input into the POC and any necessary revisions, prepares clinical documentation, and participates in in-service programs.

The physical therapist assistant is a technically educated healthcare provider who assists the PT in the provision of physical therapy. The physical therapy assistant, under the direction and supervision of the PT, is the only paraprofessional who provides physical therapy interventions.

OCCUPATIONAL THERAPIST: The occupational therapist (OT) is another important member of the home care rehabilitation team, with expertise in maximizing the patient's safety and independence in functional activities of life, including activities of daily living (ADLs [such as bathing and dressing]) and instrumental activities of daily living (IADLs [such as meal preparation or doing laundry]). In optimizing functional performance, OTs may use interventions such as upper extremity hand therapies, sensorimotor training, energy conservation, modification of the home environment, and training in the use of adaptive devices or compensatory techniques. The OT can be an excellent partner for the agency's home health aides to ensure that, whenever possible, patients maximize their functional abilities rather than increasing their dependence on others.

The OT, like all members of the interdisciplinary team, prepares clinical documentation, attends case conferences, and participates in care planning.

The occupational therapy assistant is a technically educated paraprofessional who can provide selected OT interventions under the direction and supervision of the OT.

SPEECH-LANGUAGE PATHOLOGIST (SLP): Speech-language pathology services are an important part of therapy for patients with various speech and swallowing problems and often include cognitive therapy. Home care patients who may need specialized speech-language pathology services include those with cerebral vascular accidents; tracheostomies; laryngectomies; post-radiation for throat cancers; various neurologic diseases such as Alzheimer's Disease, amyotrophic lateral sclerosis, and multiple sclerosis; and any who experience communication, swallowing, or cognitive-linguistic deficits. Like all of the team members, the SLP creates clinical documentation, provides input into the POC, and attends case conferences about the patient's status and progress on a regular basis for effective care coordination. The SLP also case manages in certain situations.

SOCIAL WORKER: The social worker (Master of Social Work [MSW] or Bachelor of Social Work [BSW]) is an important member of the home care team. Support, active listening, and resource identification are just some of the services that social workers provide to patients and family/caregivers. Problems addressed by social workers include financial concerns, housing issues, caregiver support concerns, and other patient/caregiver issues. Most home care social workers have master's degrees and clinical expertise in the counseling and other needs of home care patients and their families.

HOME HEALTH AIDE: Home health aides, or certified nursing assistants as they are called in some states, provide probably the most important service for many patients. Home health aides are the "eyes and ears" of the organization.

They often visit the patient the most, especially in the initial stages of home care, providing personal care and assistance in the activities of daily living as the patient becomes more independent, or supporting the patient in these activities to maintain them comfortably at home.

Medicare standards and most state regulations require that home health aides be specially trained and proficient in several subject areas. Home health aides are closely supervised by the RN or other appropriate team members to ensure their competence and comfort in providing the best home care to patients.

RESPIRATORY THERAPIST: Respiratory therapists, also known as respiratory care practitioners, provide evaluation, treatment, management, and monitoring services for patients with acute and chronic respiratory and cardiovascular problems (e.g., chronic obstructive pulmonary disease [COPD], asthma, emphysema, cerebrovascular accident [CVA]). Care provided by respiratory therapists may include administration of oxygen, management of mechanical ventilators, administration of respiratory drugs, and measuring and monitoring cardiopulmonary function. Respiratory therapists also provide education and training materials for other home care clinicians related to oxygen and cardiopulmonary care needs.

HOMEMAKER: Homemakers maintain the patient care area so that safe and effective home care can be provided. Homemaker services may include light housekeeping duties such as cleaning, vacuuming, and grocery shopping.

DIETITIAN: Depending on the state and licensure requirements, the dietitian may be a licensed dietitian or registered dietitian. Accreditation standards require that the patient's nutritional status be assessed and nutritional interventions implemented as appropriate. Many home care and hospice programs have dietitians available to make home visits and provide consultative services for conditions such as anorexia, mouth sores, wounds, pain, swallowing disorders, diarrhea or constipation, nausea/vomiting, and weight loss or gain. The dietitian may also make recommendations related to enteral and parenteral nutrition therapy. Other services include teaching about complex diets, identifying educational materials for use with patient teaching, and acting as an in-service educator and resource related to nutrition services.

PHARMACIST: The important role of the pharmacist is growing with the complexities of drug-drug, drug-disease, and drug-food adverse reactions. In home care, nurses are acutely aware that many patients are inappropriately medicated or overmedicated. Most home care patients are older adults and have multiple risk factors for adverse reactions related to drug therapy, including co-morbidities, multiple healthcare providers, and various functional limitations (e.g., poor eyesight, impaired hearing, arthritic fingers). The clinician in the community sees the whole picture, including the shoeboxes filled with medications given to patients by multiple physicians. Polypharmacy issues are growing and have become a real concern for the older adult population.

The clinician must address safety concerns related to medications and consult with the pharmacist for help in effectively evaluating the multiple medication regimens. The pharmacist can offer other services to the home care team, including: (1) providing in-service education and information about medications; (2) reviewing medication regimens and screening for interactions and incorrect doses or dosage forms; (3) suggesting simplifying medication regimens by altering drug delivery systems or medication administration scheduling; (4) monitoring and assessing the therapeutic or toxic effect of drugs; (5) participating in case conference as needed; and (6) acting as a resource for pain and other symptom control, especially for hospice patients. An innovative practice that some agencies are beginning to implement is to have pharmacists more involved in prescribing warfarin sodium doses, which has resulted in fewer anti-coagulation medication errors. In addition, the pharmacist provides important management of medication-related issues at end-of-life.

SPIRITUAL COUNSELOR/CHAPLAIN: A spiritual assessment should be a part of the comprehensive assessment that is performed upon evaluation and admission to home care. The spiritual care services provided should be consistent with the belief systems of the patient and family. Many home care and hospice programs have a network of community clergy who provide support and spiritual care to patients, and organizations have their own chaplain team who work with the local community spiritual representatives. Responsibilities of the chaplain team may include providing bereavement counseling, serving on ethics committees, supporting staff and attending team meetings, performing sacraments for the sick, and intervening in other ways.

The chaplain provides services that span the life continuum from birth through death. The chaplain, like the professional nurse, interacts with patients and their families and friends at some of the most difficult times of their lives. The struggle with the meaning of life, experienced by many who have significant health concerns, is the work of the chaplain, regardless of any formal religious beliefs. The role varies based on the setting, the patient and family, and other needs. It may include bereavement counseling, ethics committees, hospice staff support, and sacraments for the sick. The chaplain facilitates the patient's movement toward his or her resolution of life's questions.

Patients who may benefit from chaplaincy services include those for whom the North American Nursing Diagnosis Association-International (NANDA-I) nursing diagnosis, *spiritual distress* (distress of the human spirit), has been identified as an appropriate nursing diagnosis. Other patients may have a need for spiritual care based on their health problems. For example, the older adult patient who is temporarily homebound due to a recent fall and fracture and cannot attend church services may need a call made to the priest or minister to arrange visits to the home.

PHYSICIAN: The physician is a key member of the home care team and plays a critical role in the patient's POC. Medicare and other health insurance plans cover or pay for "medically necessary" care. They require that the physician certify that the patient needs the services and sign the POC supporting the care. All care, changes in the POC, and significant changes in the patient's condition must be reported to the physician and documented in the patient's clinical record. From legal, quality, and standards-of-practice perspectives, it is essential that the home care team members communicate and coordinate care with the patient's physician(s). Physicians can bill Medicare for these home care patient/POC services.

VOLUNTEER: Use of volunteer services varies among home care organizations, but volunteers and their supportive care and services are a unique and valued part of hospice care. The primary role of these volunteers is to offer respite for the family, but some also specialize in areas such as bereavement, spiritual support, and art or other therapies.

Box 1-8 lists and describes some professional associations for different types of home care providers.

BOX 1-8

PROFESSIONAL ASSOCIATIONS FOR HOME CARE PROVIDERS

HOME HEALTH NURSING

The Home Healthcare Nurses Association (HHNA) (www.hhna.org) is an organization involved in home healthcare practice, education, administration, and research. The HHNA became an affiliate of the National Association for Home Care & Hospice in 1999. The professional peer-reviewed journal for Home Health Care is published by Lippincott Williams & Wilkins and is *Home Healthcare Nurse*. Information about this journal can be accessed at www.marrelli.com or at www.homehealthcarenurseonline.com.

Continued

BOX 1-8

PROFESSIONAL ASSOCIATIONS FOR HOME CARE PROVIDERS—cont'd

Visiting Nurse Association

The Visiting Nurse Associations of America (VNAA) can be accessed by visiting www.vnaa.org.

Hospice Nursing

The Hospice and Palliative Nurses Association (HPNA) (www.hpna.org) was established in 1986 and is the nation's largest and oldest professional nursing organization dedicated to promoting excellence in hospice and palliative nursing care.

Psychiatric Nursing

The American Psychiatric Nurses Association (APNA) (www.apna.org) is a professional organization committed to the specialty practice of psychiatric mental health nursing, health and wellness promotion through identification of mental health issues, prevention of mental health problems, and the care and treatment of persons with psychiatric disorders.

Wound, Ostomy, Continence Nurse or Wound Care Specialist

The Wound, Ostomy and Continence Nurses Society (WOCN) (www.wocn.org) was founded in 1968 and is a professional, international nursing society for experts in the care of patients with wound, ostomy, and incontinence. It supports its members by promoting educational, clinical, and research opportunities to advance the practice and guide the delivery of expert healthcare to individuals with wounds, ostomies, and incontinence.

Certified Diabetes Educator

The American Association of Diabetes Educators (AADE) (www.aade) is a multidisciplinary organization dedicated to integrating successful self-management as a key outcome in the care of people with diabetes and related conditions. They can be accessed at www.diabetesedu cator.org.

Physical Therapist

The American Physical Therapy Association (APTA) (www.apta.org) is a national professional organization whose goal is to foster advancements in physical therapy practice, research, and education.

Occupational Therapist

The American Occupational Therapy Association (AOTA) (www.aota.org) is a professional organization committed to supporting the professional community through monitoring, responding to, and influencing healthcare, education, and community-related systems, and the way that occupational therapy is integrated into the delivery of services within those systems.

Speech-Language Pathologist

The American Speech-Language-Hearing Association (ASHA) (www.asha.org) is the professional, scientific, and credentialing association for SLPs, audiologists, and speech, language, and hearing scientists in the United States and internationally.

Medical Social Worker

The National Association of Social Workers (NASW) (www.socialworkers.org) is the largest membership organization of professional social workers in the world, and works to enhance professional growth and development, create and maintain professional standards, and advance sound social policies.

Respiratory Therapist

The American Association for Respiratory Care (AARC) (www.aarc.org) is the only professional society for respiratory therapists in hospitals, nursing homes, and home care, managers of respiratory and cardiopulmonary services, and educators who provide respiratory care training.

Continued

BOX 1-8

PROFESSIONAL ASSOCIATIONS FOR HOME CARE PROVIDERS—cont'd

Dietitian

The American Dietetic Association (ADA) (www.eatright.org) is the largest organization of food and nutrition professionals, and serves the public by promoting optimal nutrition, health and well-being.

Pharmacist

The American Pharmacists Association (APhA) (www.pharmacist.com) is the largest association of pharmacists in the United States, and provides a forum for discussion, consensus building, and policy setting for the profession of pharmacy.

The American Society of Health-System Pharmacists (www.ASHP.org).

Spiritual Counselor/Chaplain

The Association of Professional Chaplains (APC) (www.professionalchaplains.org) is an interfaith professional pastoral care association of providers of pastoral care endorsed by faith groups to serve persons in physical, spiritual, or mental need in diverse settings throughout the world.

Physician

The American Academy of Home Care Physicians (AAHCP) (www.aahcp.org) began in 1988 and serves the needs of thousands of physicians and related professionals and agencies interested in improving care of patients in the home. Members are home care physicians—physicians who make house calls, care for homebound patients, act as home health agency medical directors, or refer patients to home care agencies. Specialties include internal medicine, family practice, pediatrics, geriatrics, psychiatry, emergency medicine, and more.

Volunteers

Volunteers of America (VOA) (www.voa.org) is a national, non-profit, faith-based organization dedicated to helping those in need rebuild their lives and reach their full potential through thousands of human service programs, including housing and healthcare. Since 1896, VOA has supported vulnerable groups, including at-risk youth, the frail elderly, men and women returning from prison, homeless individuals and families, people with disabilities, and those recovering from addictions.

Team Communications and Care Coordination: Keys to Success

The essence of care coordination can be best described in the following scenario. If something happened to you and one of your colleagues had to visit your patient this morning with no verbal report, would your clinical documentation tell the story of your patient? Does it list information about the caregivers and other team members who also visit, have an accurate, up-to-date medication list, detail the current POC exactly, and contain numerous other details that provide effective documentation and clearly communicate the needs of the patient? Does it contain information related to communication and care coordination with other care providers (e.g., physicians, discharge planners) and community services (e.g., Meals-on-Wheels, Senior Housing) outside of the organization? What is the mechanism in your agency to facilitate this process? The provision of quality home care is based on care coordination activities, and ***must*** be reflected in the associated documentation.

The documentation must tell any reviewer, peer, or state or accreditation surveyor the exact details of the care for each patient—a task much easier said than done. Document in your patient's clinical records with the thought that other team members do not have the base of knowledge that you have from actually being there and providing care to the patient. Write all the information that provides the best continuity and care coordination across and among the team members. Examples of effective care coordination are listed in Box 1-9.

BOX 1-9

EXAMPLES OF EFFECTIVE CARE COORDINATION

- Calling the case manager with updates on the patient's progress and your findings
- Attending interdisciplinary team meetings and providing input
- Calling/faxing/e-mailing the physician with updates on your findings/concerns
- Validating that the patient understands the discharge instructions by being able to list the taught actions for self-care
- Planning a joint visit with another team member (e.g., nurse, aide, therapist)
- Calling in reports on the aide's or other clinician's voice mail after the visit to update team members on the patient's progress; documenting this call
- Communicating with patients, family members, and caregivers and documenting these communications
- Documenting all phone calls, meetings, and communications related to your patient's care
- Others—as numerous as the creativity of the team to facilitate this important component of quality home care

Summary

Patient care planning and related processes are the basis of the provision of home care services. The knowledge base of the first three components discussed earlier in Part One—Reimbursement/Payer Processes, Quality and Customer Service Imperatives, and Home: The Environment of Care—combine into a practical plan for patient care that will most effectively assist in the achievement of desired patient outcomes. Interdisciplinary care and the case management model are the keys to facilitating these outcomes and making home care a sought-after and viable option for the future. Box 1-10 presents a comprehensive list of the skills and knowledge needed in home care.

References

1. Warhola C: Planning for home health services: A resource handbook, DHHS Publication No. (HRA) 80-14017, Washington, D.C., 1980, U.S. Public Health Service, Department of Health and Human Resources.

BOX 1-10

SKILLS AND KNOWLEDGE NEEDED IN HOME CARE

Continuing changes in the healthcare environment make home care a challenging practice and management field for both experienced and novice healthcare professionals. The clinician and patient/family interactions, the range and diversity of clinical skills employed, and the satisfaction that accompanies caring for patients in situations in which they are equal partners in care and outcome achievement is appealing to many clinicians. The following enumerates some of the characteristics common to team members who are successful in home care.

1. KNOWLEDGE OF THE BASIC "RULES" OF HOME CARE.

Consisting of both administrative and clinical information, these "rules" are important to effective operations. For clinicians employed by Medicare-certified HHAs, a knowledge of the

Continued

BOX 1-10

SKILLS AND KNOWLEDGE NEEDED IN HOME CARE—cont'd

following is required: (1) the Medicare COPs; (2) the Medicare Program Integrity Manual provisions related to home care coverage and documentation requirements; (3) the Medicare Manual section that addresses the correct completion of the CMS POC; (4) the CMS OASIS Implementation Manual that addresses the OASIS data set requirements; and (5) state specific rules and regulations, such as licensure requirements. See Part Six of this text for further reference.Because Medicare and many states set numerous standards and licensure requirements for home care, being familiar and up-to-date with these rules is important. Other insurers may use Medicare's criteria for qualifying for coverage, the coverage itself, and the payment mechanism(s). In addition, many insurers such as state Medicaid programs and private insurers use the CMS POC data elements for their required POC or plan of treatment.

2. REPERTOIRE OF SERVICE-DRIVEN AND PATIENT-FAMILY ORIENTED INTERPERSONAL SKILLS.

Effective interpersonal skills, including community liaison and public relations activities, are an integral part of being a home care clinician. These interpersonal skills represent your organization in the community!

3. ABILITY TO PAY INCREDIBLE ATTENTION TO DETAIL—AND ENJOY IT.

This is true both in addressing complex patient needs and in documenting care and services provided. Both are equally important and go hand-in-hand. For example, the initial comprehensive assessment, including the OASIS data elements, must be completed within mandated time frames. The comprehensive assessment must be accurate and reflect the patient's true state of health and function, because HHA reimbursement and care planning are based on this assessment.

4. POSSESSION OF MULTIFACETED SKILLS ACCOMPANIED BY FLEXIBILITY.

The home care clinician is the one who must "bend" or renegotiate to meet patient needs and achieve patient-centered goals.

This flexibility usually includes visiting times, scheduling, and other aspects that center on accommodating patient and caregiver needs.

5. POSSESSION OF A RELIABLE CAR AND SAFE, EFFECTIVE DRIVING SKILLS.

The home care clinician must like—or at least not mind—driving, have a good sense of direction (and a navigation system or good map), be willing to drive in heavy traffic and/or inclement weather, and possess a spirit of adventure!

6. ABILITY TO ASSUME RESPONSIBILITY FOR THE PATIENT AND THE PATIENT'S POC.

True case management is possible in home care and essential to the achievement of outcomes. From the initial comprehensive assessment visit through the identification of needs and desired outcomes, the home care clinician assists the patient and coordinates with other team members regarding the planning and follow-through for patient care.

Because of these factors, the nurse or other team member in the community setting can directly affect the care and impact the results of that care. Often, strong communication is required between the home care organization and the case manager from the insurance company. This total patient management function, with its associated priority-setting, critical-thinking, and complex decision-making skills, and resource utilization decisions, makes home care unique. This aspect also allows team members to receive personal satisfaction and positive feedback from patients and their families, friends, and caregivers.

7. UP-TO-DATE AND PROFICIENT CLINICAL PRACTICE SKILLS, INCLUDING THE ABILITY TO FUNCTION AS BOTH A GENERALIST AND A SPECIALIST.

Home healthcare is provided for all age groups—from infancy to older adults. In addition, the diagnoses and care needs of patients may vary from day to day, or visit to visit. In home care, although the clinician may have to address a wide range of clinical problems, interventions, and desired outcomes, having an area of expertise is helpful for both the individual clinician and the organization. The special skills (e.g., certification, advanced practice credentials) are also useful when teaching, acting as a resource, case managing, or orienting clinicians new to home care. For patients with

Continued

BOX 1-10

SKILLS AND KNOWLEDGE NEEDED IN HOME CARE—cont'd

special needs, such as high-risk obstetric care, or complex infusion or wound therapy, staff must have specialized training and experience to support safety, competent practice, and other standards.

8. SELF-DIRECTION AND THE ABILITY TO FUNCTION AUTONOMOUSLY, ESTABLISH PRIORITIES, AND MANAGE DIVERSE TASKS AND RESPONSIBILITIES WHILE ADHERING TO ORGANIZATIONAL POLICIES, CLINICAL PATHS, AND OTHER STANDARDIZED PROTOCOLS.

This ability encompasses well-honed and effective time-management skills to address the many aspects of home care, including scheduling visits, completing documentation and detail-oriented administrative duties, such as making phone calls, entering required data, and completing POCs and OASIS assessments timely and accurately. The best clinicians in home care are well organized and use organizational skills in their daily routines, such as creating detailed schedules, documenting at the patient's home (unless safety concerns preclude this standard), and generally seek to *do things right the first time*. Day scheduling calendars, cellular phones, voice/e-mail, faxes, and other technology assist in this important endeavor.

9. DESIRE TO CONTINUE LEARNING AND BEING OPEN TO NEW INFORMATION AND CLINICAL SKILLS.

This is particularly true as new kinds of technologies are introduced into the home setting. Complex heart failure management, apnea monitoring, telehealth technology, innovative pain and symptom management, and ventilator care are just some of the kinds of patient care problems addressed daily by competent home care clinicians. Please refer to each clinical guideline section on evidence-based resources for a list of associations, books, and other home care resources that may be helpful to you.

10. SINCERE APPRECIATION OF PEOPLE.
Home care is a people business! This includes interacting positively with and being empathetic to physicians and patients and their families/caregivers that are often in the midst of crises. Because many traditional family caregivers continue to work outside the home, all team members use observation and assessment findings, teaching and training skills, and patient education tools to maintain patients safely in their homes. This teaching or consulting role also provides job satisfaction to home care staff and comfort and security to the patients and their families.

11. ABILITY TO BE OPEN AND SINCERELY ACCEPTING OF PEOPLE'S UNIQUE PERSONALITIES AND CHOSEN LIFESTYLES AND OF THE EFFECTS THAT THESE LIFESTYLES HAVE ON THEIR HEALTH.
Sometimes these patient choices can be difficult for the clinician. The classic example is the patient who has a tracheostomy and continues to smoke. Ethical dilemmas must be identified and addressed within the framework of the home care organization.

12. AWARENESS AND ACCEPTANCE THAT A CONSTANT BALANCE MUST BE MAINTAINED BETWEEN CLINICAL AND ADMINISTRATIVE DEMANDS.
The home care clinician knows and respects that both demands are equally important but in different ways and for different reasons. The regulatory environment mandates many processes, such as timelines for physician orders and OASIS transmission. Regulations may be promulgated by Occupational Safety and Health Administration, CMS, Centers for Disease Control, state law, professional practice acts, or other entities, such as accreditation bodies. For Medicare-certified agencies, it is important to note that one of the COPs is adherence to applicable regulations and law. It is the organization's and staff's responsibility to be aware of and compliant with these regulations—and to be aware and cooperate with changes as they occur.

13. ABILITY TO FUNCTION INDEPENDENTLY.
The home care work environment does not include the structure and "down the hall" comraderie, supervision, and peer

Continued

BOX 1-10

SKILLS AND KNOWLEDGE NEEDED IN HOME CARE—cont'd

consultation that is available in other healthcare settings, such as hospitals. Home care clinicians must be able to function independently with input from supervisors and peers.

14. POSSESSION OF A KIND SENSE OF HUMOR THAT CAN HELP PATIENTS, FAMILIES, AND PEERS GET THROUGH THE ROUGH TIMES.

This sense of humor conveys a healing power when used appropriately and is sensitive to the patient's needs.

15. KNOWLEDGE OF THE ECONOMICS OF HEALTHCARE AND THE LARGER ENVIRONMENT THAT AFFECTS HOME CARE.

Knowledge of reimbursement mechanisms in home care, including differences among payer sources, utilization, and payment mechanisms, is critical for the nurse or therapist clinician who must function as an admission and insurance specialist on the initial visit. For Medicare/Medicaid patients (and some insurance patients), the OASIS may be the basis for determining reimbursement; thus, it is imperative that clinicians have a solid understanding of the assessment process and impeccable assessment skills. As the role of case manager/care coordinator continues to evolve, it is this person who makes complex decisions authorizing limited resources based on patient needs, and rationale for the increased use of resources must be clearly stated.

16. PRACTICAL WISDOM OF HOME CARE PRACTICE.

This is information that comes with education, practice, and experience. It may be called understanding of "the best way to do things." Much of this knowledge comes from watching and learning from experienced home care clinicians, which may include learning practical tips such as always having two sets of supplies with you (the "Noah's Ark" approach to home care)—because inevitably when you do not have a second set, you will need it! Other examples include organizing paperwork, setting up schedules, and tracking physician orders. Successful agencies support their home care clinicians with these processes, including providing personal digital assistants (PDAs), laptops, or other technology to facilitate effectiveness and timely coordination and communication. As more agencies implement point-of-service and other technologies, clinicians should fight the urge to "resist" these innovations, and instead learn and choose how these technologies can help them provide better patient care!

17. KNOWLEDGE OF CASE MANAGEMENT SKILLS AND MODELS.

Certain growing patient populations in home care, such as the chronically ill or frail older adult, may not need "skilled care" but do need another level of care, such as case management services. These services may be geriatric case management or other services. As health insurers see the cost savings realized by effective case management models, home care has become more integrated with prevention efforts and community health initiatives. Telehealth, personal emergency response systems, and other technologies assist in caring for certain high-risk patient populations to keep them stable and out of high-cost hospital centers.

This is the time for care providers and managers to think "outside the box" and to be able to provide varying levels of care through innovative efforts. Case-managed care service programs may be Medicaid and other "waiver" programs for which patients do not have to meet stringent criteria for admission but are maintained in the home with the goal of keeping them safe, stable, and out of an institution. As Medicaid continues to administer increased amounts and types of home care, depending on the state, an increased number of elder service providers can be seen linking with state programs to authorize and provide "personal care only" kinds of services. These programs can be either medical or social models or a combination of both, depending on the patient populations served.

18. IMPECCABLE ASSESSMENT AND DOCUMENTATION SKILLS.

These two skills go hand-in-hand. The assessment information drives the reimbursement; the documentation of the

Continued

BOX 1-10

SKILLS AND KNOWLEDGE NEEDED IN HOME CARE—cont'd

comprehensive initial assessment must be thorough, accurate, and timely (within the defined time frames for the POC or recertification and the corresponding OASIS) because it ultimately determines reimbursement for that care. Continuing documentation of care and services needed by the patient must be determined in subsequent visits throughout the care. Some organizations have admitting clinicians (nurses and therapists) who possess a high level of assessment skills and validated credentials or a specialty certification (e.g., cardiac nurse for all cardiovascular patients). This practice may not be feasible for many organizations, depending on finances, geography, staff availability, and the size of the agency.

19. ENTHUSIASTIC AND SUCCESSFUL TEACHING SKILLS AND A KNOWLEDGE OF EVIDENCE-BASED RESOURCES.

Teaching skills are more important than ever! This includes a repertoire of evidence-based tools for patient and family teaching, including the organization's authorized and standardized teaching guides or booklets. These teaching skills are valued in the home care environment because education of the patient and family is a large part of clinical management in home care and because patients and their families usually want to, and should, achieve self-care and functioning, and as quickly as possible. Achieving patient-centered outcomes becomes important as the patient and family/caregivers understand their roles and become equal partners in care (e.g., using the information taught in their daily care routines and life). Enthusiastic teaching skills are the key to success in the home care environment.

PART TWO

2

CLINICAL PRACTICE IN HOME CARE

CLINICAL PRACTICE IN HOME CARE

This overview explains practical insights for effective home care practice; describes the basic requirements for Outcome and Assessment Information Set (OASIS); details a patient example and the corresponding comprehensive assessment with the OASIS, plan of care (POC), and Home Health Resource Group (HHRG) worksheet; and discusses home health quality initiatives including Home Health Compare, Outcome-Based Quality Monitoring (OBQM), Outcome-Based Quality Improvement (OBQI), and others.

H-O-M-E V-I-S-I-T: The Acronym in Practice

Home care is a broad term and encompasses many services, such as nursing, aides, physical therapy, speech therapy, occupational therapy, social work, infusion, and other specialties. "Home visits," or client/clinician encounters, are the most common method or unit of third-party payer-reimbursed home care. Telephone-monitoring protocols, telehealth, and other technologies have an increasing role in the provision of home care, but home visits remain the primary basis for care and reimbursement.

The acronym H-O-M-E V-I-S-I-T provides reminders about the important components of home care that are categorized into specific areas to provide the framework for effective home care:

H Holism
O Objectives
M Medications
E Environment
V Visits
I Interventions
S Standards
I Instrumental (activities of daily living)
T Teaching

H—Holistic

Home *is* the holistic site for healthcare. Much of the healthcare system is disjointed, and care is not coordinated from the perspective of the patient and family, especially in the transition from hospital to home. In home care, all aspects of care are coördinated and organized from a central site—the patient's place of residence, or *home*. The dynamics of home care are very different from those of a patient admitted to an inpatient facility—the patient, family/caregiver, home environment, and community are all integral parts of the rehabilitation process.

This holistic view of care and related care-planning processes are key components of case management. The case manager identifies patient problems and needs and requests physician orders for other team members that are identified as necessary in the care (interdisciplinary referrals). Interdisciplinary care better helps patients meet their goals timely and are more important than ever. Team members of other disciplines should be called in sooner than later in the care planning process. It is for this reason the importance of the initial assessment and its data collection cannot be overestimated. Medical necessity must be established during the initial assessment.

The Care-Planning Cycle

The patient and family/caregiver are the focus of the care-planning efforts and are equal partners in the care-planning process, including establishing goals and outcomes. The care-planning process begins with the initial comprehensive assessment, which includes the OASIS items. This comprehensive assessment is critical—it drives the POC. The information collected identifies the patient's problems and needs and determines the services needed for meeting patient goals and outcomes.

Numerous factors are evaluated as care plans are formulated and care is initiated. Box 2-1 lists alphabetically some of the patient-related considerations to be addressed when assessing and planning realistic care and outcomes. Thoughtful analysis of the OASIS data elements and other information is a valuable skill. This critical-thinking component leads to the next step, which is the thoughtful identification of services and interventions—the POC. The POC then creates the road map leading to the outcomes.

BOX 2-1

LIST OF PATIENT-RELATED CONSIDERATIONS

The following is a list of the most common patient-related considerations that are evaluated by the nurse or therapist as plans are formulated and care is begun. This list should be reviewed as a part of the admission process or packet information. This list is not all-inclusive, and other considerations may be as varied as the individual case manager's patient caseload. In addition, many of these factors are interrelated.

Absence of caregiver
Activities of daily living (ADL) limitations
Adaptive or assistive devices
Affect, such as that which is associated with depression
Behavioral or mental disorders
Caregiver support
Chemical or drug problems (e.g., alcoholism)
Chemotherapy
Chronic illnesses or co-morbidities
Cognitive function
Communication
Compliance/non-compliance
Disabilities
Discharge plan
Drug interactions
Educational level/barriers
End-of-life care

Environment
Falls/fall risk
Fatigue
Financial status
Fire safety
Functional limitations
Goals/expected outcomes
Handicaps
History
Homebound status
Home medical equipment
Home setting
Independence
Instrumental activities of daily living (IADL)
Impaired vision
Knowledge of emergency procedures
Language
Loneliness
Loss of significant other
Medical equipment or supply needs
Medications
Mobility
Motivation
Nursing assessment and reassessment findings
Nursing diagnoses
Nutritional status
Orthotic needs
Pain
Parenting
Pathology
Physical assessment findings
Polypharmacy
Probability of further complications
Prognosis
Psychopathology
Reason for prior hospitalization, for referral to home care/hospice
Rehabilitative needs
Rehabilitative potential

Continued

BOX 2-1

LIST OF PATIENT-RELATED CONSIDERATIONS—cont'd

Resources (financial, human, and other)
Risk factors
Safety
Self-care status
Skin integrity
Social factors
Social supports
Socioeconomic condition
Stability
Swallowing
Voice
Other considerations, based on patient's/family's unique needs

For example, while completing the comprehensive assessment during the initial visit, the clinician hears that the patient has concerns about finances and has prescriptions for three new medications. This information should trigger a social work referral because medications are an integral part of the POC and difficulty in affording/obtaining prescribed medications is an impediment to effective implementation of the POC. Similarly, early identification of the need for therapy and aide services should be considered and supported in documentation during the initial assessment visit. Other services may include the use of specialists such as wound, ostomy, continence nurses, respiratory therapists, dietitians, social workers, and others based on the programs offered and the patient population served.

No discussion of holistic care would be complete without emphasizing that the patient's physician is a key member of this team. Because Medicare and other health insurance plans cover or pay for medically-necessary care, a physician must certify that the patient needs the services and signs the POC supporting/authorizing the care. Medicare law requires that payment for services can be made *only* if a physician certifies the need for services and establishes a POC. All care and changes in the POC, including visit frequencies and changes in the patient's condition or diagnosis, must be reported to the physician and documented in the patient's clinical record by the home care clinician. Verbal orders or other changes must be obtained by clinicians legally authorized to take verbal orders according to state practice regulations, written, and sent to the physician for signature. Physicians look to experienced home care team members for recommendations and solutions to care for their home care patients.

The comprehensive assessment, once completed, should describe the patient to any other reader, explain why home care is involved and the plan for care and goal achievement, and other team members involved with the patient's care. Throughout this section refer to Figure 1-1 as the home care process is reviewed, step-by-step, for a thorough view of the "flow" across the home care episode.

The documentation in the clinical record provides evidence of coordinated care, the provision of holistic and comprehensive care to patients, and support to their families and caregivers. Clinicians must know the resources in the communities they serve to assist patients and families who do not meet home care admission criteria as well as to coordinate linkages for patients as discharge from home care approaches.

Practical Wisdom Tips

- Use standardized tools that include OASIS items to assist in early identification of the need for referrals to other team members. Ask, "At my organization, what triggers a referral for MSW, occupational therapist, physical therapist, speech-language pathologist, aide, or other services?"
- Integrate prevention into your care regimens (e.g., smoking cessation for those who smoke, immunizations for children, the need for Pap smears, mammograms, flu shots, prostate screening, and other covered screening).

- Ease the transition for the patient and family/caregiver if another level of care (e.g., skilled nursing facility, hospital) is needed.
- During assessments and subsequent visits, have the patient demonstrate a particular skill as much as possible (e.g., have them get up and walk to the bathroom, go into the kitchen and check for food in the refrigerator or cupboard, count/check pills)—"Show me." This means that you validate what has been reported.
- Review whether the completed assessment adequately and thoroughly describes the patient—remember that the comprehensive assessment drives reimbursement!

O—Objective

The OASIS data elements have raised the expectation for documenting objective patient findings that can be used to determine patient outcomes. OASIS is addressed in depth in the next section, but the fundamentals remain; documentation tells a story about a patient and their problems that supports optimal and appropriate reimbursement. Documentation should also support the professional standard of care and be seen as the sole legal record, the source for communication and coordination among the team, and the source for evaluation of care. All documentation must be accurate, timely, legible, concise, and specific to the patient. With the emphasis on medical review, clinicians must document every visit in a way that supports medical necessity from a medical insurer's perspective. Notes from visits and the entire record show that the patient is homebound (e.g., the reason why, specifically based on the patient's unique needs and problems), that the skill provided is clearly documented in every visit note, and (3) that the patient is responding to care and moving toward achieving goals. Documentation is addressed in more depth in Part One of this text.

Practical Wisdom Tips

- See the OASIS data elements and their collection for what they are—the basis for appropriate and optimal reimbursement and to demonstrate patient outcomes.

- Close out problems (with a date and notation) in the clinical record as patient problems are resolved.
- Support homebound status for the patient in specific functional terms.
- Ask yourself: would any other reader of this clinical note/record know why this patient is homebound and where the care is directed for goal achievement?
- Ask: does this visit note or other documentation support the OASIS and medical necessity?

M—Medications

Medications, their management, and teaching are a large part of home care clinical practice. Medicare and accreditation standards demand that home care clinicians have up-to-date medication profiles that include basic information (e.g., medication, patient, route, side effect, dose, frequency, allergies) and knowledge of more complex and problematic information (e.g., possible or observed drug/drug, drug/food, or drug/disease interactions). Polypharmacy (taking multiple medications), especially among the increasing aging population, continues to be a serious problem. Home care clinicians must also review for duplicative drug therapy and non-compliance with drug therapies. As medication therapy has become more complex, so too have the problems associated with these medications. The pharmacist is your key ally in medication safety and knowledge.

In home care, four important people are involved when home care patients receive a new drug. They are as follows (in order of the usual process): (1) the ordering physician or other ordering practitioner; (2) the pharmacist who dispenses the ordered drug; (3) the home care nurse who teaches, assesses, and monitors the drug and the patient's reaction and response to the therapy or therapist (in therapy-only cases); and, most importantly, (4) the patient, with care directed toward self-care (when possible), compliance with the medication regimen, and taking care of reporting and recording responsibilities. Because the clinician may be the last in the continuum related to medications, the nurse plays an important role in the early identification of problems. As patients become empowered and assume more responsibility for care, they will be the last link to identify a problem as an informed consumer of healthcare.

Administering and managing medications are major components of home care. The home care clinician sees the whole picture, including shoeboxes filled with medications, perhaps from multiple physicians. In these instances the home care nurse addresses safety concerns, acts as the patient's advocate, and consults with the pharmacist, who can assist in evaluating the patient's multiple medication regimens. Recent studies confirm what home care nurses have observed over the years: on the average, patients over age 65 are taking multiple medications at any given time (polypharmacy). In home care, many patients have been prescribed more than 10 medications in addition to what they may self-prescribe or purchase as over-the-counter, herbal, or home remedies. When administering medications, it is always prudent to remember the "seven R's" of medication administration:

1. Right patient
2. Right medication
3. Right dose
4. Right route
5. Right time
6. Right technique
7. Right documentation

No discussion of medications would be complete without addressing patient education and compliance. Compliance with medication and treatment regimens is a serious concern and a significant factor in rehospitalization. Clinicians must assess the level of information patients can absorb and how best to promote long-term compliance or adherence long after home care is gone. Tying new routines to long-established rituals can foster the best development of positive outcomes. Return demonstrations (such as with a patient using inhalers or self-injecting insulin or calcitonin) is a consistent method for the nurse to determine the actual level of understanding of the patient and the treatment rationale.

Practical Wisdom Tips

- Check all medications, including home remedies, herbal preparations, laxatives, vitamins, inhalers, eye medications, and other over-the-counter preparations your patient takes, including enemas—they can be found in any and all rooms!
- Carry a current home care drug reference in your visit bag or have access on your automated clinical device (point-of-service laptop, tablet, or personal digital assistant [PDA]).
- Remember that oxygen is considered a drug and must be on the POC and medication list.
- Be aware that everyone learns differently and has different knowledge.
- Always have a current list in the home for other health members and family members to refer to.
- Always ask at each visit if there are any new or changed medications—and update the list in the home and office medical record.
- Remember that you must have an order for all medications the patient is taking.
- The medication profile must be updated each time a change occurs.
- At discharge, make sure the profile is updated, accurate, and complete.

E—Environment

The environment is the basis for the major difference between inpatient healthcare and home healthcare. New clinicians are oriented to the community because organizations recognize that the environment for the patient's care extends beyond the patient's walls. A "windshield assessment" of the community can be done by driving around a new area, noting what it looks like, feels like, and what resources, such as supermarkets, drugstores, and others, are available.

A large component of the home environment is safety. In home care there are two major safety considerations: the patient's home safety and the clinician's safety in the community. Box 1-7 in Part One contains a list of the most common patient home safety concerns. This information is useful in the completion of the POC #15 (Safety Measures) and for planning care. Safety factors must be identified and assessed during the initial visit by the home care nurse or other clinician based on the home environment, setting, and other conditions. These considerations may be areas requiring education that are patient-specific (e.g., disposal of sharps, scatter rugs, oxygen safety, infection control) or that highlight safety needs for visits (e.g., personal protective equipment, infection control, standard precautions).

Personal Safety in Home Care

When going somewhere for the first time, obtain specific, detailed, and correct directions to the patient's home and validate them with the patient or caregiver. When possible, carry a detailed map of your community in the car. Be aware that other resources for directions are detailed on websites such as www.mapquest.com or www.randmcnally.com. Global positioning system technology is affordable and provides in-the-car access to maps and directions. However, local knowledge is still the most important component of getting correct directions.

If you are unsure of a neighborhood or have heard about problems, talk with your supervisor, who may have more knowledge of the communities. Be aware that local police and fire departments are great resources for community knowledge. Your organization may have contracts with security staff. Your supervisor would know of these arrangements and the process for their use. Be especially mindful of the following:

- Know your community. As you are driving, always be aware of your surroundings.
- You may want to call patients when you are en route so they can be watching for you; also ask about parking.
- Lock the car doors and keep any valuables such as purse, supplies, and any patient information out of sight; locking items in your trunk works well and keeps these items out of sight.
- Place your home care equipment where it is not visible as you drive.

- Wear seatbelts and lock your doors while driving.
- Keep emergency equipment in your car applicable to weather conditions in your area—this could include flashlight (with extra batteries), blanket, "yaktrax", shovel, water, sand, or salt to use/wear on icy walkways to prevent falls.
- Keep maps out of sight when possible, and try to avoid looking as though you are unfamiliar with the area.
- When nearing the patient's home, look for landmarks that have been described and address numbers on houses.
- Try to park in well-lit areas and in front of the home or building or as close as possible. Lock the car, identifying your route to the front door.
- Ask patients to turn on the outside lights.
- Always be cautious when entering and exiting elevators.
- When making evening or night visits, let your manager and your family know where you are going and when you expect to return.
- When walking to your car, have your keys out, ready to unlock the car.
- Before unlocking, check the back seat and floor areas.
- If you feel unsafe, you probably are—trust your feelings!
- Leave an unsafe situation immediately, and notify your supervisor.
- Speak with your supervisor about your organization's policies related to home visiting safety.
- Carry a cell phone—it is a MUST in this day and age!

Home environment and safety issues are important in all aspects of home care practice and operations. They are also key components of quality, risk management, and accreditation standards.

Practical Wisdom Tips

- Know your community and where you are going.
- Always assess the safety of the patient.
- Be careful around/with animals.
- Make sure you always have enough gas or fuel for the visits.
- Call first to verify directions and that the patient (and door opener) will be home.
- Carry a cell phone!

V—Visits

Although home care is much more than visits, the traditional face-to-face relationship and interactions between clinicians and patients and their families are the basis for home care. The following are steps to assist in reimbursement and the provision of quality care. It is important to note that this list is not all-inclusive but provides a framework for the visit.

The Initial Visit

Important points to remember on the initial visit include the following:

- Call ahead, confirm/schedule the visit, and validate directions and parking issues.
- Ask to have pets secured prior to your visit.
- Make sure you have physician orders for the assessment visit (be aware of agency policy or law).
- Explain to the patient and family in advance that this first visit will take at least 1 hour and that there are forms and other administrative tasks that must be completed. Ask that the patient have all medical insurance cards, any written instructions from the doctor or hospital, and all medications ready for your review.
- Gather all the needed equipment and forms for the visit. It is a good idea to organize the forms and complete any areas that can be done in advance.
- Arrive on time.
- Introduce yourself and explain your role. The first visit is also the time to clarify the patient's and family's expectations that significantly influence the POC.
- Spend a small amount of time making the patient comfortable. Be empathetic and use active listening skills. The initial visit is when we are most objective, and a great deal of information is being provided when coming into a new home environment.
- Verify the insurance information by asking to see the Medicare (or other insurance) card and copy the information exactly. Check the proper spelling of the patient's name including middle initial.

- Obtain patient consent, explain patient rights and responsibilities, Medicare privacy information, ask about advance directives, and complete other admission process forms. Although lengthy, they must be complete and they must be legible.
- Begin the comprehensive assessment process with OASIS data collection.
- Wash your hands.
- Perform the physical assessment and other ordered care.
- Ask your patient to walk through the home, if possible, while you survey the environment and observe how safely the patient manages it.
- Wash your hands.
- Complete remaining documentation.
- Call physician (from patient's home, if possible) to ask medication questions or to verify any information needing clarification and to obtain orders for other disciplines, if indicated.
- Determine what the patient/family expects to achieve with home health interventions.
- Complete the documentation before leaving the patient's home (unless there are safety concerns). At a minimum, complete the narrative and the objective data collection information before leaving.
- End the visit with a summary (either written or verbal) of the visit and of instructions; include when the next visit will occur.
- Initiate the care plan with the patient and family and clearly state the expectations for their care and participation.
- Discharge planning begins at the initial visit! The patient and family need to know at the time of admission that the goal is to help them become independent in their care.
- Explain your findings and other services that may be involved, based on physician orders.
- Inform patient and family of the projected frequency and duration of home care services.
- Coordinate with other disciplines for their services.
- Wash your hands.

Every Visit

For each visit, remember the following:

- Adhere to patient's rights guidelines.
- Be a role model for infection control and other procedures. (We are role models whether we want to be or not, so we need to be the best!)
- Use effective bag technique and adhere to infection control policies.
- Plan for discharge with a projected date and/or a clear idea of the goal.
- Use clinical paths as a benchmark to determine if you are on track in your discharge date/plan projection.
- Encourage the patient to maintain compliance and praise patients for their work toward goal achievement.

Practical Wisdom Tips

- Wash your hands, wash your hands, wash your hands!
- Create the care plan with the patient.
- If this is a revisit and you do not know the patient, review the previous notes.
- Use intuition and frame questions so that answers provide a variety of information (i.e., not "*did* you eat?" but "*what* did you eat?").
- Negotiate well; small agreed-upon goals are better than none.
- Evaluate retention of information given in previous visits by asking for recall of instruction and demonstration of skills.

I—Interventions

The term *interventions* refers to the six skilled interventions that are coverable by the Medicare home care program: (1) nursing, (2) home health aide, (3) physical therapy, (4) occupational therapy, (5) speech-language pathology, and (6) medical social work services. It is imperative that all clinicians and managers have an understanding of the coverage requirements related to interventions of the Medicare home care benefit. Readers are referred to Part Six of this text; this section is reprinted in its entirety and lists the coverable skilled interventions for all six services with examples.

Practical Wisdom Tips

- Memorize homebound criteria and review the six examples listed in the *Home Health Manual* (Part Six).
- Make sure the documentation demonstrates the provision of covered care. Medicare and other payers reimburse for our higher level skills (e.g., the knowledge it takes to teach, assess, provide infusion, give an injection, observe).

S—Standards

Standards of practice are an important part of home care. In fact, one of the Medicare Conditions of Participation states that organizations are in compliance with local, state, and federal laws. Nurses, therapists, and other team members must be apprised of their state practice acts, licensure, and other facets of regulation that contribute to the body of knowledge for a given profession. Readers are referred to *Part Six, Medicare Home Care Guidelines for Coverage of Services.* These standards determine what we can and cannot provide within the scope and purview of our profession.

Practical Wisdom Tips

- Know your profession's state practice act(s).
- Read *Home Healthcare Nurse* and other professional journals and publications to keep up with changing practices and standards.
- Know your state licensure law for home care (if your state has licensure).

I—Instrumental

The term *instrumental* leads into instrumental activities of daily living (IADL). The OASIS data elements have heightened the emphasis on and importance of IADL to patients' goal achievement. Such activities make all the difference in whether patients remain at home with optimal function. IADL include such activities as shopping, cooking, home cleaning, and home maintenance. Others are financial management, community access skills that require cognitive and physical abilities beyond the level of basic activities of daily living (ADL), bathing, dressing, transfers, toileting, and eating. The level of independence in IADL is an important factor in determining a patient's ability to live alone or to continue to live independently.

Practical Wisdom Tips

- Let patients continue to do what they have been doing to maintain this level of independence (after home care leaves).
- Do not make patients dependent on us; IADL support the adage "Use it or lose it." Support patients to regain functional independence or higher level functioning whenever possible; if they can do it, even if it takes a lot longer than if we do it for them, let them do it (especially if they have the motivation).

T—Teaching

Teaching is a basic tenet of home care. It is a coverable skill in the Medicare home care program. Patient education tools, handouts, and other teaching methods are the keys for patients to remain at home and independent after home care services are discontinued.

The documentation of teaching and training is important for reimbursement and coverage reasons. Assessment of the patient's knowledge base, the specific information taught, any demonstrations or feedback, and other components of patient teaching should be clearly documented in the patient's record.

Practical Wisdom Tips

- Although frustrating, be aware that there is no requirement that patient, family, or other caregivers be taught to provide a service if they cannot or choose not to provide the care.
- Patients and families can usually learn whatever we choose to teach them if we carefully evaluate their level of learning and teach to that level.
- Review the Medicare *HHA Manual* (Part Six of this text) for the teaching and training activities covered by Medicare.
- Document *who* is being taught. If your patient has significant memory loss or is not teachable, teaching should be directed toward the caregiver.
- Repetitive teaching of the same material throughout the episode of care may not be reimbursable.
- Be specific about what is taught.

OASIS: AN OVERVIEW

Development of OASIS and OBQI

Home care clinicians and administrators function in an ever-challenging and ever-changing home care arena, and few will dispute the importance of the availability of valid and standardized health and functional outcomes. In 1973 the Center for Health Services at the University of Colorado was established to analyze and review health policies and provide technical assistance on topics of quality assurance, cost containment, and regulation. One of the hallmarks of the research program resulted in the development of the OASIS, an acronym for *O*utcome and *AS*sessment *I*nformation *S*et, a discipline-neutral data set that can be used by home care clinicians (e.g., registered nurses [RNs], physical therapists, speech-language pathologists, and occupational therapists) without affecting reliability. This is not to say that there would never be a difference in response selection of a particular OASIS item by varying disciplines, but the differences demonstrated are not statistically significant. Therefore, the OASIS is appropriate for use by all home care professional team members who potentially could be the only or last skilled service provider to a home care patient.

The OASIS data items address sociodemographic, environmental, support system, health status, functional status, and health service utilization characteristics of home care patients, and form the basis for measuring patient outcomes. There will be some changes to the OASIS (e.g., versions, etc.) and readers are encouraged to keep apprised of such changes. The OASIS data items allow agencies, clinicians, payers, patients, and surveyors to analyze the impact of home care services provided in a standardized way, enabling comparison between agencies and within an agency over time. Agency outcome reports from the OASIS data are used in OBQI, OBQM, and the Home Health Compare public reporting initiative (discussed further in the next section). OASIS forms the basis of the home care prospective payment system (PPS) reimbursement mechanism and is used in the enhanced survey process for home health agency (HHA) compliance surveys. Only through these standardized data collection tools, methods, and definitions is the home care industry able to compare "apples to apples" for cost and care efficiencies. The OASIS, through its standardized collecting and reporting requirements, has contributed exponentially to the standardization of our glossary of terms and practices.

Rules for OASIS Data Collection

The Centers for Medicare and Medicaid Services (CMS) mandates OASIS data collection as part of an initial comprehensive assessment for all skilled adult (over 18 years old), non-maternity Medicare and Medicaid patients being served by a Medicare-certified HHA. In addition, OASIS data must be collected at other specified time intervals when patients are reassessed and/or at the point of discharge from home care services. Box 2-2 lists general OASIS data collection instructions found in the OASIS Implementation Manual (revised June 2006) at www.cms.hhs.gov/HomeHealthQualityInits/14_HHQIOASISUserManual.asp. Chapter 8 of the manual includes item-by-item tips for each OASIS item. Each tip contains the definition of the item, time points for the item to be completed, specific response instructions, and assessment strategies. Readers are also referred to the web-based OASIS training modules with patient examples at www.oasistraining.org/oasis11/upfront/U1.asp.

BOX 2-2

GENERAL OASIS DATA COLLECTION INSTRUCTIONS

- OASIS items can be completed by any clinician who performs the comprehensive assessment. Agency policy should determine who is responsible for completing the comprehensive assessment, including the OASIS, if individuals from more than one discipline (e.g., RN and physical therapist) are seeing the patient concurrently.

- *All the items refer to the patient's USUAL STATUS or condition at the time period or visit under consideration - unless otherwise indicated.* Though patient status can vary from day to day and during a given day, the OASIS response should be selected that describes the patient's status most of the time during the specific day under consideration.
- *OASIS items should be completed accurately and comprehensively and skip patterns should be used correctly.* Clinicians should monitor the accuracy and completeness of their own responses as they utilize the data set. Completeness of the OASIS information is critical for care planning as well as case mix reporting and performance improvement based on outcomes
- *The follow-up and discharge assessments must be done without reference to the previous values for any health status item.* It is critical for data accuracy that the clinician does not merely duplicate items from the prior assessment rather than perform a new comprehensive assessment.
- *Minimize the use of "Not Applicable" and "Unknown" answer options.* For some OASIS items, response options for "Not Applicable" or "Unknown" are available. Clinicians should limit their use of these categories to situations where no other response is possible or appropriate.
- *When items inquire about events occurring within the past 14 days or at a specified point (e.g., discharge from an inpatient facility, ADL status at 14 days prior to SOC, etc.), the specific time interval included in the item should be followed exactly.*
- *OASIS items that are scales (e.g., dyspnea, transferring, etc.) are arranged in order from least impaired to most impaired.* For example, higher values (further down the list of options) on the transferring scale refer to greater dependence in transferring. This is true whether the scale describes a functional, physiologic, or emotional health status attribute.

Continued

BOX 2-2

GENERAL OASIS DATA COLLECTION INSTRUCTIONS—cont'd

- *Collection of data through direct observation* is preferred instead of asking the patient or caregiver. However, some items (e.g., frequency of primary caregiver assistance) are most often obtained through interview. When interview data are collected, the patient should be the primary source (or a caregiver residing in the home) when at all possible. In many instances, a combined observation-interview approach is necessary.
- *The OASIS items may be completed in any order.* Since the OASIS is integrated into the clinician's usual assessment process, the clinician performing the patient assessment is responsible for determining the order in which the items are completed.
- *Each agency is responsible for monitoring the accuracy of the assessment data and the adequacy of the assessment process.*

Documentation formats for comprehensive assessments and visit notes vary across home care programs, with each discipline usually using their own specialized assessment tools and visit notes. However, OASIS has provided a degree of standardization by requiring the items embedded in the specific assessments so that OASIS data can be collected for the comprehensive assessment process. Formats may include checklists, narratives, or a combination. Often these forms are in duplicate or triplicate to facilitate communication among team members; however, more and more agencies are adopting point-of-service technology in the form of laptops or PDAs to facilitate documentation, communication, and care coordination.

CMS has emphasized the importance of OASIS accuracy. The OASIS Implementation Manual, Chapter 12, details the required OASIS data quality audits, including data entry, peer visit, and clinical record audits. The first and foremost question every clinician should ask is *"Does the comprehensive assessment, including the OASIS data elements, accurately reflect the acuity of the patient?"* The challenge for the clinician is to determine the optimal interventions/best practices and discipline mix within the organization's resource constraints.

Documenting the Comprehensive Assessment (including the OASIS) and Preparing the POC: Patient Example

Mr. Smith, an 82-year-old Caucasian male, experienced an exacerbation of heart failure and was admitted to the hospital for the fourth time in two months after examination in the emergency room revealed an O_2 saturation of 84 percent, increased apical pulse (AP) of 120, marked dyspnea, extreme weakness, blood pressure of 148/88, and a blood sugar of 280. He was diagnosed with heart failure. After four days in the hospital he was stabilized with O_2 and medication changes. He was discharged home with home care services and O_2. Ordered services include nursing and physical therapy for evaluation, home health aide for assistance with personal care, and a social work referral for an evaluation of financial and social resources.

Past Medical History: Mr. Smith has a 20-year history of type 2 diabetes (insulin-treated), which he has managed independently (self-injecting his insulin) before this hospitalization. He also has a 20-year history of hypertension and osteoarthritis in the right knee, with reports of recent exacerbation. He reports experiencing worsening dyspnea and weakness several days before he came to the emergency room.

Social History: Mr. Smith lives alone in a small studio apartment above a bar in a small town. Before this hospitalization and until several days ago, he drove his car, was independent in self-care, and mostly independent in domestic chores and other IADL. His friend, Jane, who works in the bar downstairs, visits two to three times a week, and runs errands for him occasionally, such as to the grocery store. He has a son who lives in a nearby town, but according to Mr. Smith, the son is "irresponsible and not dependable," and rarely visits.

Home Care Admission: Mr. Smith's case is assigned to an RN for case management. The admission visit is made the day after hospital discharge, with only Mr. Smith present. The RN completes the activities associated with the home care admission, including the comprehensive assessment with OASIS, and prepares the POC (See Figure 2-2). Box 2-1 lists patient-related considerations that are evaluated by the home care clinician as the POC is formulated and care is begun. The clinical supervisor (or the computer program the supervisor is using) calculates Mr. Smith's HHRG score using a Case-Mix Grouper Worksheet based on the clinician's OASIS scoring (See Figure 2-3), and determines the approximate reimbursement for the 60-day episode of care. In this way, the clinician and the supervisor can plan the use of available resources efficiently and effectively to provide quality care for Mr. Smith.

Competency Assessment: Key to OASIS Success

OASIS data collection activities are within the scope of all professional home care clinicians; however, the OASIS items may cover several specific clinical and health-related domains that may not have been routinely addressed by all disciplines. Competence in assessing the domains related to OASIS in the comprehensive assessment of the patient should be established for all disciplines involved in data collection and become part of organizations' policies and procedures.

Figures 2-1 to 2-3 present sample OASIS Competency Assessment tools, and allow clinicians, peers, and clinical

PATIENT TRACKING SHEET

1. **(M0010) Agency Medicare Provider Number:** 123456
2. **(M0012) Agency Medicaid Provider Number:** _______________

Branch Identification

3. **(M0014) Branch State:** ____
4. **(M0016) Branch ID Number:** __________

5. **(M0020) Patient ID Number:** 111-08

6. **(M0030) Start of Care Date:** 08-15-2008 (mm dd yyyy)
7. **(M0032) Resumption of Care Date:** __-__-____ (mm dd yyyy) ☒ NA - Not Applicable

8. **(M0040) Patient Name:** Mortimer P. Smith ____ ____ (First) (MI) (Last) (Suffix)
9. **Patient Address:** 690 Sunset Dr. — Street, Route, Apt. Number - not P.O. Box; Any Town (City) USA **(M0050)** State 54321-1234 **(M0060)** Zip Code

10. **Patient Phone:** (444) 666-9876

11. **(M0063) Medicare Number:** 123456789A (including suffix if any) ☐ NA - No Medicare
12. **(M0064) Social Security Number:** 123 45 6789 ☐ UK - Unknown or Not Available

13. **(M0065) Medicaid Number:** _____________ ☒ NA - No Medicaid
14. **(M0066) Birth Date:** 08-01-1926 (mm dd yyyy)

15. **(M0069) Gender:** ☒ 1-Male ☐ 2-Femal

16. **(M0072) Primary Referring Physician ID:** 5882234338 (UPIN#) ☐ UK-Unknown or Not Available
Name Patrick McDreamy, MD — Phone (444) 888-9999
Address 5555 Main St, Any Town, USA — Fax (444) 888-9999

17. **Marital Status:** ☒ Not Married ☐ Married ☐ Widowed ☐ Divorced ☐ Separated ☐ Unknown

18. (M0140) **Race/Ethnicity** (as identified by patient): **(Mark all that apply.)**
☐ 1 - Americal Indian or Alaska Native ☐ 3 - Black or African-American ☐ 5 - Native Hawaiian or Pacific Islander ☐ UK - Unknown
☐ 2 - Asian ☐ 4 - Hispanic or Latino ☒ 6 - White

19. **Emergency Contact (Name and Relationship):** JANE CRANE (friend)
20. **Emergency Contact Address:** 170 Magnolia Lane, Any Town, USA
21. **Emergency Contact Telephone No:** c) (444) 321-4567 w) 444 987-1234

22. **(M0150) Current Payment Sources for Home Care:**
(Mark all that apply.)
- ☐ 0 - None; no charge for current services
- ☒ 1 - Medicare (traditional fee-for-service)
- ☐ 2 - Medicare (HMO/managed care)
- ☐ 3 - Medicaid (traditional fee-for-service)
- ☐ 4 - Medicaid (HMO/managed care)
- ☐ 5 - Workers' compensation
- ☐ 6 - Title programs (e.g., Title III, V or XX)
- ☐ 7 - Other government (e.g., CHAMPUS, VA, etc.)
- ☐ 8 - Private insurance
- ☐ 9 - Private HMO/managed care
- ☐ 10 - Self-pay
- ☐ 11 - Other (specify) ____________________
- ☐ UK - Unknown

OASIS-B1 PTS (1/2008)

Figure 2-1 Comprehensive assessment with OASIS.

2

STAR OF CARE ASSESSMENT (Also used for Resumption of Care Following Inpatient Stay (Page 1 of 15)	Client's Name: Mortimer P. Smith Client's Record No. 111-08

A. DEMOGRAPHIC INFORMATION - Update Patient Tracking Sheet at ROC

1. **(M0080) Discipline of Person Completing Assessment:**
   - ☒ 1 - RN
   - ☐ 2 - PT
   - ☐ 3 - SLP/ST
   - ☐ 4 - OT

2. **(M0090) Date Assessment Completed:**
   08 - 16 - 2008
   mm dd yyyy

3. **(M0100) This Assessment is Currently Being Completed for the Following Reason:**

   Start/Resumption of Care
   - ☒ 1 - Start of care—further visits planned
   - ☐ 3 - Resumption of care(after inpatient stay)

   Follow - Up
   - 4 - Recertification (follow-up reassessment)
   - 5 - Other follow-up

   Transfer to an Inpatient Facility
   - 6 - Transferred to an inpatient facility—patient not discharged from agency
   - 7 - Transferred to an inpatient facility—patient discharged from agency

   Discharge from Agency—Not to an Inpatient Facility
   - 8 - Death at home
   - 9 - Discharge from agency

4. **(M0110) Episode Timing:** Is the Medicare home health payment episode for which this assessment will define a case mix group an "early" episode or a "later" episode in the patient's current sequence of adjacent Medicare home health payment episodes?
   - ☒ 1 - Early
   - ☐ 2 - Later
   - ☐ UK - Unknown
   - ☐ NA - Not Applicable: No Medicare case mix group to be defined by this assessment.

5. **Economic/Financial Problems of Needs** (describe):

   Monthly income = $600
   Social security - just barely covers expense (housing, food, meds)

6. **(M0175)** From which of the following Inpatient Facilities was the patient discharged during the past 14 days? **(Mark all that apply.)**
   - ☒ 1 - Hospital
   - ☐ 2 - Rehabilitation facility
   - ☐ 3 - Skilled nursing facility
   - ☐ 4 - Other nursing home
   - ☐ 5 - Other (specify) ______
   - ☐ NA - Patient was not discharged from an inpatient facility **[If NA, go to *#9, Medical or Treatment Regimen Change*]**

7. **(M0180) Inpatient Dischare Date** (most recent):
   08 - 14 - 2008
   mm dd yyyy
   - ☐ UK - Unknown

8. **(M0190) Inpatient Diagnoses** and ICD-9-CM code categories (three digits required; five digits optional) for only those conditions treated during an inpatient facility stay within the last 14 days (no surgical or V-codes):

	Inpatient Facility Diagnosis	ICD-9-CM
a.	Heart Failure	(428.9)
b.	Type 2, Diabetes, not stated as complicated or uncontrolled	(250.00)

9. **(M0200) Medical or Treatment Regimen Change Within Past 14 Days:** Has this patient experienced a change in medical or treatment regimen (e.g., medication, treatment, or service change due to new or additional diagnosis, etc.) within the last 14 days?
   - ☐ 0 - No **[If No, go to *#11 - M0220, Conditions Prior*]**
   - ☒ 1 - Yes

10. **(M0210)** List the patient's **Medical Diagnoses** and ICD-9-Cm code categories (three digits required; five digits optional) for those conditions requiring changed medical or treatment regimen (no surgical or V-codes):

	Changed Medical Rgimen Diagnosis	ICD-9-CM
a.	Heart Failure	(428.9)
b.	Type 2, Diabetes	(250.00)
c.		
d.		

OASIS-B1 SOC/ROC (1/2008)

Figure 2-1, cont'd

STAR OF CARE ASSESSMENT **(Also used for Resumption of Care Following Inpatient Stay** (Page 2 of 15)	Client's Name: M. P. Smith Client's Record No. 111-08

11. **(M0220) Conditions Prior to Medical or Treatment Regimen Change or Inpatients Stay Within Past 14 Days:** If this patient experienced an inpatient facility discharge or change in medical or treatment regimen within the past 14 days, indicate any conditions which existed prior to the inpatient stay or change in medical or treatment regimen. **(Mark all that apply.)**

- ☐ 1 - Urinary incontinence
- ☐ 2 - Indwelling/suprapubic catheter
- ☐ 3 - Intractable pain
- ☐ 4 - Impaired decision-making
- ☐ 5 - Disruptive or socially inappropriate behavior
- ☐ 6 - Memory loss to the extent that supervision required
- ☒ 7 - None of the above
- ☐ NA - No inpatient facility discharge and no change in medical or treatment regimen in past 14 days
- ☐ UK - Unknown

B. CURRENT ILLNESS

1. **M0230/240/246 Diagnoses, Severity Index, and Payment Diagnoses:** List each diagnosis for which the patient is receiving home care (Column 1) and enter its ICD-9-CM code at the level of highest specificity (no surgical/procedure codes) (Column 2). Rate each condition (Column 2) using the severity index. (Choose one value that represents the most severe rating appropriate for each diagnosis.) V code (for M0230 or M0240) or E codes (for M0240 only) may be used. ICD-9-CM sequencing requirements must be followed if multiple coding is indicated for any diagnoses. If a V code is reported in place of a case mix diagnosis, then optional item M0246 Payment Diagnoses (Columns 3 and 4) may be completed. A case mix diagnosis is a diagnosis that determines the Medicare PPS case mix group.

Code each row as follows:

(Column 1): Enter the description of the diagnosis.

(Column 2): Enter the ICD-9-Cm code for the diagnosis described in Column 1;
Rate the severity of the condition listed in Column 1 using the following scale:

0 - Asymptomatic, no treatment needed at this time
1 - Symptoms well controlled with current therapy
2 - Symptoms controlled with difficulty, affecting daily functioning; patient needs ongoing monitoring
3 - Symptoms poorly controlled; patient needs frequent adjustment in treatment and dose monitoring
4 - Symptoms poorly controlled; history of re-hospitalizations

(Column 3): (OPTIONAL) If a V code reported in any row in Column 2 is reported in place of a case mix diagnosis, list the appropriate case mix diagnosis (the description and the ICD-9-CM code) in the same row in Column 3. Otherwise, leave Column 3 blank in that row.

(Column 4): (OPTIONAL) If a V code in Column 2 is reported in place of a case mix diagnosis that requires multiple diagnosis codes under ICD-9-CM coding guidelines, enter the diagnosis descriptions and the ICD-9-CM codes in the same row in Column 3 and 4. For example, if the case mix diagnosis is a manifestation code, record the diagnosis description and ICD-9-CM code for the underlying condition in Column 3 of that row and the diagnosis description and ICD-9-CM code for the manifestation in Column 4 of that row. Otherwise, leave Column 4 blank in that row.

(M0230) Primary Diagnosis & (M0240) Other Diagnoses		**(M0246) Case Mix Diagnoses (OPTIONAL)**	
Column 1	Column 2	Column 3	Column 4
	ICD-9-CM and severity rating for each condition	Complete **only if** a V code in Column 2 is reported in place of a case mix diagnosis.	Complete **only if** the V code in Column 2 is reported in place of a case mix diagnosis that is a multiple coding situation (e.g., a manifestation code).
Description	ICD-9-CM/ Severity Rating	Description/ ICD-9-CM	Description/ ICD-9-CM
(M0230) Primary Diagnosis	**(V codes are allowed)**	**(V or E codes are NOT allowed)**	**(V or E codes NOT allowed)**
a. Heart failure	a. (428.9) ☐0 ☐1 ☐2 ☐3 ☒4	a. ______ (___•___)	a. ______ (___•___)
(M0240) Other Diagnoses	**(V or E Codes are allowed)**	**(V or E codes are NOT allowed)**	**(V or E codes NOT allowed)**
b. Type 2 Diabetes	b. (250.00) ☐0 ☐1 ☒2 ☐3 ☐4	b. ______ (___•___)	b. ______ (___•___)
c. Osteoarthritis Rt Knee	c. (715.96) ☐0 ☐1 ☒2 ☐3 ☐4	c. ______ (___•___)	c. ______ (___•___)
d. Hypertension	d. (401.9) ☐0 ☐1 ☒2 ☐3 ☐4	d. ______ (___•___)	d. ______ (___•___)

OASIS-B1 SOC/ROC (1/2008)

Figure 2-1, cont'd

2

START OF CARE ASSESSMENT (Also used for Resumption of Care Following Inpatient Stay (Page 3 of 15)	Client's Name: M. P. Smith Client Record No. 111-08

(M0230) Primary Diagnosis & (M0240) Other Diagnoses		(M0246) Case Mix Diagnoses (OPTIONAL)	
Column 1	Column 2	Column 3	Column 4
e. Abnormality of gait	e. (781.2) ☐0 ☐1 ☐2 ☐3 ☐4	e. ____ (___•__)	e. ____ (___•__)
f. Cataracts	f. (366.9) ☐0 ☐1 ☐2 ☐3 ☐4	f. ____ (___•__)	f. ____ (___•__)

C. **SIGNIFICANT PAST HEALTH HISTORY:** Hx of Type 2 diabetes x 20 yrs & independent in self-injecting insulin prior to this hospitalization; dx. of HF x 5-6 yrs; frequent ER visits & rehospitalizations in p̄ 2-3 mo. due to ↑ dyspnea & exacerbation of HF; osteoarthritis in Rt. Knee & c̄ recent exacerbation & pain on ambulation; recent exacerbation of hypertension

D. **(M0250) THERAPIES** the patient receives at home: **(Mark all that apply.)**
- ☐ 1 - Intravenous or infusion therapy (excludes TPN)
- ☐ 2 - Parenteral nutrition (TPN or lipids)
- ☐ 3 - Enteral nutrition (nasogastric, gastrostomy, jejunostomy, or any other artificial entry into the alimentary canal)
- ☑ 4 - None of the above

E. **PROGNOSIS**

1. **(M0260) Overall Prognosis:** Best description of patient's overall prognosis of recovery from this episode of illness.
   - ☐ 0 - Poor: little or no recovery is expected and/or further decline is imminent
   - ☑ 1 - Good/Fair: partial of full recovery is expected
   - ☐ UK - Unknown
2. **(M0270) Rehabilitative Prognosis:** Best description of patient's prognosis for functional status.
   - ☑ 0 - Guarded: minimal improvement in functional status is expected; decline is possible
   - ☐ 1 - Good: marked improvement in functional status is expected
   - ☐ UK - Unknown
3. **(M0280) Life Expectancy:** (Physician documentation is not required.)
   - ☐ 0 - Life expectancy is greater than 6 months
   - ☑ 1 - Life expectancy is 6 months or fewer

F. **ALLERGIES:** (Environmental, drugs, food, etc.)
SULFA
ASA

G. **IMMUNIZATION/SCREENING TESTS**

1. **Immunizations:**
   - Flu Yes X No __ Date 10/07
   - Tetanus Yes X No __ Date ? not sure
   - Pneumonia Yes X No __ Date 1998 ? not sure
   - Other: ____ Date ____
2. **Screening:**
   - Cholesterol level Yes X No __ Date 2006 ? not sure
   - Mammogram Yes __ No __ Date ____
   - Colon cancer screen Yes __ No X Date 2000 ? not sure
   - Prostate cancer screen Yes X No __ Date ____
3. **Self-Exam Frequency**
   - Breast self-exam frequency ____
   - Testicular self-exam frequency Doesn't do/doesn't want to be taught

OASIS-BI SOC/ROC (1/2008)

Figure 2-1, cont'd

START OF CARE ASSESSMENT
(Also used for Resumption of Care Following Inpatient Stay
(Page 4 of 15)

Client's Name: *M. P. SMITH*
Client Record No. *111-08*

11. **(M0290) HIGH RISK FACTORS** characterizing this patient: **(Mark all that apply.)**
- ☒ 1 - Heavy smoking
- ☐ 2 - Obesity
- ☐ 3 - Alcohol dependency
- ☐ 4 - Drug dependency
- ☐ 5 - None of the above
- ☐ UK - Unknown

Hx of smoking 2-3 packs/day when young—quit 40+ years ago although probably impacting current health status

1. **LIVING ARRANGEMENTS**

1. **(M0300) Current Residence:** *studio*
   - ☒ 1 - Patient's owned or (rented) residence (house, (apartment), or mobile home owned or rented by patient/couple/significant other)
   - ☐ 2 - Family member's residence
   - ☐ 3 - Boarding home or rented room
   - ☐ 4 - Board and care or assisted living facility
   - ☐ 5 - Other (specify) ______

2. **(M0340) Patient Lives With: (Mark all that apply.)**
   - ☒ 1 - Lives alone
   - ☐ 2 - With spouse or significant other
   - ☐ 3 - With other family member
   - ☐ 4 - With a friend
   - ☐ 5 - With paid help (other than home care agency staff)
   - ☐ 6 - With other than above

3. **Physical Environment:** (Check to indicate presence of problem or check, "No problems identified.")
   - ☐ 1 - No problems
   - ☒ 2 - High crime area
   - ☐ 3 - Electrical hazards
   - ☒ 4 - Structural hazards *narrow hallway/gm rooms*
   - ☒ 5 - Stairs *narrow steep, uncovered stairs outside leading to apt*
   - ☐ 6 - Water supply problems
   - ☐ 7 - Sewage disposal problems
   - ☒ 8 - (Insect)/rodent problems
   - ☐ 9 - Food storage or preparation problems
   - ☐ 10 - Telephone access problem
   - ☐ 11 - Other

COMMENTS: *lives in a small studio apt above a noisy bar in a low-income, high-crime section of town; narrow stairs from side of bar outside are narrow & steep to apt; building is run-down but Mr. S. states "its home-I like it here".*

J. OTHERS LIVING IN HOUSEHOLD: *ϕ*

Name	Age	Sex	Relationship	Able and willing to assist?	Name	Age	Sex	Relationship	Able and willing to assist?

OASIS-B1 SOC/ROC (1/2008)

Figure 2-1, cont'd

START OF CARE ASSESSMENT **(Also used for Resumption of Care Following Inpatient Stay** (Page 5 of 15)	Client's Name: M. P. Smith Client Record No. 111-08

K. SUPPORTIVE ASSISTANCE

1. **Names of Persons/Organizations Providing Assistance:**

   Jane Crane - works in bar below his apt + helps MR. S. w/IADL's - checks on him 2-3x/wk by phone or in person but is willing to help out more

2. **(M0350) Assisting Persons) Other than Home Care Agency Staff: (Mark all that apply.)**
   - ☒ 1 - Relative, friends, or neighbors living outside the home
   - ☐ 2 - Person residing in the home (EXCLUDING paid help)
   - ☐ 3 - Paid help
   - ☐ 4 - None of the above **[If None of the above, go to *Section L - Review of Systems/Physical Assessment*]**
   - ☐ UK - Unknown **[If Unknown, go to *Section L - Review of Systems/Physical Assessment*]**

3. **(M0360) Primary Caregiver** taking lead responsibility for providing or managing the patient's care, providing the most frequent assistance, etc. (other than home care agency staff):
   - ☐ 0 - No one person **[If No one person, go to *Section L - Review of Systems/Physical Assessment*]**
   - ☐ 1 - Spouse or significant other
   - ☐ 2 - Daughter or son
   - ☐ 3 - Other family member
   - ☒ 4 - Friend or neighbor or community or church member
   - ☐ 5 - Paid help
   - ☐ UK - Unknown **[If Unknown, go to *Section L - Review of Systems/Physical Assessment*]**

4. **(M0370) How often** does the patient receive assistance from the primary caregiver?
   - ☐ 1 - Several times during day and night
   - ☐ 2 - Several times during day
   - ☐ 3 - Once daily
   - ☒ 4 - Three or more times per week
   - ☐ 5 - One to two times per week
   - ☐ 6 - Less often than weekly
   - ☐ UK - Unknown

5. **(M0380) Type of Primary Caregiver Assistance: (Mark all that apply.)**
   - ☐ 1 - ADL assistance (e.g., bathing, dressing, toileting bowel/bladder,eating/feeding)
   - ☒ 2 - IADL assistance (e.g., meds, meals [occasionally], housekeeping, laundry, telephone, shopping, finances)
   - ☐ 3 - Environmental support (housing, home maintenance)
   - ☒ 4 - Psychosocial support (socialization, companionship, recreation)
   - ☐ 5 - Advocates or facilitates patient's participation in appropriate medical care
   - ☐ 6 - Financial agent, power of attorney, or conservator of finance
   - ☐ 7 - Health care agent, conservator of person, or medical power of attorney
   - ☐ UK - Unknown

Comments regarding assistance available to patient:

Son lives in nearby town but is not involved in any aspect of care & rarely visits - no other family

L. REVIEW OF SYSTEMS/PHYSICAL ASSESSMENT

(Mark S for subjective, O for objectively assessed problem. If no problem present or if not assessed, mark NA.)

1. **Head:** S/O Dizziness When gets up   NA Headache (describe location, duration) ______

2. **Eyes:** Has Glasses S/O   NA Blurred/double vision   NA Glaucoma
   Has Cataracts S/O   NA PERRL   X Other (specify) Admits to difficulty seeing markings on the insulin syringe

   (M0390) Vision with corrective lenses if the patient usually wears them:
   - ☐ 0 - Normal vision: sees adequately in most situations; can see medication labels, newsprint.
   - ☒ 1 - Partially impaired: cannot see [well] medication labels or newsprint, but can see obstacles in path, and the surrounding layout; can count fingers at arm's length.
   - ☐ 2 - Severely impaired: cannot locate objects without hearing or touching them or patient nonresponsive.

3. **EARS:** NA Hearing Aid   NA Tinnitus   X Other (specify) had to speak louder at times

   (M0400) Hearing and Ability to Understand Spoken Language in patient's own language (with hearing aids if the patient usually uses them):
   - ☐ 0 - No observable impairment. Able to hear and understand complex or detailed instructions and extended or abstract conversation.
   - ☒ 1 - With minimal difficulty, able to hear and understand most multi-step instructions and ordinary conversation. May need occasional repetition, extra time, or louder voice.
   - ☐ 2 - Has moderate difficulty hearing and understanding simple, one-step instructions and brief conversation; needs frequent prompting or assistance.
   - ☐ 3 - Has severe difficulty hearing and understanding simple greetings and short comments. Requires multiple repetitions, restatements, demonstrations, additional time.
   - ☐ 4 - Unable to hear and understand familiar words or common expressions consistently, or patient nonresponsive.

OASIS-B1 SOC/ROC (1/2008)

Figure 2-1, cont'd

START OF CARE ASSESSMENT
(Also used for Resumption of Care Following Inpatient Stay (Page 6 of 15)

Client's Name: *M. P. Smith*
Client Record No. *111-08*

4. **ORAL:** *S/O* Gum problems *S/O* Chewing problems *S/O* Dentures ____ Other specify *Needs dental f.u. - loose dentures/sore gum*

(M0410) Speech and Oral (Verbal) Expression of Language (in patient's own language):
- ☐ 0 - Expresses complex ideas, feelings, and needs clearly, completely, and easily in all situations with no observable impairment.
- ☒ 1 - Minimal difficulty in expressing ideas and needs (may take extra time; makes occasional errors in word choice, grammar or speech intelligibility; needs minimal prompting or assistance).
- ☐ 2 - Express simple ideas or needs with moderate difficulty (needs prompting or assistance, errors in word choice, organization or speech) Intelligibility). Speaks in phrases or short sentences.
- ☐ 3 - Has severe difficulty expressing basic ideas or needs and requires maximal assistance or guessing by listener. Speech limited to single words or short phrases.
- ☐ 4 - Unable to express basic needs even with maximal prompting or assistance but is not comatose or unresponsive (e.g., speech is nonsensical or unintelligible).
- ☐ 5 - Patient nonresponsive or unable to speak.

5. **NOSE AND SINUS:** *NA* Epistaxis ___ Other (specify) ____

6. **NECK AND THROAT:** *NA* Hoarseness *NA* Difficulty swallowing ___ Other (specify) ____

7. **MUSCULOSKELETAL, NEUROLOGICAL:**

✓ Hx arthritis	✓ Joint pain	___ Syncope	___ Paralysis (describe) ____
___ Gout	✓ Weakness	___ seizure	___ Amputation (where) ____
✓ Stiffness *Rt. Knee*	___ Leg cramps	✓ Tenderness *Rt Knee*	___ Tremor
✓ Swollen joints	___ Numbness	___ Deformities	___ Aphasia/inarticulate speech
___ Unequal grasp	___ Temp changes	___ Comatose	___ Other (specify) ____

Coordination, gait, balance (describe):
Hx of falls x 2-3 in p̄ 6 mo - "I slipped on this darn rug" (throw rug; walks w/walker but slow, unsteady due to weakness and painful Rt knee

COMMENTS: (Prostheses, appliances)
Had been using cane-came home from hospital w/walker

Patient;s Perceived Pain Level: *6-7* (Scale 0-10) *Rt. Knee*

(M0420) Frequency of Pain interfering with patient's activity or movement:
- ☐ 0 - Patient has no pain or pain does not interfere with activity or movement
- ☐ 1 - Less often than daily
- ☐ 2 - Daily, but not constantly
- ☒ 3 - All of the time

(M0430) Intractable Pain: Is the patient experiencing pain that is not easily relieved, occurs at least daily, and affects the patient's sleep, appetite, physical or emotional energy, concentration, personal relationships, emotions, or ability or desire to perform physical activity?
- ☐ 0 - No
- ☒ 1 - Yes

Comments on pain management: *"Frequent pain in my knees slows me down"- When it gets too bad, sits in recliner & puts his legs up & it usually gets better; worse @ night, wakes him up & it is hard for him to get back to sleep & then nothing seems to make pain better- "I take pain medicine only when I have to"*

OASIS-BI SOC/ROC (1/2008)

Figure 2-1, cont'd

START OF CARE ASSESSMENT (Also used for Resumption of Care Following Inpatient Stay) (Page 7 of 15)	Client's Name: M. P. Smith Client Record No. 111 - 08

8. **INTEGUMENT:**

a. NA Hair changes (where)________ NA Pruritus ___ Other (specify) ________

b. Skin condition (Record type # on body area. Indicate size to right of numbered category.)

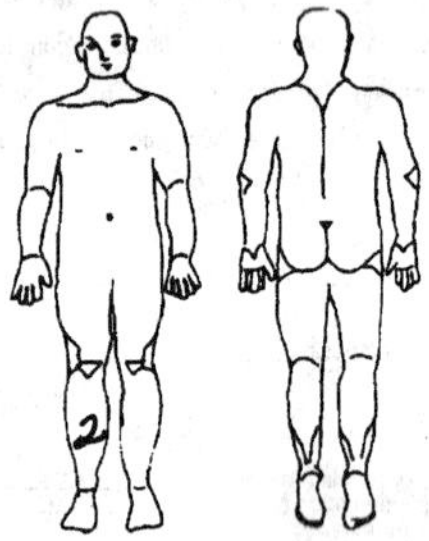

Type	Size
1. Lesions	
(2. Bruises)	quarter-size bluish bruises-Mr.S. hadn't noticed them
3. Masses	
4. Scars	
5. Stasis Ulcers	
6. Pressure Ulcers	
7. Surgical Wounds	
8. Other (specify)________	

c. **(M0440)** Does this patient have a **Skin Lesion** or an **Open Wound**? This excludes "OSTOMIES."
- ☐ 0 - No **[If no, go to *Section 9 - Cardiorespiratory*]**
- ☒ 1 - Yes

d. **(M0445)** Does this patient have a **Pressure Ulcer**?
- ☒ 0 - No **[If no, go to #8.e - *Stasis Ulcer*]**
- ☐ 1 - Yes

(M0450) Current Number of Pressure Ulcers at Each Stage: (Circle one response for each stage.)

Pressure Ulcer Stages	Number of Pressure Ulcers				
a) Stage 1: Nonblanchable erythema of intact skin; the heralding of skin ulceration. In darker-pigmented skin, warmth, edema, hardness or discolored skin may be indicators.	0	1	2	3	4 or more
b) Stage 2: Partial thickness skin loss involving epidermis and/or dermis. The ulcer is superficial and presents clinically as an abrasion, blister, or shallow crater	0	1	2	3	4 or more
c) Stage 3: Full-thickness skin loss involving damage or necrosis of subcutaneous tissue which may extend down to, but not through, underlying fascia. The ulcer presents clinically as a deep crater with or without undermining of adjacent tissue.	0	1	2	3	4 or more
d) Stage 4: Full-thickness skin loss with extensive destruction, tissue necrosis, or damege to muscle, bone, or supporting structures (e.g., tendon, joint capsule, etc.).	0	1	2	3	4 or more
e) In addition to the above, is there at least one pressure ulcer that cannot be observed due to the presence of eschar or a nonremovalbe dressing including casts? ☐ 0 - No ☐ 1 - Yes					

(M0460) Stage of Most Problematic (Observable) Pressure Ulcer:
- ☐ 1 - Stage1
- ☐ 2 - Stage2
- ☐ 3 - Stage3
- ☐ 4 - Stage4
- ☐ NA - No observable pressure ulcer

(M0464) Status of Most Problematic (Observable) Pressure Ulcer:
- ☐ 1 - Fully granulating
- ☐ 2 - Early/partial granulation
- ☐ 3 - Not healing
- ☐ NA - No observable pressure ulcer

Describe current treatment approach(es) for pressure ulcer(s):

OASIS-B1 SOC/ROC (1/2008)

Figure 2-1, cont'd

START OF CARE ASSESSMENT
(Also used for Resumption of Care Following Inpatient Stay)
(Page 8 of 15)

Client's Name: M. P. Smith
Client Record No. 111-08

e. **(M0468)** Does this patient have a **Stasis Ulcer?**
- ☒ 0 - No **[If No, go to #8.*f - Surgical Wound*]**
- ☐ 1 - Yes

(M0470) Current Number of Observable Stasis Ulcer(s):
- ☐ 0 - Zero
- ☐ 1 - One
- ☐ 2 - Two
- ☐ 3 - Three
- ☐ 4 - Four or more

(M0474) Does this patient have at least one **Stasis Ulcer that Cannot be Observed** due to the presence of a nonremovable dressing?
- ☐ 0 - No
- ☐ 1 - Yes

(M0476) Status of Most Problematic (Observable) Stasis Ulcer:
- ☐ 1 - Fully granulating
- ☐ 2 - Early/partial granulation
- ☐ 3 - Not healing
- ☐ NA - No observable stasis ulcer

Describe current treatment approach(es) for stasis Ulcer(s):

f. **(M0482)** Does this patient have a **Surgical Wound?**
- ☒ 0 - No **[If No, go to *Section 9 - Cardiorespiratory*]**
- ☐ 1 - Yes

(M0484) Current Number of Observable Surgical Wounds: (If a wound is partially closed but has more than one opening, consider each opening as a separate wound.)
- ☐ 0 - Zero
- ☐ 1 - One
- ☐ 2 - Two
- ☐ 3 - Three
- ☐ 4 - Four or more

(M0486) Does this patient have at least one **Surgical wound that Cannot be Observed** due to the presence of a nonremovable dressing?
- ☐ 0 - No
- ☐ 1 - Yes

(M0488) Status of Most Problematic (Observable) Surgical Wound:
- ☐ 1 - Fully granulating
- ☐ 2 - Early/partial granulation
- ☐ 3 - Not healing
- ☐ NA - No observable surgical wound

Describe current treatment approach(es) for surgical wound(s):

Other Wounds Requiring Treatment

Type of Wound:

Status:

Current treatment Approach(es):

9. **CARDIORESPIRATORY:** Temperature 98.2° Respirations 18

BLOOD PRESSURE: Lying 136/82 Sitting 142/86 Standing 150/88

PULSE: Apical rate 102 Radial rate 100 Rhythm IRREG Quality Strong

CARDIOVASCULAR:

___ Palpitations	✓ Dyspnea on exertion	✓ BP problems	___ Murmurs
___ Claudication	✓ Paroxysmal nocturnal dyspnea	___ Chest pain	✓ Edema
✓ Fatigues easily	✓ Orthopnea (# of pillows 2)	✓ Cardiac problems (specify) HF	___ Cyanosis
___ Pacemaker ______ (Date of last battery change)		___ Other (specify) ______	___ Varicosities

COMMENTS:

Bilateral +1 edema lower calf & ankle

OASIS-B1 SOC/ROC (1/2008)

Figure 2-1, cont'd

START OF CARE ASSESSMENT
(Also used for Resumption of Care Following Inpatient Stay
(Page 9 of 15)

Client's Name: M. P. Smith
Client Record No. 111-08

RESPIRATORY:

History of: ____ Asthma ✓ Bronchitis (Every yr) ✓ Pneumonia (2000?) ____ Other (specify) ____
____ TB ____ Pleurisy ____ Emphysema

Present Condition:

NA Cough (describe) ____
S/O Breath sounds (describe) rales in LLL
NA Sputum (character and amount) ____
____ Other (specify) ____

(M0490) When is the patient dyspneic or noticeably **Short of Breath?**

- ☐ 0 - Never, patient is not short of breath
- ☐ 1 - When walking more than 20 feet, climbing stairs
- ☐ 2 - With moderate exertion (e.g., while dressing, using commode or bedpan, walking distances less than 20 feet)
- ☒ 3 - With minimal exertion (e.g., while eating, talking or performing other ADLs) or with agitation
- ☐ 4 - At rest (during day or night)

COMMENTS:

(M0510) Respiratory Treatments utilized at home: **(Mark all that apply.)**

- ☒ 1 - Oxygen (intermittent or (continuous)) 2L/min N/C
- ☐ 2 - Ventilator (continually or at night)
- ☐ 3 - Continuous positive airway pressure
- ☐ 4 - None of the above

10. **GENITOURINARY TRACT:**

NA Frequency
↓ Pain
↓ Hematuria
↓ Vaginal discharge/bleeding
S/O Nocturia 3-4x/night
S/O Urgency sometimes
? Prostate disorder
____ Other (specify) ____
NA Dysmenorrhea
↓ Lesions
↓ Hx hysterectomy
X Gravida/Para
X Date last PAP test
X Contraception

(M0510) Has this patient been treated for a **Urinary Tract Infection** in the past 14 days?

- ☒ 0 - No
- ☐ 1 - Yes
- ☐ NA - Patient on prophylatic treatment
- ☐ UK - Unknown

(M0520) Urinary Incontinence or Urinary Catheter Presence:

- ☒ 0 - No incontinence or catheter (includes anuria or ostomy for urinary drainage) [**If No, go to *Section 11-Gastrointestinal Tract***]
- ☐ 1 - Patient is incontinent
- ☐ 2 - Patient requires a urinary catheter (i.e., external, indwelling, intermittent, suprapubic) [**Go to *Section 11-Gastrointestinal Tract***]

(M0530) When does **Urinary Incontinence** occur?

- ☐ 0 - Timed-voiding defers incontinence
- ☐ 1 - During the night only
- ☐ 2 - During the day and night

COMMENTS: (e.g., appliances and care, bladder programs, catheter type and care)

11. **GASTROINTESTINAL TRACT:**

S/O Indigestion once in a while-every wk or so
____ Nausea, vomiting
____ Ulcers
____ Pain
____ Hernias (where) ____
____ Diarrhea/constipation
____ Rectal bleeding
____ Hemorrhoids
____ Gallbladder problems
____ Jaundice
____ Tenderness
____ Other (specify) ____

(M0540) Bowel Incontinence Frequency:

- ☒ 0 - Very rarely or never has bowel incontinence
- ☐ 1 - Less than once weekly
- ☐ 2 - One to three times weekly
- ☐ 3 - Four to six times weekly
- ☐ 4 - On a daily basis
- ☐ 5 - More often than once daily
- ☐ NA - Patient has ostomy for bowel elimination
- ☐ UK - Unknown

COMMENTS: (bowel function, use of laxatives or enemas, bowel program, GI status)

Occasionally takes a dose of MOM but very rarely needs to

(M0550) Ostomy for Bowel Elimination: Does this patient have an ostomy for bowel elimination that (within the last 14 days): a) was related to an inpatient facility stay, or b) necessitated a change in medical or treatment regiment?

- ☒ 0 - Patient does not have an ostomy for bowel elimination.
- ☐ 1 - Patient's ostomy was not related to an inpatient stay did not necessitate change in medical or treatment regimen.
- ☐ 2 - The ostomy was related to an inpatient stay or did necessitate change in medical or treatment regimen.

OASIS-B1 SOC/ROC (1/2008)

Figure 2-1, cont'd

START OF CARE ASSESSMENT
(Also used for Resumption of Care Following Inpatient Stay
(Page 10 of 15)

Client's Name: M. P. Smith
Client Record No. 111-08

12. **NUTRITIONAL STATUS:** ± 6-7lbs c̄ HF episodes in p̄ 3-4mos. 1800 cal ADA
S/O Weight (loss/gain) last 3 mos. Give amount ____) ____ Over/under weight ____ Change in appetite Diet 2gm NA
____ Other (specify) Weight = 165lbs Meals prepared by Self/sometimes Jane brings a sandwich
COMMENTS:
Does not follow diet! Needs dental F.U. & dietary consult to help c̄ food choices.

13. **BREASTS:** (For both male and female)
NA Lumps NA Tenderness NA Discharge NA Pain ____ Other (specify) ____
COMMENTS:
No pbs noted in physical assessment

14. **NEURO/EMOTIONAL/BEHAVIORAL STATUS:**
NA Hx of previous psych.illness No pbs noted Other (specify) ____

(M0560) Cognitive Functioning: (Patient's current level of alertness, orientation, comprehension, concentration, and immediate memory for simple commands.)
- ☐ 0 - Alert/oriented, able to focus and shift attention.
- ☑ 1 - Required prompting (cueing, repetition, reminders) only under stressful or unfamiliar conditions.
- ☐ 2 - Requires assistance and some direction in specific situations (e.g., on all tasks involving shifting of attention), or consistently requires low stimulus environment due to distractibility.
- ☐ 3 - Requires considerable assistance in routine situations. Is not alert and oriented or is unable to shift attention and recall directions more than half the time.
- ☐ 4 - Totally dependent due to disturbances such as constant disorientation, coma, persistent vegetative state, or delirium.

(M0570) When Confused (Reported or Observed):
- ☐ 0 - Never
- ☑ 1 - In new or complex situations only
- ☐ 2 - On awakening or at night only
- ☐ 3 - During the day and evening, but not constantly
- ☐ 4 - Constantly
- ☐ NA - Patient nonresponsive

(M0580) When Anxious (Reported or Observed)
- ☐ 0 - None of the time
- ☑ 1 - Less often than dialy
- ☐ 2 - Daily, but not constantly
- ☐ 3 - All of the time
- ☐ NA - Patient nonresponsive

(M0590) Depressive Feelings Reported or Observed in Patient: (Mark all that apply.)
- ☑ 1 - Depressed mood (e.g., feeling sad, tearful)
- ☐ 2 - Sense of failure or self reproach
- ☐ 3 - Hopelessness
- ☐ 4 - Recurrent thoughts of death
- ☐ 5 - Thoughts of suicide
- ☐ 6 - None of the above feelings observed reported

(M0610) Behaviors Demonstrated at Least Once a Week (Reported or Observed): (Mark all that apply.)
- ☐ 1 - Memory deficit: failure to recognize familiar persons/places, inability to recall events of past 24 hours, significant memory loss so that supervision is required
- ☐ 2 - Impaired decision-making: failure to perform usual ADLs or IADLs, inability to appropriately stop activities, jeopardizes safety through actions
- ☐ 3 - Verbal disruption: yelling, threatening, excessive profanity, sexual references, etc.
- ☐ 4 - Physical aggression: aggressive or combative to self and others (e.g., hits self, throws objects, punches, dangerous maneuvers with wheelchair or other objects)
- ☐ 5 - Disruptive, infantile, or socially inappropriate behavior (**excludes** verbal actions)
- ☐ 6 - Delusional, hallucinatory, or paranoid behavior
- ☑ 7 - None of the above behaviors demonstrated

(M0620) Frequency of Behavior Problems (Reported or Observed): (e.g., wandering episodes, self abuse, verbal disruption, physical aggression, etc.):
- ☐ 0 - Never
- ☐ 1 - Less than once a month
- ☐ 2 - Once a month
- ☐ 3 - Several times each month
- ☑ 4 - Several times a week Anxious and depressed
- ☐ 5 - Atleast daily

(M0630) Is this patient receiving **Psychiatric Nursing Services** at home provided by a qualified psychiatric nurse?
- ☑ 0 - No
- ☐ 1 - Yes

COMMENTS: (describe other related behaviors or symptoms, e.g., weight loss, sleep disturbances, coping skills)
Sleep disturbances often due to dyspnea, nocturia, noisy bar downstairs; naps during day; somewhat anxious & depressed now b/c he's afraid of having to give up apt & go to nursing home; minimal outside support & coping skills presently; does not like being tied to his O_2

OASIS-B1 SOC/ROC (1/2008)

Figure 2-1, cont'd

START OF CARE ASSESSMENT (Also used for Resumption of Care Following Inpatient Stay) (Page 11 to 15)	Client's Name: M. P. Smith Client Record No. 111 - 08

15. ENDOCRINE AND HEMATOPOIETIC:

S/O Diabetes ___ Polyuria ___ Polydipsia ___ Thyroid problem ___ Excessive bleeding or bruising

Fractionals: Usual results 110 - 120 ___ Intolerance to heat and cold

Frequency checked q am ✓ Other (specify) AIC - 7.4(05/08)

COMMENTS: Dx of Type 2 Diabetes x 20yrs; ✓s BS q am & self-injects insulin (until last hospitalization)

M. LIFE SYSTEM PROFILE: For M0640-M0800, complete the "Current" column for all patients. For these same items, complete the "Prior" column only at start of care and at resumption of care; mark the level that corresponds to the patient's condition 14 days prior to start of care date (M0030) or resumption of care date (M0032). In all cases, record what the patient is able to do.

1. **(M0640)** Grooming: Ability to lend to personal hygiene needs (i.e., washing face and hands, hair care, shaving or make up, teeth or denture care, fingernail care).

Prior	Current	
☒	☐	0 - Able to groom self unaided, with or without the use of assistive devices or adapted methods.
☐	☐	1 - Grooming utensils must be placed within reach before able to complete grooming activities.
☐	☒	2 - Someone must assist the patient to groom self.
☐	☐	3 - Patient depends entirely upon someone else for grooming needs.
☐		UK - Unknown

2. **(M06500 Ability to Dress Upper Body** (with or without dressing aids) including undergarments, pullovers, front-opening shirts and blouses, managing zippers, buttons, and snaps:

Prior	Current	
☒	☐	0 - Able to get clothes out of closets and drawers, put them on and remove them from the upper body without assistance.
☐	☐	1 - Able to dress upper body without assistance if clothing is laid out or handed to the patient.
☐	☒	2 - Someone must help the patient put on upper body clothing.
☐	☐	3 - Patient depends entirely upon another person to dress the upper body.
☐		UK - Unknown

3. **(M0660) Ability to Dress Lower Body** (with or without dressing aids) including undergarments, slacks, socks or nylons, shoes:

Prior	Current	
☒	☐	0 - Able to obtain, put on, and remove clothing and shoes without assistance.
☐	☐	1 - Able to dress lower body without assistance if clothing and shoes are laid out or handed to the patient.
☐	☒	2 - Someone must help the patient put on undergarments, slacks, socks, or nylons, and shoes.
☐	☐	3 - Patient depends entirely upon another person to dress lower body.
☐		UK - Unknown

4. **(M0670) Bathing:** Ability to wash entire body. **Excludes grooming)washing face and hands only).**

Prior	Current	
☐	☐	0 - Able to bathe self in shower or tub independently.
☒	☐	1 - With the use of devices, is able to bathe self in shower or tub independently.
☐	☐	2 - Able to bathe in shower or tub with the assistance of another person: (a) for intermittent supervision or encouragement or reminders, OR (b) to get in and out of the shower or tub, OR (c) for washing difficult to reach areas.
☐	☒	3 - Participates in bathing self in shower or tub, but requires presence of another person throughout the bath for assistance or supervision.
☐	☐	4 - Unable to use the shower or tub and is bathed in bed or bedside chair.
☐	☐	5 - Unable to effectively participate in bathing and is totally bathed by another person.
☐		UK - Unknown

5. **(M0680) Toileting: Ability to get to and from the toilet or bedside commode.**

Prior	Current	
☒	☐	0 - Able to get to and from the toilet independently with or without a device.
☐	☒	1 - When reminded, assisted, or supervised by another person, able to get to and from the toilet.
☐	☐	2 - Unable to get to and from the toilet but is able to use a bedside commode (with or without assistance).
☐	☐	3 - Unable to get to and from the toilet or bedside commode but is able to use a bedpan/urinal independently.
☐	☐	4 - Is totally dependent in toileting.
☐		UK - Unknown

OASIS- B1 SOC/ROC (1/2008)

Figure 2-1, cont'd

START OF CARE ASSESSMENT **(Also used for Resumption of Care Following Inpatient Stay** (Page 12 of 15)	Client's Name: M. P. Smith Client Record No. 111-08

6. **(M0690) Transferring:** Ability to move from bed to chair, on and off toilet or commode, into and out of tub or shower, and ability to turn and position self in bed if patient is bedfast.

Prior Current
- ☐ ☐ 0 - Able to independently transfer.
- ☒ ☒ 1 - Transfers with minimal human assistance or with use of an assistive device. *Very slowly*
- ☐ ☐ 2 - Unable to transfer self but is able to bear weight and pivot during the transfer process.
- ☐ ☐ 3 - Unable to transfer self and is unable to bear weight or pivot when transferred by another person.
- ☐ ☐ 4 - Bedfast, unable to transfer but is able to turn and position self in bed.
- ☐ ☐ 5 - Bedfast, unable to transfer and is unable to turn and position self.
- ☐ UK - Unknown

7. **(M0700) Ambulation/Locomotion:** Ability to SAFELY walk, once in a standing position, or use a wheelchair, once in a seated position, on a variety of surfaces.

Prior Current
- ☐ ☐ 0 - Able to independently walk on even and uneven surfaces and climb stairs with or without railings (i.e., needs no human assistance or assistive device).
- ☒ ☐ 1 - Requires use of a device (e.g., cane, walker) to walk alone or requires human supervision or assistance to negotiate stairs or steps or uneven surfaces.
- ☐ ☒ 2 - Able to walk only with the supervision or assistance of another person at all times. *weak, recent falls, painful gait*
- ☐ ☐ 3 - Chairfast, unable to ambulate but is able to wheel self independently.
- ☐ ☐ 4 - Chairfast, unable to ambulate and is unable to wheel self.
- ☐ ☐ 5 - Bedfast, unable to ambulate or be up in a chair.
- ☐ UK - Unknown

8. **( ) Feeding or Eating:** Ability to feed self meals and snacks. **Note: This refers only to the process of eating, chewing, and swallowing, not preparing the food to be eaten.**

Prior Current
- ☒ ☐ 0 - Able to independently feed self.
- ☐ ☒ 1 - Able to feed independently but requires:
  - (a) meal set-up; OR
  - (b) intermittent assistance or supervision from another person; OR
  - (c) a liquid, pureed or ground meat diet.
- ☐ ☐ 2 - Unable to feed self and must be assisted or supervised throughout the meal/snack.
- ☐ ☐ 3 - Able to take in nutrients orally and receives supplemental nutrients through a nasogastric tube or gastrostomy.
- ☐ ☐ 4 - Unable to take in nutrients orally and is fed nutrients through a nasogastric tube or gastrostomy.
- ☐ ☐ 5 - Unable to take in nutrients orally or by tube feeding.
- ☐ UK - Unknown

9. **(M0720) Planning and Preparing Light Meals** (e.g., cereal, sandwich) or reheat delivered meals:

Prior Current
- ☒ ☐ 0 - (a) Able to independently plan and prepare all light meals for self or reheat delivered meals; OR
  (b) Is physically, cognitively, and mentally able to prepare light meals on a regular basis but has not routinely performed light meal preparation in the past (i.e., prior to this home care admission).
- ☐ ☒ 1 - Unable to prepare light meals on a regular basis due to physical, cognitive, or mental limitation.
- ☐ ☐ 2 - Unable to prepare light meals or reheat any delivered meals.
- ☐ UK - Unknown

10. **(M0730) Transportation:** Physical and mental ability to safely use a car, taxi, or public transportation (bus, train, subway).

Prior Current
- ☒ ☐ 0 - Able to independently drive a regular or adapted car; OR uses a regular or handicap-accessible public bus.
- ☐ ☒ 1 - Able to ride in a car only when driven by another person; OR able to use a bus or handicap van only when assisted or accompanied by another person.
- ☐ ☐ 2 - Unable to ride in a car, taxi, bus, or van, and requires transportation by ambulance.
- ☐ ☐ UK - Unknown

11. **(M0740) Laundry:** Ability to do own laundry -- carry laundry to and from washing machine, to use washer and dryer, to wash small items by hand.

Prior Current
- ☐ ☐ 0 - (a) Able to independently take care of all laundry tasks; OR
  (b) Physically, cognitively, and mentally able to do laundry and access facilities, but has not routinely performed laundry tasks in the past (i.e., prior to this home care admission).
- ☒ ☐ 1 - Able to do only light laundry, such as minor hand wash or light washer loads. Due to physical, cognitive, or mental limitations, needs assistance with heavy laundry such as carrying large loads of laundry.
- ☐ ☒ 2 - Unable to do any laundry due to physical limitation or needs continual supervision and assistance due to cognitive or mental limitation.
- ☐ ☐ UK - Unknown

OASIS-B1 SOC/ROC (1/2008)

Figure 2-1, cont'd

2

START OF CARE ASSESSMENT **(Also used for Resumption of Care Following Inpatient Stay)** (Page 13 of 15)	Client's Name: M. P. Smith Client Record No. 111-08

12. **(M0750) Housekeeping:** Ability to safely and effectively perform light housekeeping and heavier cleaning tasks.

Prior Current
- ☐ ☐ 0 - (a) Able to independently perform all housekeeping tasks: OR
  (b) Physically, cognitively, and mentally able to perform all housekeeping tasks but has not routinely participated in housekeeping tasks in the past (i.e., prior to this home care admission).
- ☐ ☐ 1 - Able to perform only light housekeeping (e.g., dusting, wiping kitchen counters) tasks independently.
- ☒ ☐ 2 - Able to perform housekeeping tasks with intermittent assistance or supervision from another person.
- ☐ ☐ 3 - Unable to consistently perform any housekeeping tasks unless assisted by another person throughout the process.
- ☐ ☒ 4 - Unable to effectively participate in any housekeeping tasks.
- ☐ UK - Unknown

13. **(M0760) Shopping:** Ability to plan for, select, and purchase items in a store and to carry them home or arrange delivery.

Prior Current
- ☐ ☐ 0 - (a) Able to plan for shopping needs and independently perform shopping tasks, including carrying packages; OR
  (b) Physically, congnitively, and mentally able to take care of shopping, but has not done shopping in the past (i.e., prior to this home care admission).
- ☒ ☐ 1 - Able to go shopping, but needs some assistance:
  (a) By self is able to do only light shopping and carry small packages, but needs someone to do occasional major shopping; OR
  (b) Unable to go shopping alone, but can go with someone to assist.
- ☐ ☒ 2 - Unable to go shopping, but is able to identify items needed, place orders, and arrange home delivery.
- ☐ ☐ 3 - Needs someone to do all shopping and errands.
- ☐ UK - Unknown

14. **(M0770) Ability to Use Telephone:** Ability to answer the phone, dial numbers, and effectively use the telephone to communicate.

Prior Current
- ☐ ☐ 0 - Able to dial numbers and answer calls appropriately and as desired.
- ☒ ☒ 1 - Able to use a specially adapted telephone (i.e., large numbers on the dial, teletype phone for the deaf) and call essential numbers.
- ☐ ☐ 2 - Able to answer the telephone and carry on a normal conversation but has difficulty with placing calls.
- ☐ ☐ 3 - Able to answer the telephone only some of the time or is able to carry on only a limited conversation.
- ☐ ☐ 4 - Unable to answer the telephone at all but can listen if assisted with equipment.
- ☐ ☐ 5 - Totally unable to use the telephone.
- ☐ ☐ NA - Patient does not have a telephone.
- ☐ UK - Unknown

15. **(M0780) Management of Oral Medications:** Patient's ablity to prepare and take all prescribed oral medications reliably and safely, including administration of the correct dosage at the appropriate times/intervals. **Excludes injectable and IV medications. (NOTE: This refers to ability, not compliance or willingness.)**

Prior Current
- ☐ ☐ 0 - Able to independently take the correct oral medication(s) and proper dosage(s) at the correct times.
- ☒ ☒ 1 - Able to take medication(s) at the correct times if:
  (a) individual dosages are prepared in advance by another person; OR *pharmacist will set up medi-planner*
  (b) given daily reminders; OR
  (c) someone develops a drug diary or chart.
- ☐ ☐ 2 - Unable to take medication unless administered by someone else.
- ☐ ☐ NA - No oral medications prescribed.
- ☐ UK - Unknown

16. **(M0790) Management of Inhalant/Mist Medications:** Patient's ablity to prepare and take all prescribed inhalant/mist medications (nebulizers, metered dose devices) reliably and safely, including administration of the correct dosage at the appropriate times/intervals. **Excludes all other forms of medication (oral tablets, injectable and IV medications).**

Prior Current
- ☐ ☒ 0 - Able to independently take the correct medication and proper dosage at the correct times.
- ☐ ☐ 1 - Able to take medication at the correct times if:
  (a) individual dosages are prepared in advance by another person; OR
  (b) given daily reminders.
- ☐ ☐ 2 - Unable to take medication unless administered by someone else.
- ☒ ☐ NA - No inhalant/mist medications prescribed.
- ☐ UK - Unknown

OASIS-B1 SOC/ROC (1/2008)

Figure 2-1, cont'd

START OF CARE ASSESSMENT **(Also used for Resumption of Care Following Inpatient Stay** (Page 14 of 15)	Client's Name: M. P. Smith Client Record No. 111-08

17. **(M0800) Management of Injectable Medications:** Patient's ability to prepare and take all prescribed injectable medications reliably and safely, including administration of correct dosage at the appropriate times/intervals. **Excludes IV medications.**

Prior Current
☒ ☐ 0 - Able to independently take the correct medication and proper dosage at the correct times.
☐ ☒ 1 - Able to take injectable medication at correct times If:
(a) individual syringes are prepared in advance by another person, OR *having a hard time seeing so Jane Crane is coming to fill syringes*
(b) given daily reminders.
☐ ☐ 2 - Unable to take injectable medications unless administered by someone else.
☐ ☐ NA - No injectable medications prescribed.
☐ UK - Unknown

18. **(M0810) Patient Management of Equipment** (includes ONLY oxygen, **IV/infusion therapy, enteral/parenteral nutrition equipment or Supplies):** Patient's ability to set up, monitor and change equipment reliably and safely, add appropriate fluids or medication, clean/store/dispose of equipment or supplies using proper technique. **(NOTE: This refers to ability, not compliance or willingness.)**

☐ 0 - Patient manages all tasks related to equipment completely independently.
☐ 1 - If someone else sets up equipment (i.e., fills portable oxygen tank, provides patient with prepared solutions), patient is able to manage all other aspects of equipment
☐ 2 - Patient requires considerable assistance from another person to manage equipment, but independently completes portions of the task
☒ 3 - Patient is only able monitor equipment (e.g., liter flow, fluid in bag) and must call someone else to manage the equipment.
☐ 4 - Patient is completely dependent on someone else to manage all equipment.
☐ NA - No equipment of this type used in care **[If NA, go to *Section N-Therapy Need*]**

19. **(M0820) Caregiver Management of Equipment (Includes ONLY oxygen, IV/infusion therapy, enteral/parenteral nutrition, ventilator therapy equipment or supplies):** Caregiver's ability to set up, monitor and change equipment reliably and safely, add appropriate fluids or medication, clean, store/dispose of equipment or supplies using proper technique. **(NOTE: This refers to ability, not compliance or willingness.)**

☐ 0 - Caregiver manages all tasks related to equipment completely independently.
☐ 1 - If someone else sets up equipment, caregiver is able to manage all other aspects.
☐ 2 - Caregiver requires considerable assistance from another person to manage equipment, but independently completes significant portions of task
☐ 3 - Caregiver is only able to complete small portions of task (e.g., administer nebulizer treatment clean/store/dispose of equipment or supplies).
☐ 4 - Caregiver is completely dependent on someone else to manage all equipment. supplies).
☒ NA - No caregiver *-if Jane is willing to learn, will teach her care of O_2 equip*
☐ UK - Unknown

N. **THERAPY NEED**

1. **(M0826) Therapy Need:** In the home health plan of care for the Medicare payment episode for which this assessment will define a case mix group, what is the indicated need for therapy visits (total of reasonable and necessary physical, occupational, and speech-language pathology visits combined)? **(Enter Zero ["000"] if no therapy visits indicated.)**

(0 0 7) Number of therapy visits indicated (total of physical, occupational and speech-language pathology combined).
☐ NA - Not Applicable: No case mix group defined by this assessment.

O. **EQUIPMENT AND SUPPLIES:**

1. Equipment Needs: (check appropriate box)

	Has	Needs
a. Oxygen/Respiratory Equip.	X	
b. Wheelchair		
c. Hospital Bed		
d. Other (specify) *Walker*	X	

2. Supplies Needed and Comments Regarding Equipment Needs:
Respiratory Services, Inc (444-596-9966) supplies O_2

3. Financial Problems/Needs:
$600 social security income/mo-barely covers housing & food expenses-SW referral

P. **SAFETY MEASURES RECOMMENDED TO PROTECT PATIENT FROM INJURY:**

Remove throw rugs
Grab bars in shower

OASIS-B1 SOC/ROC (1/2008)

Figure 2-1, cont'd

2

START OF CARE ASSESSMENT (Also used for Resumption of Care Following Inpatient Stay (Page 15 of 15)	Client's Name: *M. P. Smith* Client Record No. *111-08*

Q. EMERGENCY PLANS

Able to dial 911 in emergency
Friend Jane Crane to ✓ on Mr. S. daily
** Recommend PERS*

R. CONCLUSIONS/IMPRESSIONS AND SKILLED INTERVENTIONS PERFORMED THIS VISIT:

Anxiety & depression due to fear of nursing home placement
Dyspnea c̄ minimal exertion due to worsening HF
Limited endurane, weakness, unsteady gait due to HF & RT knee osteoarthritis pain
Pateint education to medication schedule & med changes - set up med chart for pt to follow in large print - ✓ on medi - planner
Instruct on 1800 cal ADA/2 gm Na diet - food choices discussed
Instruct on energy conservation - avoid overexertion, importance of frequent rest periods & pacing activities
Instruct basic home safety precautions
Instruct safe use of O_2 & equip set-up - placed 'No smoking' signs on door & in living room
Instruct to weigh daily & notify nurse if weight >168lbs - weigh @ same time of day (when doing BS✓)
Appeared to understand instruction - will review on next vs.

To do - call Jane Crane re: More frequent ✓ on Mr. S. & teach help c̄ meds & insulin syringe prep

- Also needs dental F.U. & dietary consult

Date of assessment: *08152008* Signature of Assessor: *Bonnie Brown, RN*

OASIS-B1 SOC/ROC (1/2008)

Figure 2-1, cont'd

Department of Health and Human Service
Health Care Financing Administration

Form Approved
OMB No 0938-0357

HOME HEALTH CERTIFICATION AND PLAN OF CARE

1. Patient's HI Claim No.	2. Start of Care Date	3. Certification Period	4. Medical Record No.	5. Provider No.
123456789A	08/15/2008	From: 08/15/2008 To: 10/14/2008	111-08	123456

6. Patient's Name and Address	7. Provider's Name, Address and Telephone Number
Mortimer P. Smith 690 Sunset Dr. Any Town, USA 54321-1234 444-666-9876	Any Town Home Health 2222 Main Street Any Town, USA 54321-4321 444-555-6666

8. Date of Birth 08/01/1926 9. Sex X M ☐ F

11. ICD-9-CM	Principal Diagnosis	Date
428.9	Heart Failure	08102008
12. ICD-9-CM	Surgical Procedure	Date
13. ICD-9-CM	Other Pertinent Diagnoses	Date
250.00	Type 2 Diabetes	00001987
715.96	Osteoarthritis Rt Knee	07012008
401.9	Hypertension	00001987
781.2	Abnormality of gait	07012008
366.9	Cataracts	00002006

10. Medications: Dose/Frequency/Route (N)ew (C)hanged
Oxygen 2L/min per N/C continuously (N)
Coreg 25 mg BID PO (C)
Lasix 40 mg daily PO
Spironolactone 25 mg BID PO
Lisinopril 20 mg daily PO (N)
Lantus Insulin 20 units subq daily (C)
Celebrex 200mg daily PO (N)

14. DME and Supplies
Walker

15. Safety Measures: PERS, fall precautions, remove throw rugs, add nightlight, smoke detectors, fire plan

16. Nutritional Req. 2 Gm NA, 1800 cal ADA

17. Allergies: Sulfa, ASA

18.A. Functional Limitations
1 ☐ Amputation
2 ☐ Bowel/Bladder (Incontinence)
3 ☐ Contracture
4 ☐ Hearing
5 ☐ Paralysis
6 X Endurance
7 X Ambulation
8 ☐ Speech
9 ☐ Legally Blind
A X Dyspnes With minimal Exertion
B X Other (Specify) pain right knee

18.B. Activities Permitted
1 ☐ Complete Bedrest
2 ☐ Bedrest BRP
3 X UP As Tolerated
4 ☐ Transfer Bed/Chair
5 ☐ Exercises Prescribed
6 ☐ Partial Weight Bearing
7 ☐ Independent At Home
8 ☐ Crutches
9 ☐ Cane
A ☐ Wheelchair
B X Walker
C ☐ No Restrictions
D ☐ Other (Specify)

19. Mental Status: 1 X Oriented 2 ☐ Comatose 3 ☐ Forgetful 4 X Depressed 5 ☐ Disoriented 6 X Lethargic 7 ☐ Agitated 8 ☐ Other

20. Prognosis: 1 ☐ Poor 2 X Guarded 3 ☐ Fair 4 ☐ Good 5 ☐ Excellent

21. Orders for Discipline and Treatments (Specify Amount/Frequency/Duration)

SN 1w1; 3w1 2w2; 1w1 Assessment and observation of cardiovascular status, teaching and training of disease process and management, diet and medication management as appropriate, how to take pulse; assess pain and teach pain management strategies; perform pulse oximetry PRN for s/s cardiorespiratory distress and notify physician if<94%; draw blood for hemoglobin A1C (may use butterfly needle if needed) wk of 8/18 and call results to physician; O2 @ 2L/min continuously per N/C; instruct O2 use, safety issues (including use of "No Smoking" sign), storage, reordering and need for fire plan; may also accept orders from Dr. Tom Jones

PT 2w1; 2w2; 1w1 Home safety assessment; evaluation; home exercise program for energy conservation,strengthening, mobility safety

HHA 2w5 Personal care; ADL assistance, support home safety program needs

SW 1w1 Evaluate for social and financial support

OT 2w1; 1w1 Evaluation, home safety assessment, work simplification, energy conservation techniques, low vision assessment for insulin management

22. Goals/Rehabilitation Potential/Discharge Plans

By end of episode, pt will demonstrate knowledge of disease process, trt goals, and self-care management; demonstrate knowledge of trt plan, diet, medications, exercise; achieve adequate symptom control within normal limits for patient; verbalize s/s to report to appropriate health care provider and what to do in emergency situation; demonstrate ability to administer O2safely/ Rehab potential fair to return to previous level of function/D/C to community with comm resource support in 5-7 wks goals met

23. Nurse's Signature and Date of Verbal SOC Where Applicable: [signature] RN 08/15/08

25. Date HHA Received Signed POT 08/30/08

24. Physician's Name and Address
Patrick Mc Dreamy, MD
5555 Main Street
Any Town, USA 54321-4444
444-888-9999

26. I certify that this patient needs intermittent skilled nursing care, physical therapy and/or speech therapy or continues to need occupational therapy. The patient is under my care, and I have authorized the services on this plan of care and will periodically review the plan.

27. Attending Physician's Signature and Date Signed
Dr. P. McDreamy MD 8/21/08

28. Anyone who misrepresents, falsifies, or conceals essential information required for payment of Federal funds may be subject to fine, imprisonment, or civil penalty under applicable Federal laws.

Figure 2-2 Home Health Certification and POC.

Patient M.P. Smith
Date 08 15 2008

Clinical Dimension CASE - MIX GROUPER WORKSHEET

M0 Item	Response	Points Earned			
	Episode #	1 or 2	1 or 2	3+	3+
	Therapy Visits	0-13	14+	0-13	14+
1st or 2nd = Blindness/Low Vision		3	3	3	3
1st or 2nd = Blood Disorders		2	5		
1st or 2nd = CA, Selected Benign Neoplasms		4	7	3	10
Primary = Diabetes		5	12	1	8
2nd =Diabetes		(2)	4	1	4
1st or 2nd = Dysphagia AND Neuro 3 – Stroke		2	6		6
1st or 2nd = Dysphagia AND M0250 (therapy at home) = 3 (Enteral)			6		
1st or 2nd = Gastrointestinal Disorders		2	6	1	4
1st or 2nd = Gastrointestinal Disorders AND M0550 (Ostomy) = 1 or 2		3			
1st or 2nd = Gastrointestinal Disorders AND 1st or 2nd Neuro 1, 2, 3 or 4				2	
1st or 2nd = Heart Disease OR Hypertension		(3)	7	1	8
Primary = Neuro 1 – Brain Disorders and Paralysis		3	8	5	8
1st or 2nd = Neuro 1 – Brain Disorders and Paralysis AND M0680 (toileting) = 2 or more		3	10	3	10
1st or 2nd = Neuro 1 – Brain Disorders and Paralysis OR Neuro 2 – Peripheral Neurological disorders AND M0650 or M0660 (Dressing ↑ and ↓ body) = 1, 2 or 3		2	4	2	2
1st or 2nd = Neuro 3 – Stroke			1		
1st or 2nd = Neuro 3 – Stroke AND M0650 or M0660 (Dressing ↑ and ↓ body) = 1, 2 or 3		1	3	2	8
1st or 2nd = Neuro 3 – Stroke AND M0700 (Ambulation) = 3 or more		1	5		
1st or 2nd = Neuro 4 – MS AND at least 1 of the following: M0670 (bathing) = 2 or more or M0680 (toileting) = 2 or more or M0690 (transfer) = 2 or more or M0700 (ambulation) = 3 or more		3	3	12	18
1st or 2nd = Ortho 1 – Leg or Gait Disorders AND M0460 (problem PU) = 1, 2, 3 or 4		2			
1st or 2nd = Ortho 1 – Leg or Gait Disorders OR Ortho 2 – Other orthopedic disorders AND M0250 (Therapy at home) = 1 (IV/Infusion) or 2 (Parenteral)		5	5		
1st or 2nd = Psych 1 – Affective and other psychoses, depression		3	5	2	5
1st or 2nd = Psych 2 – Degenerative and organic psychiatric disorders		1	2		2
1st or 2nd = Pulmonary disorders		1	5	1	5
1st or 2nd Pulmonary disorders AND M0700 (Ambulation) = 1 or more		1			
Primary = Skin 1 – traumatic wounds, burns & post-op complications		10	20	8	20
2nd = Skin 1 – traumatic wounds, burns & post-op complications		6	6	4	4
2nd = Skin 1 – traumatic wounds, burns & post-op OR Skin 2 – Ulcers and other skin conditions AND M0250 (therapy at home) = 1 (IV/Infusion) or 2 (Parenteral)		2		2	
1st or 2nd = Skin 2 – Ulcers and other skin conditions		6	12	5	12
1st or 2nd = Tracheostomy		4	4	4	
1st or 2nd = Urostomy/Cystostomy		6	23	4	23
M0250 (Therapy at home) = 1 (IV/Infusion) or 2 (Parenteral)		8	15	5	12
M0250 (Therapy at home) = 3 (Enteral)		4	12		12
M0390 (Vision) = 1 or more		(1)			1
M0420 (Pain) = 2 or 3		(1)			
M0450 = 2 or more pressure ulcers at Stage 3 or 4		3	3	5	5
M0460 (Most problematic pressure ulcer) = 1 or 2		5	11	5	11
M0460 (Most problematic pressure ulcer) = 3 or 4		16	26	12	23
M0476 (Stasis ulcer) = 2		8	8	8	8
M0476 (Stasis ulcer) = 3		11	11	11	11
M0488 (Surgical wound status) = 2			2	3	
M0488 (Surgical wound status) =3		4	4	4	4
M0490 (Dyspnea) = 2, 3 or 4		(2)	2		
M0540 (Bowel incontinence) = 2, 3, 4 or 5		1	2	1	
M0550 (Ostomy) = 1 or 2		5	9	3	9
M0800 (Injectable drugs) = 0, 1 or 2		(1)	1	2	4
TOTAL FOR CLINICAL DIMENSION		10			

Figure 2-3 Case-Mix Grouper Worksheet.

Functional Dimension

M0 Item	Response	Points Earned			
	Episode #	1 or 2	1 or 2	3+	3+
	Therapy Visits	0-13	14+	0-13	14+
M0650 or M0660 (Dressing UB and LB) = 1,2, or 3		(2)		2	2
M0670 (Bathing) = 2 or more		(3)	3	6	6
M0680 (Toileting) = 2 or more		2	3	2	
M0690 (Transferring) = 2 or more			2		
M0700 (Ambulation) = 1 or 2		(1)		• 1	
M0700 (Ambulation) = 3 or more		3	4	4	5
TOTAL FOR FUNCTIONAL DIMENSION		6			

Number of Therapy Vs: 10

CFS Scoring			**1st and 2nd Episodes**		**3rd + Episodes**		**All Episodes**
	Severity Levels	***HIPPS Value***	***THERAPY VISITS MADE FOR EPISODE***				
Dimension			***0 to 13***	***14 to19***	***0 to 13***	***14 to19***	***20+ vs***
Clinical	C1	A	0 to 4	0 to 6	0 to 2	0 to 8	0 to 7
	C2	B	5 to 8	7 to 14	3 to 5	9 to 16	8 to 14
	(C3)	(C)	(9+)	15+	6+	17+	15+
Functional	F1	F	0 to 5	0 to 6	0 to 8	0 to 7	0 to 6
	(F2)	(G)	(6)	7	9	8	7
	F3	H	7+	8+	10+	9+	8+
Service	S1	K	0 to 5	14 to 15	0 to 5	14 to 15	20+
	S2	L	6	16 to 17	6	16 to 17	
	S3	M	7 to 9	18 to 19	7 to 9	18 to 19	
	(S4)	(N)	(10)		10		
	S5	P	11 to 13		11 to 13		

Non-Routine Supply

Severity level	Points	HIPPS value w/NRS	HIPPS value w/o NRS	Payments
1	0	S	1	14.12
2	1-14	T	2	51.00
3	15-27	U	3	139.84
4	28-48	V	4	207.76
5	49-98	W	5	320.76
6	99+	X	6	551.00

Final Scoring

Scoring	Dimension	Value	HIPPS Value	Dollar Amt
	Clinical	C3	C	722.64
	Functional	F2	G	201.15
	Service	S4	M	1570.40
	NRS			

Constant = $1322.92
722.64
201.15
1570.40
$ 3817.11

CASE - MIX WEIGHT = 1.6813

Figure 2-3, cont'd

supervisors to identify knowledge or skill deficits that may affect OASIS data integrity and patient outcomes. Areas of OASIS data collection that appear to be most problematic for therapists are those items assessing medication administration or integumentary assessment, and nurses may have more problems assessing functional status items. Use the particular strength of a discipline to train other clinicians—for example, physical therapists should train nurses in the best approaches to assess functional status, and nurses should train therapists on good assessment techniques for dyspnea and medication administration. Instructing staff in areas of weakness is essential to achieve the cross-discipline reliability of the OASIS data and is necessary to identify the multidisciplinary needs of the patient and facilitate appropriate care plan development and interdisciplinary referral.

OASIS Tips for Documentation

- Know that OASIS is the driver – impacts case mix, patient outcomes, and reflects your competence
- Check that diagnosis codes are properly assigned
- Check that they are properly sequenced
- Check that co-morbidities are listed (painting that picture!)
- Check that M0 items are consistent with diagnoses (congruent) and other assessemt items (like homebound)
- Collaborate with the therapist if unsure of the functional activity findings
- Check that findings flow to the POC/485
- Check that the information is consistent from one assessment to the next
- Remember that you are painting a picture of the patient and your risk adjustment

Summary

With OASIS comes increased opportunity for the interdisciplinary team to work collaboratively, sharing the unique and specialized knowledge that each discipline possesses for the benefit of maximizing patient outcomes. Interdisciplinary teams should discuss assessment strategies and develop skills to improve the validity and reliability of the OASIS data collected. The OASIS is expected to change with the next version, "OASIS C." As OASIS data collection practices become more consistent within and between team members, the value of the OASIS data for outcome purposes is enhanced, with associated benefits to patients, providers, and payers.

EVALUATING CLINICAL PRACTICE

Quality of healthcare is more important than ever, and evaluating clinical practice is essential to every successful home care organization. Medicare, Medicaid, managed care plans, and other payers, in addition to consumers themselves, demand to know what they are getting for the dollars they spend. Home care agencies must co-manage resources and quality of care in the context of today's market realities.

The emphasis on clinical outcomes has increased with the requirement for OASIS data collection and reporting for Medicare (and other) patients. Accreditation programs, such as the Joint Commission (JC), Community Health Accreditation Program (CHAP), and state surveys also focus on clinical outcomes. In addition, patients and their families are demanding accountability for their healthcare and the financial implications of the outcome of the care provided; they are becoming more educated and asking more questions as they have better access to internet and other resources.

Additionally, PPS has moved home care toward the achievement of predetermined, positive goals in a more detailed way. The newest CMS reimbursement initiative, Pay For Performance or P4P, is gaining increased momentum as the reimbursement mechanism for healthcare, including inpatient and skilled nursing facilities, physician practices, and home care. The basic premise of P4P is reimbursement of care based on the provider's "performance" in achieving specified clinical, functional, and healthcare utilization outcomes known as *quality indicators*. The emphasis is clearly directed toward quality, outcomes, and their measurement.

No matter what new reimbursement system is implemented in the future, home care has become more objective, data-driven, and sophisticated, and clinicians now routinely collect and analyze patient data in the course of providing quality clinical care.

OBQM and OBQI

The OASIS is a standardized tool for measuring patient outcomes in home health—what happens to patients as a result of our care. To measure patient outcomes, we must examine health status changes between two or more time points. These changes could be a result of the care provided, natural progression of the disease and disability, or both. Improvement outcomes measure how many patients improved of those who could have improved. Stabilization outcomes measure how many patients stayed the same or improved of those who could have.

OBQM is a systematic approach home care agencies implement and follow to *continuously monitor* the quality of care they provide (www.cms.hhs.gov/HomeHealthQualityInits/18_HHQIOASISOBQM.asp#TopOfPage). Two reports—the *Case Mix Report* and *Adverse Event Outcome Report*—are part of the report series produced by CMS for home care agencies to use in the OBQM process. The *Case Mix Report* provides a descriptive overview of the types of patients admitted to an agency and reports patient attributes present at start of care (SOC) or resumption of care (ROC), that may impact health status (such as patient's demographics, baseline health status). These reports are derived from agencies' submitted OASIS data for a specific time period and are compared with a risk-adjusted national reference sample.

The information listed in the *Adverse Event Outcome Report* is low-frequency negative or untoward events that potentially reflect serious health problems or a decline in health status for individual patients. The reports are derived from OASIS data for a specific time period and are compared with a national reference sample. Examples of adverse events include "emergent care for injury caused by fall or accident at home," "emergent care for improper medication administration/medication side effects," and "emergent care for hypo/hyperglycemia." Adverse events are important to include in an agency's overall quality program because they are seen as serious, but potentially preventable, "markers" of quality care.

OBQI is a systematic and ongoing approach home care agencies implement and follow to *continuously improve* the quality of care they provide (www.cms.hhs.gov/HomeHealthQualityInits/16_HHQIOASISOBQI.

asp#TopOfPage). Three reports are produced by CMS for agency use in OBQI—the *Case Mix, Outcome*, and *Patient Tally Reports*. The *Case Mix Report* provides a descriptive overview of the types of patients admitted to an agency and reports patient attributes present at SOC or ROC that may impact health status (such as patient's demographics, baseline health status). These reports are derived from agencies' submitted OASIS data for a specific time period and are compared with a risk-adjusted national reference sample. Risk-adjusted *Outcome Reports* are provided based on OASIS data submitted and include the individual agency's observed outcome rate and a risk-adjusted national reference rate for specific OASIS-derived outcomes—currently there are 29 risk-adjusted outcomes and 13 descriptive outcomes that are reported. This may change and readers should keep apprised of such Medicare changes related to the OASIS, its data, and its collection. The *Patient Tally Report* provides descriptive information for each individual case included in the outcome report analysis and can be used to select patients for process-of-care investigations to identify specific care processes that can be remedied or reinforced. These specific clinical actions and corresponding best practices become the basis for the plan of action to improve care. Web-based OBQI training and other valuable OBQI resources are available at www.medqic.org under the Home Health tab.

State surveyors for Medicare-certified home care agencies routinely follow a protocol to examine selected adverse events from the OBQM reports and outcomes from the OBQI Outcome Report. If selected adverse events for an agency are significantly different from the national reference value, either a record review, home visit, or both will be conducted for selected patients with the adverse event. Selected OBQI outcomes are also compared with the national reference values and, if one falls below a certain level and is statistically significant, one or two patients with this outcome may be selected for home visits and record reviews. Therefore, it is critical that agencies study their OBQI Outcome Reports and select patients for process-of-care investigations to identify specific care processes that can be remedied or reinforced.

These specific clinical actions and corresponding best practices become the basis for the plan of action to improve care. It is also crucial for agencies to perform quarterly investigations of adverse events. Review each patient event to determine if a true adverse outcome has occurred, and then tally the adverse events by separating true adverse events from those that are not true adverse events. Tracking adverse events in this way can help identify trends that may need to be addressed in an agency's quality improvement program. Together, OBQM and OBQI help an agency evaluate the care they provide and develop methods to improve or reinforce care and care processes for their patients.

Home Health Compare

The CMS Home Health Quality Initiative began in 2003 with the publication of Home Health Compare information on its website www.medicare.gov/HHCompare/Home.asp. The objectives of this initiative are twofold: empower consumers with quality of care information so that they can make more informed decisions about their home healthcare and stimulate and support providers and clinicians to improve the quality of healthcare.

There are currently 12 quality measures derived from OASIS data that are posted on the Home Health Compare website and updated quarterly. The Home Health Compare website is primarily for consumers; thus, the outcome measures are worded in consumer language. Table 2-1 lists the OASIS-based outcome measures and the corresponding consumer language found on the Home Health Compare website. Readers are encouraged to keep apprised of Medicare changes related to the outcome measures/indicators, as these may change or additional items may be added.

Other Home Health Quality Initiatives

The Medicare Quality Improvement Community (www.medqic.org) supported Quality Improvement Organizations (QIOs) and providers in finding, using, and sharing quality

TABLE 2-1

HOME HEALTH QUALITY MEASURES/INDICATORS

OASIS Outcome Measures	Consumer Language
Improvement in Ambulation/Locomotion	Patients who get better at walking or moving around
Improvement in Transferring	Patients who get better at getting in and out of bed
Improvement in Pain Interfering with Activity	Patients who have less pain when moving around
Improvement in Urinary Incontinence	Patients whose bladder control improves
Improvement in Bathing	Patients who get better at bathing
Improvement in Management of Oral Meds	Patients who get better at taking their medicines correctly (by mouth)
Improvement in Dyspnea	Patients who are short of breath less often
Improvement in Status of Surgical Wound	Patients whose surgical wound(s) gets better
Discharge to Community	Patients who stay at home after an episode of home health care ends
Acute Care Hospitalization	Patients who had to be admitted to the hospital
Any Emergent Care provided	Patients who need urgent, unplanned medical care
Emergent Care for Wound Infections/ Deteriorating Wound Status	Patients who need urgent, unplanned medical care for wound infections and/or deteriorating wound status

improvement resources. Medicare QIOs work with consumers, HHAs, hospitals, physicians, and other providers to refine care delivery systems and assure patients the right care at the right time, particularly among underserved populations. The program also safeguards the integrity of the Medicare trust fund by ensuring payment is made only for medically-necessary services and investigates beneficiary complaints about quality of care. Under the direction of CMS, the program consists of a United States national network of QIOs responsible for each state, territory, and the District of Columbia. For a listing of individual QIOs, visit www.medqic.org.

One important home health quality initiative was the development of the Home Health Quality Improvement National Campaign 2007 (www.homehealthquality.org). This campaign was a grassroots, collaborative quality improvement effort that arose from the home health community and QIOs with the goal of decreasing avoidable hospitalizations for home care patients. Each month through its website the Home Health Quality Improvement initiative disseminated Best Practice Intervention Packages designed for use by any HHA to support reducing avoidable acute care hospitalizations. Each package contained background information, leadership guidance, implementation tools, discipline-specific education, and application materials relevant to the targeted best practice of the month. Packages included hospitalization risk assessment, patient emergency plan, medication management, phone monitoring and front-loading visits, teletriage, telemonitoring, immunization, physician relationships, fall prevention, patient self-management, disease management, and transitional care coordination.

Challenges

Evaluating clinical quality in home care remains a daunting, yet exciting, challenge. Quality indicators, such as hospital readmission or improvement in dyspnea rates, are only as good as the data that clinicians collect on their patients. Therefore, the biggest challenge that clinicians face in relation to evaluating the quality of their care is to ensure the accuracy of their assessments, whether OASIS or another form of assessment. Does the OASIS and other assessment data accurately reflect the acuity of the patient? With this accomplished, clinicians can focus on determining optimal interventions and discipline mix within financial constraints for the patient and participate in the on-going quest for "best practices."

SUMMARY

Home care clinical practice requires excellence—clinicians who continue to learn, remain flexible, perform accurate, quality assessments, and provide up-to-date, evidence-based clinical interventions in the delivery of care to their patients. This care and the underlying rationale need to be communicated clearly to the patient and family, the home care manager, and perhaps a third-party payer representative who is responsible for tracking and approving or denying visits. As payers continue to provide incentives to decrease the number of patient visits, clinicians must articulate the specific clinical and other needs of the patient and family. This advocacy role will ensure high-quality care for the patient at home. Because patients need management of peripherally inserted central catheter lines or ventilators in the home, home care clinicians will be providing these services. Those who can explain needs based on objective information and patient findings to numerous reimbursement gatekeepers will be successful in home care. The increasing complexity of the situations of patients who are sent home with limited resources and coverage demands these skills for safe, effective patient care.

PART THREE

3

ADULT CLINICAL GUIDELINES

A Systems Approach for Assessment, Care Planning, and Documentation

CARE OF OLDER ADULTS: A TEMPLATE FOR QUALITY CARE

The following is a template based on the care of older adults to be used for each of the following systems-based clinical guidelines.

1. General Considerations

According to the Centers for Disease Control and Prevention (CDC), by 2030 the number of older Americans will have more than doubled to 70 million, or one in every five Americans. Chronic diseases exact a particularly heavy health and economic burden on older adults due to associated long-term illness, diminished quality of life, and greatly increased health care costs. Much of the illness, disability, and death associated with chronic disease is avoidable through known prevention measures. Key measures include practicing a healthy lifestyle (e.g., regular physical activity, healthy eating, and avoiding tobacco use) and the use of early detection practices (e.g., screening for breast, cervical, and colorectal cancers, diabetes and its complications, and depression).

Older adults are the primary population of many home care agencies due to coverage by the Medicare program (44 million individuals) and their higher risk of multiple chronic conditions necessitating home care services. Even though persons over the age of 65 comprise only 12 percent of the population, they account for 38 percent of the hospitalizations. Even so, the length of stay continues to decline, making them more vulnerable on discharge. Of special concern is the high incidence of fractures in this population, accounting for over one-half of the 1 million discharges hospitalized for fractures (526,000) (DeFrances, C.J., & Hall, M.J. 2005 National Hospital Discharge Survey. Advance data from vital and health statistics; no. 385. Hyattsville, MD: National Center for Health Statistics. 2007.).

The availability, cost and quality of health care is one of the major concerns of all age groups in the United States today. Preventable admissions—inpatient stays that could potentially be prevented with high quality primary and preventive care—are an area where higher quality care can save dollars, particularly in the older adult population. Data from the Healthcare Cost and Utilization Project (HCUP) indicates that from 1997–2004, total hospital expenditures for potentially preventable admissions rose 31 percent, while the number of admissions increased by only 3 percent. In 2004, preventable hospitalizations cost $29 billion, or one out of every 10 dollars spent on hospitalizations. Nearly 4.4 million hospital stays could possibly have been prevented with better access to health education, care and treatment (Russo, C.A. [Thomson Healthcare], Jiang, H.J. [AHRQ], and Barrett, M. [Thomson Healthcare]. *Trends in Potentially Preventable Hospitalizations among Adults and Children, 1997–2004*. HCUP Statistical Brief #36. August 2007. Agency for Healthcare Research and Quality, Rockville, MD. http://www.hcup-us.ahrq.gov/reports/statbriefs/sb36.pdf).

Also of interest from the HCUP data is that costs increased for preventable admissions related to diabetes (44 percent), circulatory diseases (26 percent), chronic respiratory diseases (16 percent), and acute conditions (38 percent) *even though admissions declined.* These diseases primarily affect older adults, and the rise in costs associated with these admissions suggests more complex care and treatment was required.

Better discharge planning and early referral to home care could perhaps have prevented these admissions. Studies have shown that discharge planning and care coordination are woefully lacking, and follow–up care after discharge is sporadic at best. The health care and insurance maze can be overwhelming for older adult patients and families alike.

The home care clinician's efforts are directed *first and foremost* toward educating the patient and family/caregivers—teaching them to identify and manage: (1) safety issues, including specific signs and symptoms that necessitate calling emergency services or other follow-up (such as 911 or their health care provider); (2) symptomatology; (3) medication regime; (4) recommended lifestyle changes, including diet, activity/exercise, etc; (5) importance of follow-up with health care providers; and (6) other information specific to the patient/caregivers. Not all disease is reversible, and some patients with end-stage disease need skilled, compassionate hospice or palliative care through death, with support also provided to their family/caregivers. For patients with end-stage disease, readers are also referred to the Hospice and Palliative Care guideline.

2. Potential Diagnoses and Codes

The diagnoses listed under each system addressed in the following guidelines include some of the most common conditions in home care, and have been alphabetized for easy identification. Keep in mind that the ICD-9-CM system requires a focused review of the patient's medical information in addition to the physician-assigned diagnoses. Accuracy in coding is critical for PPS reimbursement in home care. OASIS items M0230/M0240/M0246 (diagnoses, severity index, and payment diagnoses) are used for many diagnoses to determine case mix classification and reimbursement. Should additional information be needed, refer to the coding books or a qualified coder.

3. OASIS and Assessment Considerations

The complete, accurate, and timely completion of the comprehensive assessment, including the OASIS data elements, is the primary basis for determining the patient's case-mix assignment (HHRG), and subsequent reimbursement, in the PPS model. With this in mind, clinicians must assess the patient and choose the response that *best* reflects the patient at a given point in time as specified in the OASIS Implementation Manual. The OASIS items (referred to as *M0*) that specifically target the system addressed in the following guidelines are listed. Please keep in mind that these lists are not all-inclusive, since patient comorbidities vary, as do other variables unique to the patient's situation.

4. Associated Nursing Diagnoses (see Part Seven)

Nursing diagnoses are used in many home care agencies, and the most up-to-list is listed in Part Seven.

5. Supportive Factors for the Determination and Documentation of Homebound Status

The definition of homebound as found in the Home Health Agency Medicare Manual is found in Box 3-1.

The OASIS M0640-M0820 items document the patient's functional status—the patient's activities of daily living (ADLs) and instrumental activities of daily living (IADLs)—and assist in supporting homebound status. Pain (M0420/M0430) and dyspnea (M0490) also assist in supporting homebound status, as do M0350–M0380, caregiver availability and assistance. Other supportive factors for determining and documenting homebound status for specific disease processes are addressed in each of the following system guidelines.

6. Potential Interdisciplinary Goals and Outcomes

Patient-centered goals/outcomes are a required component of the POC and help the clinician project what will be achieved by the end of care as a result of the clinical care and interventions with the patient and family/caregiver. Progress toward the goals determined at the start of care should be documented on each visit so that the clinician can project

BOX 3-1

HHA MANUAL **DEFINITION OF HOMEBOUND**

204.1 (Cont.)

COVERAGE OF SERVICES

07-02

A. Patient Confined to The Home.—In order for a patient to be eligible to receive covered home health services under both Part A and Part B, the law requires that a physician certify in all cases that the patient is confined to his/her home. (See §240.I.) An individual does not have to be bedridden to be considered as confined to the home. However, the condition of these patients should be such that there exists a normal inability to leave home and, consequently, leaving home would require a considerable and taxing effort. If the patient does in fact leave the home, the patient may nevertheless be considered homebound if the absences from the home are infrequent or for periods of relatively short duration, or are attributable to the need to receive health care treatment. Absences attributable to the need to receive health care treatment include, but are not limited to, attendance at adult day centers to receive medical care, ongoing receipt of outpatient kidney dialysis, and the receipt of outpatient chemotherapy or radiation therapy. Any absence of an individual from the home attributable to the need to receive health care treatment, including regular absences for the purpose of participating in therapeutic, psychosocial, or medical treatment in an adult day-care program that is licensed or certified by a State, or accredited, to furnish adult day-care services in a State shall not disqualify an individual from being considered to be confined to his home. Any other absence of an individual from the home shall not so disqualify an individual if the absence is of an infrequent or of relatively short duration. For purposes of the preceding sentence, any absence for the purpose of attending a religious service shall be deemed to be an absence of infrequent or short duration. It is expected that in most instances, absences from the home that occur will be for the purpose of receiving health care treatment. However, occasional absences from the home for nonmedical purposes, e.g., an occasional trip to the barber, a walk around the block, a drive, attendance at a family reunion, funeral, graduation, or other infrequent or unique event would not necessitate a finding that the patient is not homebound if the absences are undertaken on an infrequent basis or are of relatively short duration and do not indicate that the patient has the capacity to obtain the health care provided outside rather than in the home. The examples provided above are not all-inclusive and are meant to be illustrative of the kinds of infrequent or unique events a patient may attend.

Generally speaking, a patient will be considered to be homebound if he/she has a condition due to an illness or injury that restricts his/her ability to leave his/her place of residence except with the aid of supportive devices such as crutches, canes, wheelchairs, and walkers, the use of special transportation, or the assistance of another person or if leaving home is medically contraindicated. Some examples of homebound patients that illustrate the factors used to determine whether a homebound condition exists would be: (1) a patient paralyzed from a stroke who is confined to a wheelchair or requires the aid of crutches in order to walk; (2) a patient who is blind or senile and requires the assistance of another person to leave his/her residence; (3) a patient who has lost the use of his/her upper extremities and, therefore, is unable to open doors, use handrails on stairways, etc., and requires the assistance of another individual to leave his/her residence; (4) a patient who has just returned from a hospital stay involving surgery suffering from resultant weakness and pain and, therefore, his/her actions may be restricted by his/her physician to certain specified and limited activities such as getting out of bed only for a specified period of time, walking stairs only once a day, etc.; (5) a patient with arteriosclerotic

Continued

BOX 3-1

HHA MANUAL DEFINITION OF HOMEBOUND—CONT'D

heart disease of such severity that he/she must avoid all stress and physical activity; (6) a patient with a psychiatric problem if the illness is manifested in part by a refusal to leave home or is of such a nature that it would not be considered safe to leave home unattended, even if he/she has no physical limitations; and (7) a patient in the late stages of ALS or neurodegenerative disabilities.

In determining whether the patient has the general inability to leave the home and leaves the home only infrequently or for periods of short duration, it is necessary (as is the case in determining whether skilled nursing services are intermittent) to look at the patient's condition over a period of time rather than for short periods within the home health stay. For example, a patient may leave the home (under the conditions described above, e.g., with severe and taxing effort, with the assistance of others) more frequently during a short period when, for example, the presence of visiting relatives provides a unique opportunity for such absences, than is normally the case. So long as the patient's overall condition and experience is such that he or she meets these qualifications, he or she should be considered confined to the home.

14

REV.302

07-02

COVERAGE OF SERVICES

204.1 (Cont.)

The aged person who does not often travel from home because of feebleness and insecurity brought on by advanced age would not be considered confined to the home for purposes of receiving home health services unless he/she meets one of the above conditions. A patient who requires skilled care must also be determined to be confined to the home in order for home health services to be covered.

Although a patient must be confined to the home to be eligible for covered home health services, some services cannot be provided at the patient's residence because equipment is required that cannot be made available there. If the services required by a patient involve the use of such equipment, the HHA may make arrangements or contract with a hospital, skilled nursing facility, or a rehabilitation center to provide these services on an outpatient basis. (See §§200.2 and 206.5.) However, even in these situations, for the services to be covered as home health services, the patient must be considered confined to his/her home; and to receive such outpatient services a homebound patient will generally require the use of supportive devices, special transportation, or the assistance of another person to travel to the appropriate facility.

If a question is raised as to whether a patient is confined to the home, the HHA will be asked to furnish the intermediary with the information necessary to establish that the patient is homebound as defined above.

when the patient can be discharged, and the patient and family are part of the discharge planning.

Listed below are generic, interdisciplinary goals that should always be individualized according to the patient and family/caregiver assessed needs. Each goal/outcome begins with the statement "By the end of the projected episode of care, the patient and/or family/caregiver will:"

Demonstrate knowledge of disease process, treatment goals, and self-care management

Demonstrate knowledge of treatment plan, diet, medication regimen, exercise, other _____ (specify)

Achieve adequate symptom control through use of medications and/or other therapies/treatments within normal limits for patient (specify)

State signs/symptoms to report to physician or other health care provider and what to do in emergency situations

Demonstrate ability to remain safe in home environment

Achieve and maintain optimal weight (specify)

Demonstrate stable fluid and nutritional status

Demonstrate improvement in self-care status to level of independence experienced prior to hospitalization

Obtain a thorough work-up appointment to determine underlying causes of _____ (specify)

List appropriate measures for managing changes in body image/lifestyle

Identify appropriate community services available and how to contact them

Demonstrate satisfaction with care as written or verbalized

Achieve regulation of medication regimen as demonstrated by lab values within acceptable ranges _____ (specify)

Identify medication dosages and rationale of needing medications for _____ regimen (specify)

Perform at desired activity level

Experience care in line with patient/family wishes, dignity, and privacy

State medication dosages, verbalize monitoring test frequency/schedule _____ (specify) and how to follow-up on dosage and other safety considerations (e.g., missed doses, foods to avoid)

Demonstrate compliance with medications, exercises, self-observational skills, and other therapeutic regimens

Demonstrate effective self-care management and who to call for questions, changes, concerns

Demonstrate safe use of energy conservation techniques to increase functional activity level

Demonstrate safe use of adaptive techniques (and/or assistive devices) for increased independence in ADLs

Demonstrate compliance/adherence to _______ program/ regimen (specify)
Achieve stable _______ status (specify) as defined by designated clinical path (specify parameters)
Implement plan for home modifications for safety and optimal function
State and demonstrate understanding of care (e.g., medications, ADLs, etc.)
Achieve effective regulation of medications to maximize function
Access community resources to continue plan after discharge
Be supported with skilled and compassionate palliative care for end-stage disease through death
Other goals/outcomes as appropriate for patient

7. Skills, Interventions/Services, and Management

Home care clinicians must exercise acute and effective critical thinking, observation, technical, teaching, and evaluation skills when performing clinical assessments, interventions, and management of home care patients. Listed below are generic, interdisciplinary skills and interventions/services that can be selected based on clinician competency and appropriate scope of practice, and individualized according to the patient/caregiver assessed needs. Also included are generic interventions for Home Health Aide, Medical Social Services, Dietary Counseling, and Pharmacy Services.

Critical Thinking/Assessment Components

Observation and complete systems assessment of patient with _____ (specify problem necessitating care)
Assess and monitor patient's pain (specify), implement pain control/relief measures, and assess patient's response to interventions

Assess, monitor for presence of, fluid retention and measure amount of lower leg (or other site) edema
Weigh ____ (specify)
Measure vital signs, obtaining baseline values every visit
Assess bilateral BP; measure for postural changes
Telephone follow-up related to care plan compliance and medication management
Assessment and observation of patient status after ______ surgery (specify) for signs/symptoms of infection, other complications
Skilled observation and assessment of patient with surgical site due to ______ surgery (specify)
Assess _____ wound (specify site), change dressings (specify orders and frequency), and teach patient/caregiver wound care, infection control, and symptoms that necessitate additional care
Assess patient/caregiver anxiety level and coping skills and support use of positive coping skills
Assess patient response to care and interventions, and report changes and undesired responses to physician

Teaching

Assess learning readiness, learning barriers, specific educational needs, how the patient may best learn (reading, pictures, listening, etc.) and the patient/caregiver's desire/assessed ability to learn
Comprehensive _________ patient education protocol (specify) initiated
Instruct patient in specific symptoms that necessitate calling the nurse, physician, or 911
Instruct patient on lifestyle modifications needed
Teach and provide educational materials about diet, sexual activity, exercise, smoking cessation, substance abuse, other _____ (specify) and monitoring of _____ (specify)
Instruct on preventive measures to maintain health, such as immunizations (flu, pneumonia), regular check-ups, regular mammograms for women, etc.

Instruct on relaxation techniques
Instruct on activities that promote a positive self-concept
Instruct family/caregivers to encourage patient to be as independent as possible
Teach patient/family to weight ____ (specify); use of weight documentation form; weight parameters to report (per physician orders)

Medication/Therapeutic Regimens

Instruct patient/caregiver regarding complex medication management, including schedule, functions, routes, rationale for compliance, possible side effects, drug-drug and drug-food interaction, and when and what to report to whom
Venipuncture for monitoring ________ (specify test and frequency per physician
Instruct patient/caregiver about the need to have prescriptions filled before the last dose(s) of medications
Telephone follow-up related to medication regimen

Nutrition/Hydration/Elimination

Assess hydration and nutrition status and provide nutritional information/education
Monitor intake and output, patient to report weight gain of under/over __ lbs.
Implement bowel management/constipation prevention program
Initiate plan for _____ diet (specify)
Instruct on appropriate food choices for prescribed diet (spe cify) and provide rationale
Provide sample menu plans and review food choices for prescribed diet

Activity

Teach patient energy conservation techniques, such as daily rest periods and pacing of activities

Provide patient/caregiver recommended instructions related to exercise, sexual and other activities (such as lifting/pulling, climbing stairs, or shoveling snow during the postoperative or recuperative period), and other monitoring of _____ (specify)
Instruct on use of assistive devices

Safety

Instruct patient/caregiver specific signs/symptoms that necessitate calling nurse, physician, or 911
Assess patient need for a personal emergency response system (PERS) or other community safety resource
Assess patient/caregiver emergency plan and instruct as indicated
Provide patient/caregiver with home safety information and instructions related to _____ (specify)
Initiate fall protocol in patient with history of falls, postural hypotension, or decreased sensation in feet
Instruct on adaptations to accommodate for visual loss

Care Coordination/Case Management/ Discharge Planning

Develop mutual goals/outcomes and discharge plan with patient/caregiver at initial visit
Initiate _____ pathway/clinical path (specify) per organizational protocol and provide patient with corresponding educational tools/information on admission
Assess need and initiate referral(s) for other agency/community services, including aide, PT/OT/SLP, social worker, dietitian, clinical specialist, pharmacist, wound specialist, and others
Instruct regarding applicable available community resources
Evaluate knowledge of, and agreement with, discharge plan
Assess ability to purchase necessary supplies, food, etc., for treatment
Evaluate knowledge of plan/barriers of care for home care services

Interdisciplinary communication with _____ (specify)
Management and evaluation of the POC
Implement _______ (specify) telehealth protocol
Telephone follow-up related to care plan compliance/adherence
Communicate with insurance company or payer about patient status, reporting information in quantifiable terms
Assess for long-term ability of the patient and family to comply with therapeutic regimen

Other Considerations

Other interventions, care management, etc. based on patient's unique condition and needs

Home Health Aide

Personal care
ADL assistance
Assist with exercises/activities per case manager and prescribed plan
Observation, record-keeping, and reporting
Monitor medication compliance
Other activities/tasks as assigned

Medical Social Services

Evaluation/assessment of how patient's problems adversely impact the POC and impede progress toward identified goals (e.g., cannot afford medications or ordered nutritional supplements, depressed, noncompliant, others)
Assess the patient/caregiver adjustment post-hospitalization, post-diagnosis, etc. and associated problems
Provide linkage to community resources as indicated
Other interventions

Dietary Counseling

Nutritional evaluation of patient with ___ (specify) for achievement of optimal nutrition/hydration

Comprehensive nutritional assessment and plan
Assessment of diet history, calculation of nutrient intake, others
Other interventions

Pharmacy Services
Assessment of medication regimens for safety, efficacy, and drug/drug, drug/food interactions
Assessment of medication regimen and plan for team and patient education related to medications/drug therapies
Other interventions

8. Tips to Support Medical Necessity, Quality, and Reimbursement

Medicare and other insurers seek to pay for value. Part of what determines value is reviewing the documentation to determine if it supports medical necessity and quality so that the entity providing the care can receive the appropriate reimbursement. Did the organization provide the right care to the right patient at the right time? The following documentation tips help provide support for medical necessity, quality, and reimbursement.

- Document the specific care provided, the patient's response, and the plan for the next visit.
- Documentation throughout the clinical record must be congruent—that is, the initial comprehensive assessment including the OASIS, the POC, and the daily visit notes must contain *congruent* information where appropriate.
- Demonstrate the patient's progress toward goals through the episode of care, while also indicating the patient's continued need for home care.
- Document the specific reason(s) the patient is homebound in functional terms.
- Document laboratory and other objective findings that assist in painting a picture of the progress toward goals (e.g., patient's SOB improving and when reaches _____ [specified goal] will discharge).

- Document any medication or other changes to the POC (and obtain physician orders for these changes).
- Document any identified barriers to learning or performance, such as arthritic hands or poor eyesight.
- Document care coordination in the record: communication, including phone calls, with the physician or other health care provider, other team members, team meetings, community resources, and the patient/caregiver.
- Present other objective, measurable information that assists in supporting skilled care and the need for intervention (oximetry results, etc.).
- Document oxygen information (orders) on the medication list.
- Document any variance to the goals/outcomes.
- If the patient receives therapy services, the nursing documentation must be congruent with the therapy documentation, and support the need for therapy.
- Document all medical supplies required during the period under home care even if it is not part of the skilled service needs (e.g., a patient with HF has an old ostomy and is independent in its care; while on service for the HF-related care and teaching however, the HHA also provides ostomy supplies needed during each visit for the duration of the episode—this is a consolidated billing requirement under PPS).
- Document discharge plan each visit that was mutually agreed upon at admission, and any changes.
- Document if the family/patient is unable or unwilling to provide care, such as wound care to site.
- If you are providing daily care for longer than 21 days, there must be a realistic and projected endpoint (specific date) to the daily care (exception is insulin, discussed in more detail in Part One in section, Daily Care).
- Obtain prn visit orders (1 to 2) for problems which may necessitate an extra visit such as for wound care, infusion problems, Foley complications (e.g., dysuria, hematuria, dislodgement, the catheter comes out), and others.

3

QUERIES FOR QUALITY

1. What signs/symptoms is the patient experiencing?
2. Is patient's pain managed effectively?
3. Is patient's and/or caregiver's anxiety managed effectively?
4. Is patient's functional ability/status (ADLs/IADLs) clearly documented?
5. Are infection control and safety measures implemented as needed?
6. Do patient and/or caregiver have access to appropriate community and other needed resources?
7. What progress is the patient making toward reaching established goals and discharge?
8. Have you documented all of the above and other pertinent information in the interdisciplinary plan of care?

9. Evidence-Based and other Resources for Practice and Education

Each of the following systems-based clinical guidelines lists 5–6 of the most important evidence-based and other resources for practice and education. The following are general evidence-based and other resources for practice and education particularly related to prevention and wellness in the older adult population, as well as other aspects of geriatric care.

The Agency for Healthcare Research and Quality (AHRQ) (www.ahrq.gov or 1-800-358-9295) offers numerous resources and clinical guidelines.

The Arthritis Foundation (www.arthritis.org or 1-404-872-7100 offers many resources for older adults.

BenefitsCheckUp (www.benefitscheckup.org) was developed by the National Council on Aging (NCOA) and assists seniors and their families in determining benefit eligibility for services in their area.

The Centers for Disease Control and Prevention (www.cdc.gov/healthyliving) offers numerous resources related to healthy living for all age groups, including older adults (www.cdc.gov/aging).

Elder Care Online (www.ec-online.net) is an internet community of caregivers for older adults which includes information on education and support for caregivers, safety advice, and resources.

Eldercare Locator (www.eldercare.gov or 1-800-677-1116) is a public service of the U.S. Administration on Aging and helps older adults and their caregivers find service in their area.

First for Seniors (www.usa.gov/topics/seniors.shtml) offers a wide range of information related to government services and provides information on a number of topics including health, housing, and consumer protection for older Americans.

Geriatrics At Your Fingertips—Online Edition (2007–2008) (www.geriatricsatyourfingertips.org) from the American Geriatrics Society offers current evidence-based assessment and intervention information for a variety of geriatric syndromes (falls, anxiety, incontinence, malnutrition, etc). Also included are the most utilized and up-to-date geriatric assessment instruments for a variety of conditions, including pain, mental status, depression, etc. The hard cover copy of the book is also available to order through the website.

The John A. Hartford Foundation Institute for Geriatric Nursing (www.hartfordign.org) has a series of geriatric assessment tools available and provides information for nurses on geriatric topics, certifications, geriatric nursing news, and upcoming conferences.

The National Academy of Elder Law Attorneys (NAELA) (www.naela.org) provides a national registry of attorneys specializing in elder law and a Q&A section related to finding and working with an elder law attorney.

The National Association of Area Agencies on Aging (www.n4a.org or 1-202-872-0888) offers reports such as the "Maturing Americans Report," as well as information sheets including "Background on Flu Shots" and publications like "Making the Link: Connecting Caregivers with Services Through Physicians."

The National Family Caregivers Association (NFCA) (www.thefamilycaregiver.org or 1-800-896-3650) offers information and support through their website for caregivers with resources like "Family Caregiving 101" and "A Home Healthcare Primer."

The National Institute on Aging (www.nia.nih.gov or 1-800-222-4225) offers research and health information resources for consumers and providers, including "Working With Your Older Patient: A Clinician's Handbook."

The National Institutes of Health (NIH) (www.nihseniorhealth.gov) have a website devoted to senior citizens with sections on specific problems, such as high blood pressure, Alzheimer's disease, and stroke, including facts on risk factors, prevention, symptoms, and treatment as well as resources on exercise for older adults, sleeping well, and taking medicines. The site also provides information on depression including facts about depression, symptoms of depression, and treatment.

The U.S. Administration on Aging (AoA) (www.aoa.gov or 1-202-619-0724) is an agency of the U.S. Department of Health and Human Services that provides resources and information for older adults and their caregivers.

The U.S. Food and Drug Administration (www.otcsafety.org) has publications from the Council on Family Health available for download in both English and Spanish including "Medicines and You: A Guide for Older Adults" and "Drug Interactions: What You Should Know."

CARDIOVASCULAR SYSTEM CARE

1. General Considerations

The high costs and numbers of cardiac disease in the United States reflected in morbidity and mortality rates are well documented. Heart disease, specifically coronary artery disease (CAD), is the number one cause of death in men and women in the United States. Each year, over one million persons have heart attacks, and almost 500,000 die from heart disease. About one-half of those who die do so within one hour of the start of symptoms and before reaching the hospital.

According to the National Institutes of Health, heart failure (HF) is the number one reason for hospitalization for people over age 65. HF is more common in African-Americans. Also, men have a higher rate of heart failure than women. In addition, the National Heart Lung and Blood Institute reports that about 5 million people in the United States have heart failure and the number is growing.

According to the National Heart Lung and Blood Institute nearly 1 in 3 American adults has high blood pressure, resulting in a higher risk for strokes and other chronic, debilitating diseases.

This Cardiovascular System Care guideline encompasses cardiac pathology and related problems, and includes care related to angina, post-myocardial infarction, cardiac surgery, heart failure, and hypertension. Not all cardiac disease is reversible, and some patients with end-stage cardiac disease need skilled, compassionate hospice or palliative care through death, with support also provided to their family/caregivers. For patients with end-stage cardiac disease, readers are also referred to the Hospice and Palliative Care guideline.

2. Potential Diagnoses and Codes

The diagnoses and codes listed here include some of the most common cardiovascular conditions in home care, and have been alphabetized for easy identification. The ICD-9-CM system requires a focused review of the patient's medical information in addition to the physician-assigned diagnoses. Should additional information be needed, refer to the coding books or a qualified coder.

Abdominal aortic aneurysm (no mention of rupture)	441.4
Acute myocardial infarction (AMI)	410.9X
Angina, pectoris	413.9
Angina, unstable	411.1
Anticoagulants, long term use of	V58.61
Aortic stenosis	424.1
Aortic valve disorder	424.1
Arterial insufficiency	447.1
Arterial occlusive disease, lower extremity	444.22
Arrhythmia, unspecified	427.9
Arterial thromboembolic disease, unspecified site	444.9
Atherosclerosis (coronary)	414.00
Atrial fibrillation	427.31
Atrial flutter	427.32
Bacterial endocarditis	421.0
Cardiac dysrhythmia	427.9
Cardiomegaly	429.3
Cardiomyopathy	425.4
Cerebrovascular accident (CVA) (M0246 only)	434.91
Cerebrovascular accident (CVA) with hemiplegia (M0246 only)	434.91 and 342.90
Cerebrovascular disease (CVD)	437.9
Cerebrovascular disease with aphasia, late effect	438.11
Cerebrovascular disease with hemiplegia, late effect	438.20
Cerebrovascular disease with dysphagia, late effect	438.82

Cerebrovascular disease, unspecified late effect	438.9 and 787.20
Chronic ischemic heart disease	414.9
Congestive heart failure (CHF)	428.0
Cor pulmonale	416.9
Coronary artery disease (CAD)	414.00
Coronary atherosclerosis	414.00
Coronary insufficiency syndrome	411.1
Deep vein thrombosis of leg	453.4X
Deep vein thrombosis of unspecified site	453.9
Digoxin toxicity	972.1 and E980.4
Digoxin toxicity, due to accumulative effect	995.2 and E942.1
Edema	782.3
Electrolyte and fluid imbalance	276.9
Endocarditis, unspecified	424.90
Endocarditis, bacterial	421.0
Hypertensive cardiovascular disease (HCVD), with CHF	402.91
Heart block, unspecified	426.9
Heart disease, chronic ischemic, unspecified	414.9
Hyperlipidemia	272.4
Hypertension, unspecified	401.9
Hypertension, malignant	401.0
Hypertension with heart involvement	402.9X
Hypertensive nephrosclerosis	403.9X
Infected CABG/heart valve/pacemaker (chronic)	996.61
Ischemic heart disease, chronic	414.9
Left heart failure	428.1
Long-term use O_2	V46.2
Lung edema, acute, with heart disease or failure, congestive	428.0
Mechanical complications, pacemaker	996.01
Mechanical complications, heart valve prosthesis	996.02
Mechanical complication, coronary bypass graft	996.03
Mediastinitis	519.2
Mitral stenosis	394.0
Mitral valve disease	394.9
Mitral valve disorder	424.0

Continued

Muscle disuse, atrophy/weakness	728.2
Myocardial infarction (MI)	410.92
Myocardial infarction (OLD)	412
Myocardial infarction, history of	412
Pericardial disease/effusion	423.9
Peripheral vascular disease	443.9
Pleural effusion	511.9
Pulmonary edema	514
Pulmonary edema with cardiac disease or failure	428.1
Pulmonary edema with cardiac disease or failure, congestive	428.0
Pulmonary hypertension, primary	416.0
Respiratory arrest (S/P)	799.1
Therapeutic drug monitoring	V58.83
Thrombophlebitis, unspecified site	451.9
Venous thromboembolic disease, unspecified site	453.9
Venous thrombosis	453.9
Others	

3. OASIS and Assessment Considerations

The following are some of the OASIS items (referred to as *M0*) that specifically target or affect the system addressed in this guideline. Please keep in mind that this list is not all-inclusive, since patient comorbidities vary, as do other variables unique to the patient's situation. OASIS items that may be used in determining the case-mix index are highlighted.

M0230/M0240/M0246—Diagnoses, Severity Index, and Payment Diagnoses
M0420—Pain
M0430—Intractable Pain
M0468/M0470/M0474—Stasis Ulcer
M0476—Stasis Ulcer Status
M0482/M0484/M0486—Surgical Wound

M0488—Surgical Wound Status
M0490—Dyspnea
M0500—Respiratory treatments
M0580—Anxiety
M0650/M0660—Ability to dress upper/lower body
M0670/M0680/M0690—Bathing, toileting, transferring ability
M0700—Ambulation/locomotion
M0780/M0790—Management of oral, inhalant medications
M0810/M0820—Equipment Management
M0826—Therapy Need

4. Associated Nursing Diagnoses (see Part Seven)

5. Supportive Factors for the Determination and Documentation of Homebound Status

Review the generic recommendations for documenting homebound status, and Medicare's definition of homebound in #5 of the template located at the beginning of this Part of this text. Other supportive factors for determining and documenting homebound status for patients with cardiovascular problems may include:

Taxing effort as evidenced by severe SOB (M0490), other (specify in functional terms)
Post-surgery and pacemaker insertion, on activity restrictions
Need for walker and/or assistance to ambulate post-cardiac event/surgery
Inability to negotiate stairs inside/outside of home
Infected postoperative chest site (M0488), on infection precautions with intravenous antibiotics post cardiac surgery
Pain (M0420/M0430) at level _____ (specify) when _____ (specify activity)
Chest pain (M0420/M0430) caused by minimal exertion

Infected pacemaker site (M0488); needs assistance with all activities
Severe SOB (M0490) on any exertion; awaiting heart transplant
Activity restricted due to HF, COPD, and asthma—patient SOB (M0490) and temperature outside is 90 degrees with humidity and smog alert
Post-CABG surgery with cardiac restrictions _____ (specify) through _____ (specify date in physician orders)
Other reasons, including non-cardiac

6. Potential Interdisciplinary Goals and Outcomes

The template presented at the beginning of this Part lists patient-centered goals/outcomes that can be individualized according to the identified needs of the patient and family. The goals/outcomes listed below are specific examples related to cardiovascular system care, and each begins with the statement "By the end of the projected episode of care, the patient and/or family/caregiver will:"

Demonstrate ability to administer oxygen as ordered and manage equipment safely
Demonstrate improvement in dyspnea (as evidenced by _____ (specify)
Demonstrate adequate oxygenation as evidenced by _____ (specify) (e.g., decreased dyspnea)
Achieve replacement of electrolytes lost secondary to medication therapies (or other reasons)
Demonstrate improvement in angina
Achieve effective regulation of medications to maximize optimal cardiac function (e.g., blood pressure, activity tolerance, urine output, SOB, chest pain)
Demonstrate diaphragmatic breathing techniques to decrease SOB and increase functional activity level

Demonstrate pulse measurement and signs/symptoms which require physician notification
Other goals/outcomes as appropriate for patient

7. Skills, Interventions/Services, and Management

The template presented at the beginning of this Part lists generic skills, interventions, and management of the different home care services that can be individualized according to the identified needs of the patient and family. Skills and interventions utilized by home care clinicians specific to cardiovascular system care include:

Assessment

Observe for signs/symptoms of SOB, DOE, and/or chest/leg pain
Observe color of skin, oral mucosa and nail beds; note pallor or cyanosis
Assess vital signs
- Radial and apical pulses; note regular/irregular
- Lying/sitting/standing blood pressures on both arms

Assess for postural hypotension in patient complaining of dizziness on standing or _____ (specify)
Auscultate lung fields, especially posterior bases, for signs/symptoms of fluid retention (fine crackles)
Palpate fingernails for capillary refill
Assess lower extremities for:
- Edema
- Arterial or venous stasis ulcers
- Signs/symptoms of impaired circulation by assessing:
  - Pedal pulses
  - Color/temperature of skin
  - Capillary refill of great toenail

Obtain daily weights, observing for weight gain of 2 or more pounds in a day or 5 or more pounds in a week; precise weight monitoring and management

Assess patient status post-cardiac surgery for signs/symptoms infection, other complications

Assess surgical site

Medication/Therapeutic Regimens

Assessment of medications, especially OTC and herbal

Teach patient/caregiver about anticoagulation therapy, including schedule, need for blood tests, side effects to observe for, interactions with foods/medications, and missed dose management

Measure pulse oximetry q _____ for signs/symptoms cardiorespiratory distress (specify frequency and parameters—at rest, with oxygen, past activity, or room air); report saturation < _____ percent (specify) and when to report to physician

Teach patient/family to measure/record pulse in patient taking digitalis

Teach patient to focus on prevention measures

Observe for signs, symptoms of digoxin toxicity, including nausea, vomiting, diarrhea, neurological changes such as visual disturbances, headache, or C-V manifestations

Monitor nitroglycerin use, including storage, frequency, amount, relief patterns

Obtain vital signs (by clinician) and follow-up by patient

Nutrition/Hydration/Elimination

Teach signs/symptoms of potassium (K^+) loss and food choices high in K^+, including dried fruit, orange juice, bananas, and leafy green vegetables

Teach patient about avoiding/managing constipation, stool softeners, dietary recommendations, and need for adequate hydration for optimal bowel function

Safety

Instruct patient/family regarding postural hypotension and safety implications

Initiate fall protocol for patient with history of falls or postural hypotension

Teach safe and correct use of home oxygen therapy, including safety/exit plan, working smoke detector(s) and fire extinguisher(s), O2 sign on door, and provide written information on safe use of oxygen

Care Coordination/Case Management/ Discharge Planning

Assess need and initiate referral(s) for other agency/ community services, including aide, PT/OT/SLP, social worker, dietitian, cardiac clinical specialist, pharmacist, wound specialist, and others

Physical Therapy

Assessment

Vital signs at rest, during and after activity or exercise

Perceived exertion or dyspnea scale during activities or exercise

Physiologic response to position change

Edema/girth measurements

Cardiovascular signs/symptoms in response to increased oxygen demand of activity/exercise

Interventions/Teaching

Progressive endurance training/reconditioning/exercise prescription

Functional mobility retraining

Therapeutic exercises for strengthening and ROM for specific deficits

Instruct in diaphragmatic breathing and other breathing techniques as related to mobility retraining

Educate patient/caregiver(s) on home programs for all instructions provided

Instruct on normal/abnormal responses to exercise/activity
Perform lymphatic drainage techniques
Teach application of compression bandages, garments
Other interventions

Speech-Language Pathology
Evaluation
Swallowing problems post-surgery or post-AMI
Other interventions

Occupational Therapy
Evaluation, including vital signs at rest and during/after activity
Instruct in safety and use of assistive and adaptive devices techniques and assistive devices for maximum support and independence in ADLs
Instruct in energy conservation, work simplification, and breathing techniques for maximum functional activity level
Teach graded resumption/progression of self-care tasks
Assess and instruct in home modification as needed for maximum safety and independence
Teach therapeutic exercise for strength, ROM and coordination of UE as needed for ADL and functional mobility
Educate patient/caregiver(s) on home programs for all instructions provided
Teach modification of tasks to accommodate cardiac/sternal precautions
Other interventions

Other Considerations
Out-patient Cardiac Rehabilitation program (per physician order)
Other interventions, care management, etc. based on patient's unique condition and needs

8. Tips to Support Medical Necessity, Quality, and Reimbursement (see Care of Older Adults Template at the beginning of this Part)

9. Evidence-based and other Resources for Practice and Education

The Agency for Healthcare Research and Quality (AHRQ) (www.ahrq.gov or 1-800-358-9295 or 1-410-381-3150) offers free resources, including a *Quick Reference Guide for Clinicians, Cardiac Rehabilitation, Clinical Practice Guideline No. 17* and the *Consumer Version*. Patient guides are available in English and Spanish.

The American Heart Association (www.americanheart.org or 1-800-AHA-USA1 [1-800-242-8721]) offers numerous professional and patient resources, including the American College of Cardiology/American Heart Association Practice Guideline: *Guidelines for the Management of Patients with Acute Myocardial Infarction*. Cardiac pharmacology is discussed in depth, as is the long-term management of the patient to facilitate a return to prior levels of activity. Other resources include: "Know the Facts, Get the Stats," a guide to heart disease, stroke, and risks, "Heart Insight," a monthly publication for professionals and consumers, and *Answers by Heart*, patient information sheets on a variety of topics related to heart care. They are split up into three categories, cardiovascular conditions, treatments and tests, and lifestyle and risk reduction, and include titles such as "How Can I Live With Heart Failure?," "How Do I Manage My Medicines?," "How Can I Handle the Stress of Not Smoking?," "What is High Blood Pressure Medicine?," and "How Do I Follow A Healthy Diet?"

Heart Failure Online (www.heartfailure.org) is available in both English and Spanish with information about the heart, specifics of heart failure, and prevention and treatment information, including frequently asked questions page and a glossary of heart-related terms.

The Heart Failure Society of America (www.abouthf.org or 1-651-642-1633) offers information on heart failure and cardiac care guidelines, including the New York Heart Association Classification for the stages of heart failure, with related symptoms to patient's daily activities and quality of life.

The National Heart, Lung, and Blood Institute (www.nhlbi.nih.gov or 1-301-592-8573) has information about heart failure (what it is, the signs and symptom, treatment options, how it is diagnosed) and cardiac care, including "Your Guide to Lowering Your Blood Pressure with DASH" which explains the DASH eating plan and how it can help control blood pressure, "High Blood Cholesterol—What You Need to Know" brochure, and "Live Healthier, Live Longer" which offer helpful tips and information for prevention and management of heart failure.

ENDOCRINE SYSTEM CARE

1. General Considerations

The most common endocrine system problem seen in home care is diabetes mellitus, although thyroid problems, hypoglycemia, and other metabolic/hormonal syndromes are also part of the endocrine system. Diabetes is a syndrome in which hyperglycemia results from a deficiency of insulin secretion, a reduction of its effectiveness, or both. Diabetes is classified into two types, Type 1 (juvenile-onset) and Type 2 (late-onset). Type 1 diabetes, which is the most severe form, occurs primarily in juveniles and results when circulating insulin is virtually absent. Patients with Type 1 diabetes require insulin injections. Type 2 diabetes, which occurs primarily in adults but occasionally in children, results when endogenous insulin circulates but is inadequate or ineffective in meeting the total needs of the body. Insulin may be required in later stages of Type 2 diabetes.

According to the Agency for Healthcare Research and Quality, diabetes is the leading cause of cardiovascular disease, stroke, blindness, and lower limb amputations. In the last 15 years, the number of people in the United States diagnosed with diabetes more than doubled to 20.6 million (9.6 percent) persons aged 20 and older. Of those aged 60 and over, 10.3 million (20.9 percent) have diabetes.

Between 1996 and 2003, data indicates that diabetes patients were hospitalized more often than other patients. The American Heart Association lists diabetes as a major risk factor for heart disease, ranking it with smoking and hypertension. The total cost of diabetes for 2002 was estimated to be $132 billion, with direct medical costs of $92 billion, and indirect costs (disability, work loss, premature death).

Intensive control is the answer to decrease the incidence of sequelae of the long-term effects of diabetes. Glycated hemoglobin tests are essential for validating that treatment objectives are being achieved. Observation and assessment of the myriad effects of diabetes on other systems, teaching and training related to numerous skills needed for self-care, and management of this problematic diagnosis and its long-term implications for patients, require skill and costly resources. Unfortunately, diabetes is the most common cause of blindness, kidney failure, and amputations in adults. Should your patient with diabetes be admitted to home care after an amputation, refer to the Musculoskeletal System guideline for care related to amputations.

2. Potential Diagnoses and Codes

The diagnoses and codes listed here include some of the most common endocrine conditions in home care, and have been alphabetized for easy identification. The ICD-9-CM system requires a focused review of the patient's medical information in addition to the physician-assigned diagnoses. Should additional information be needed, refer to the coding books or a qualified coder.

Diagnosis	Code
Amputee, bilateral	V49.70
Arterial occlusive disease	444.22
Blindness, due to diabetes, type 1	250.51 and 369.00
Cellulitis and abscess	682.9
Diabetes glaucoma	250.50 and 365.44
Diabetes insipidus	253.5
Diabetes mellitus, with unspecified complications, type 2, NIDDM	250.90
Diabetes mellitus, with unspecified complications, type 1 IDDM	250.91
Diabetes mellitus with neurological manifestations	250.60
Diabetic neuropathy	250.60 and 357.2
Diabetic retinopathy (type 2)	250.50 and 362.01
Diabetic retinopathy (type 1)	250.51 and 362.01

Gangrene, right or left foot, in diabetic	250.70 and 785.4
Hyperglycemia	790.6
Hypoglycemia	251.2
Hypoglycemia, in diabetic	250.80
Ketoacidosis, type 1	250.11
Ketoacidosis, type 2	250.10
Long-term current use of insulin	V58.67
Others	

3. OASIS and Assessment Considerations

The following are some of the OASIS items (referred to as *M0*) that specifically target or affect the system addressed in this guideline. Please keep in mind that this list is not all-inclusive, since patient comorbidities vary, as do other variables unique to the patient's situation. OASIS items that may be used in determining the case-mix index are highlighted.

M0230/M0240/M0246—Diagnoses, Severity Index, and Payment Diagnoses
M0350/M0360/M0370/M0380—Caregiver availability/assistance (for insulin injection assistance)
M0390—Vision
M0420—Pain
M0430—Intractable Pain
M0468/M0470/M0474—Stasis Ulcer
M0476—Stasis Ulcer Status
M0650/M0660—Ability to dress upper/lower body
M0670/M0680/M0690—Bathing, toileting, transferring ability
M0700—Ambulation/locomotion
M0780/M0790—Management of oral, inhalant medications
M0800—Management of injectable medications
M0826—Therapy Need

3

4. Associated Nursing Diagnoses (see Part Seven)

5. Supportive Factors for the Determination and Documentation of Homebound Status

Review the generic recommendations for documenting homebound status, and Medicare's definition of homebound in #5 of the template located at the beginning of this Part of this text. Other supportive factors for determining and documenting homebound status for patients with endocrine problems may include:

Patient has a ____ AKA (specify) and admitted to home care for ____ (specify) and has problems ambulating (specify)
Need for walker and/or assistance to ambulate post ____ (specify)
Pain (M0420/M0430) on ambulation due to peripheral neuropathy
Patient is blind, has renal failure, and needs assistance for ambulation and activities
Taxing effort as evidenced by severe SOB (M0490), other (specify in functional terms)
Other reasons, including non-endocrine related

6. Potential Interdisciplinary Goals and Outcomes

The template presented at the beginning of this Part lists patient-centered goals/outcomes that can be individualized according to the identified needs of the patient and family. The goals/outcomes listed below are specific examples related to endocrine system care, and each begins with the statement "By the end of the projected episode of care, the patient and/or family/caregiver will:"

List signs/symptoms of low/high blood sugar levels and needed interventions
Demonstrate appropriate foot care, including inspections, footwear, etc.

Identify "sick day" activities and what to do if insulin, meal, or medication dose missed
Maintain HbA1c (glycated hemoglobin) at _____ (specify)
Maintain blood sugar within ____ (specify range)
Self-administer medications (insulins, oral hypoglycemic agents, etc.)
Demonstrate understanding of diet, exercise, foot care, other aspects of successful self-care (specify)
Assume self-care responsibilities and activities related to effective diabetes management
Demonstrate no active complications of diabetes
Other goals/outcomes as appropriate for patient

7. Skills, Interventions/Services, and Management

The template presented at the beginning of this Part lists generic skills, interventions, and management of the different home care services that can be individualized according to the identified needs of the patient and family. Skills and interventions utilized by home care clinicians specific to endocrine system care include:

Thyroid Assessment

Assess pulse, noting bradycardia or tachycardia
Assess BP, noting abnormal pulse pressure
Assess eyes for sign/symptoms of exophthalmic or periorbital puffiness
Palpate for nodules on thyroid gland
Assess skin texture for signs of dryness/coarseness/coolness or moistness/smoothness/warmth
Determine bowel movement frequency

Diabetes Assessment

Assess for signs/symptoms of hypo and hyperglycemia
Assess and monitor patient's pain (neuropathy and other)

Assess lower extremities for signs of skin breakdown, stasis ulcers, cellulitis

Determine nutritional intake and level of activity

Assess patient's technique for glucose testing and insulin administration

Test fasting and pre-prandial blood glucose

Test urine for ketones if blood glucose elevated

Determine patient's last glucolated Hemoglobin level

Teaching

Initiate comprehensive patient education protocol, including signs/symptoms and actions to take related to hypo/hyperglycemia, insulin preparation, administration, and storage, "sick day" care, who to call with questions, and other educational components to support self-management

Teach patient/caregiver how to use flow sheet for tracking of labs, capillary blood glucose checks, sites of injections, and other self-observational information to be tracked/trended

Instruct patient and caregiver on the long-term consequences/complications to other body systems (e.g., C-V, renal, vision) if diabetes not well-controlled

Medication/Therapeutic Regimens

Glucometer testing q _____; call physician if over _____ or less than _____ (specify parameters)

Teach patient/family safe home glucose monitoring and the correct disposal of sharps

Instruct patient/caregiver basics of insulin administration: drawing up, administration, rotating sites, record-keeping, etc.

Administer insulin _____ as ordered (specify)

Teach patient/caregiver how to mix insulins and their actions

Teach patient/caregiver use and care of auto-inject insulin infusion pump

Initiate fall protocol for patient with history of falls, postural hypotension, or decreased sensation in feet
Instruct on adaptations to accommodate for visual loss

Nutrition/Hydration/Elimination
Instruct patient about specific nutritional therapy as determined by blood glucose levels
Teach patient/caregiver regarding diet and the need to eat meals at consistent times and actions to take when a meal is missed

Care Coordination/Case Management/ Discharge Planning
Assess need and initiate referral(s) for other agency/ community services, including aide, PT/OT/SLP, social worker, dietitian, diabetes educator, pharmacist, wound specialist, and others

Physical Therapy
Evaluation, including sensory assessment of feet/hands
Therapeutic exercises for strengthening, ROM, or balance
Functional mobility retraining
Instruct patient on reconditioning and endurance retraining as needed for daily functioning
Assess for adaptive footwear
Assessment and instructions in wheelchair and/or prosthetic training if needed
Instruct patient/caregiver in safety in balance, gait/ ambulation and transfer training
Modalities for neuropathy-related sensory deficits, if indicated
Other interventions

Occupational Therapy
Evaluation, including sensory assessment of hands and visual testing
Instruct in safety and use of adaptive techniques and assistive devices for maximum independence in ADL

Instruct in energy conservation and task modifications for maximum functional activity level
Assess and instruct in home modification as needed for maximum safety and independence
Teach therapeutic exercise for strength, ROM, and coordination of UE as needed for ADL and functional mobility
Instruct patient/caregiver on splints and/or prosthesis for functional positioning
Instruct on compensatory techniques for UE neuropathy
Educate patient/caregiver(s) on home programs for all instructions provided
Instruct on devices/techniques to accommodate low vision (magnifiers, writing aids, injection devices to facilitate independent administration of insulin, etc.)
Other interventions

Pharmacy Services
Coordination/delivery of pre-filled insulin syringes
Other interventions

Other Considerations
Diabetes education program
Foot clinic/program
Other interventions, care, management, based on the patient's condition and unique need

8. Tips to Support Medical Necessity, Quality, and Reimbursement (see Care of Older Adults Template at the beginning of this Part)

Insulin administration is the ONLY exception to the "daily" coverage rules of Medicare—"insulin is customarily self-injected by patients or is injected by their families. However, where a patient is either physically or mentally unable to self-inject insulin and there is no other person able and willing to inject the patient, the injections would be considered a reasonable and necessary skilled nursing service" (205.1 of Chapter 7—Home Health Services of the Medicare Benefit Policy Manual). Readers are encouraged to read the entire text of the insulin section with the accompanying example and the specific information about prefilling syringes. Remember, the prefilling of insulin syringes by an RN must have a qualifying skill.

In the rare instance that a patient receives daily (or BID) insulin injections, clearly document the specific reasons the patient is unable or unwilling to self-inject. Most patients will say they cannot give themselves an injection when they are first prescribed insulin for treatment. Part of the clinician's role is to support the patient through this challenging time. Teach patients use of devices available to facilitate self-injection. Guide patients toward learning and accepting self-injection and insulin management.

Be aware that the monochromatic infrared energy modality, sometimes used to treat neuropathy, is not covered by Medicare. For a visit to be covered, a covered skill must be provided in addition to this modality.

9. Evidence-Based and other Resources for Practice and Education

The American Diabetes Association (ADA) (www.diabetes.org, or 1-800-DIABETES [1-800-342-2383]) offers many resources for patients, families, and professionals including themed research summaries on topics such as "Blood Glucose Control," "Attitudes Toward Insulin Therapy' and others. They also offer information about "Diabetic Heart and Blood Vessel Disease" with articles on "Lifestyle Changes Improve Artery Health" and others.

The Center for Disease Control and Prevention (CDC) (www.cdc.gov/diabetes or 1-800-CDC-INFO [1-800-232-4636]) offers a Public Health Resource page on diabetes with information on diabetes, eating right, and publications including fact sheets and statistics in both English and Spanish.

The Diabetes Action Research and Education Foundation (www.diabetesaction.org or call 1-202-333-4520) offers numerous resources on their website including healthy recipes, frequently asked questions, an "Ask the Diabetes Educator" page, news updates on research and funding projects, and more.

The Joslin Diabetes Center (www.joslin.org or 1-617-732-2400) has educational resources on managing diabetes and a "Diabetes Words and Phrases" page as well as research information and professional education programs.

The National Amputation Foundation (www.nationalamputation.org or 1-516-887-3600) has information and support available.

The National Diabetes Information Clearinghouse (www.diabetes.niddk.nih.gov or 1-800-860-8747) offers many fact sheets, information packets, and professional publications.

The National Federation of the Blind (NFB) (www.nfb.org or 1-410-659-9314) publishes *Voice of the Diabetic* four times a year as a free service to those with diabetes, clinicians, and others, including health care programs. It is available on the web or in standard print.

GASTROINTESTINAL SYSTEM CARE

1. General Considerations

Patients in home care often have varying disease processes affecting the gastrointestinal (GI) system, including ostomies, anemias and other conditions. Older adults may have less efficient digestion and absorption of nutrients and need vitamin B-12 injections long-term. Other GI patients have colostomies or ostomies, have had cancer or another pathology that necessitates an ostomy, or have feeding tubes for various reasons. GI disorders may be caused by poor food choices, inadequate food and fluid intake, poor dentition, chewing and/or swallowing problems, and some medications. GI disorders often result in poor digestion and malabsorption of nutrients, which may present as diarrhea and be the cause of serious loss of water, electrolytes, and minerals. Constipation is another common problem in older adults that demands ongoing management and prevention of future episodes.

Because ostomy care also has implications for skin care, readers are referred to the Integumentary System Care guideline. Similarly, for some colon cancer patients with ostomies, palliative care may be appropriate, and readers are referred to the Oncology/Hematology System and Hospice and Palliative Care guidelines, respectively.

2. Potential Diagnoses and Codes

The diagnoses and codes listed here include some of the most common gastrointestinal conditions in home care, and have been alphabetized for easy identification. The ICD-9-CM system requires a focused review of the patient's medical information in addition to the physician-assigned diagnoses. Should additional information be needed, refer to the coding books or a qualified coder.

3

Aftercare following surgery to digestive system	V58.75
Alcoholic neuropathy	357.5
Anal fissure	565.0
Anemia, pernicious	281.0
Anemia (unspecified)	285.9
Appendicitis	541
Appendicitis, acute	540.9
Attention to colostomy	V55.3
Attention to G-tube	V55.1
Attention to ileostomy	V55.2
Attention to PICC line	V58.81
B-12 deficiency	281.1
Bowel impaction	560.30
Bowel obstruction	560.9
Bowel perforation	569.83
Cancer of the colon	153.9
Cancer, rectosigmoid	154.0
Cancer of the rectum	154.1
Colitis	558.9
Colitis, ulcerative	556.9
Colon cancer	153.9
Colostomy (surgical)	46.10
Complication of colostomy, enterostomy, unspecified	569.60
Constipation	564.0
Crohn's disease	555.9
Dehydration	276.51
Diarrhea	787.91
Diverticulitis	562.11
Diverticulosis	562.10
Dressing change, surgical	V58.31
Dysphagia	787.2
Esophagitis	530.10
Esophageal reflux	530.81
Esophageal stricture	530.3
Fish tapeworm anemia	123.4
Fissure, anal	565.0
Gastric ulcers	531.90
Gastritis	535.50
Gastrointestinal hemorrhage	578.9
Hemorrhoids	455.6

Hernia, unspecified	553.9
Ileus, paralytic	560.1
Ileus, following surgery	997.4
Impaction, bowel	560.30
Impaction, bowel, fecal	560.39
Infection of colostomy, enterostomy, unspecified	569.61
Jaundice	782.4
Jaundice, newborn	774.6
Mechanical malfunction of colostomy, enterostomy, unspecified	569.62
Malnutrition	263.9
Nasogastric tube, insertion, with feeding tube (surgical)	96.35
Obstruction, intestinal	560.9
Other vitamin B-12 deficiency	281.1
Peristomal rash	782.1
Peritonitis	567.9
Pneumonia, aspiration	507.0
Polyps, bowel	211.3
Radiation enteritis	558.1
Short bowel syndrome	579.3
Skin, excoriation	919.8
Suture removal	V58.32
Ulcerative colitis	556.9
Umbilical hernia	553.1
Others	

3. OASIS Considerations

The following are some of the OASIS items (referred to as *M0*) that specifically target or affect the system addressed in this guideline. Please keep in mind that this list is not all-inclusive, since patient comorbidities vary, as do other variables unique to the patient's situation. OASIS items that may be used in determining the case-mix index are highlighted.

M0230/M0240/M0246—Diagnoses, Severity Index, and Payment Diagnoses
M0250—Therapy at home
M0420—Pain
M0430—Intractable Pain
M0540—Bowel incontinence
M0550—Ostomy for bowel elimination
M0650/M0660—Ability to dress upper/lower body
M0670/M0680/M0690—Bathing, toileting, transferring ability
M0700—Ambulation/locomotion
M0780/M0790—Management of oral, inhalant medications
M0800—Management of injectable medications
M0810/M0820—Management of equipment
M0826—Therapy Need

4. Associated Nursing Diagnoses (see Part Seven)

5. Supportive Factors for the Determination and Documentation of Homebound Status

Review the generic recommendations for documenting homebound status, and Medicare's definition of homebound in #5 of the template located at the beginning of this Part of this text. Other supportive factors for determining and documenting homebound status for patients with gastrointestinal problems may include:

New/recent ostomy (M0550) surgery with pain (M0420/M0430) on movement, needs assistance with ambulation and ADLs/IADLs (specify)
Need for walker and/or assistance to ambulate (M0700)
Pain M0420/M0430) at level ____ (specify) when _____ (specify activity)
Problems with balance, walking _____ feet (specify)

Gastrostomy tube s/p surgical repair of _____ (specify, functional limits)
Taxing effort as evidenced by severe SOB (M0490), other (specify in functional terms)
Feeding tube (M0250); is bedbound/chair-bound (M0700)
Other reasons, including non-GI related

6. Goals and Potential Interdisciplinary Outcomes

The template presented at the beginning of this Part lists patient-centered goals/outcomes that can be individualized according to the identified needs of the patient and family. The goals/outcomes listed below are specific examples related to gastrointestinal system care, and each begins with the statement "By the end of the projected episode of care, the patient and/or family/caregiver will:"

Minimize weight loss; achievement and maintenance of optimal weight
Provide optimal nutrition, water, vitamins, and minerals per order
Demonstrate/perform accurate B-12 injections and care
Demonstrate appropriate management of ostomy/tube feeding
Describe relationship between activity levels and nutritional/fluid needs
Maintain optimal hematologic status through B-12 therapy as evidenced by decreased symptoms, increased absorption, and lab values within prescribed limits
Maintain patent tube with correct placement and infection-free site
Exhibit safe swallowing skills, understandable speech, and increased strength of oral-motor movements
Other goals/outcomes as appropriate for patient

7. Skills, Interventions/Services, and Management

The template presented at the beginning of this Part lists generic skills, interventions, and management of the different home care services that can be individualized according to the identified needs of the patient and family. Skills and interventions utilized by home care clinicians specific to cardiovascular system care include:

Assessment

Determine height, weight, BMI

Assess skin turgor

Assess mouth and throat; note wetness of oral mucosa, condition of teeth, presence of lesions in mouth or throat

Observe contours of abdomen

Auscultate 4 quadrants of abdomen for bowel sounds

Palpate abdomen for areas of pain or masses

Assess bowel movements; color, consistency, amount, frequency

Assess nutrition and fluid intake:

- Perform 24-hour dietary recall
- Ask patient to keep record of foods eaten with amounts
- Record fluid intake

Obtain and track daily weights

If vomiting or diarrhea, assess:

- Color, consistency, amount
- Onset and frequency
- Intake of fluids/electrolytes, amount "staying down"
- Signs/symptoms of dehydration (poor skin turgor, dry or sticky oral mucosa)

If enteral feedings, determine:

- Type of tube, if tube can be changed, dressing to tube entry site
- Name of feeding, amount, frequency, rate (if given by pump)

- Post-feeding/medication flush; fluid, amount
- If the patient is NPO or can take food/fluids by mouth
- If pills delivered through feeding tube, determine with pharmacist if pills can be crushed

Assess skin and tube/ostomy site for movement, discomfort, excoriation, redness, tenderness, swelling, purulent or other leaking drainage (e.g., stool, etc.), and other problems/changes

Observe and assess patient for complications related to aspiration, diarrhea, distention, impaction, others

Teaching

Comprehensive patient education protocol initiated, including identifying tube displacement, dislodgement, or clogging; administration of feeding; preparation, storage, placement, and safety checks; and who should be called with questions

Medication/Therapeutic Regimens

Venipuncture for monitoring blood levels (electrolytes for tube feeding, CEA for colon cancer with ostomy, serum test for B-12, etc.) and frequency per doctor orders

Teach care and management of ostomy

Teach modification of appliance to preserve wound/skin integrity and the need to protect site from irritation/ infection

Teach care and management of pumps used for administration of nutritional formulas

Teach patient/caregiver how to use flow sheet for tracking of feedings, water intake, I & O feeding schedule, and other self-observational information

Teach site care to insertion area

Teach regarding ordered irrigation procedures

Teach the importance and methods of checking tube placement before every feeding

Teach the importance of oral/mouth care

Teach patient/caregiver observational skills, including record-keeping of intake and output, nutritional solution, supplement, or prescription, rate, frequency, and amount and times of feedings

Teach patient/caregiver S/S of obstruction of tube, actions to take, and whom to call

Teach procedure for changing feeding bags/tubing per orders/protocol

Administer/teach administration of prescribed medications via tube

Hang and administer tube feeding per physician order

Administer B-12 injection per physician order

Nutrition/Hydration/Elimination

Initiate plan for new tube-feeding regimen as prescribed by physician, and in collaboration with nutritionist/dietitian and SLP

Teach care and management of nutritional formulas

Teach regarding diet and the need to eat meals/receive feedings at consistent times and actions to take when a meal/feeding is missed

Weigh q _____ per order and notify physician if above ____ or below ____ (specify parameters)

Implement bowel management/constipation prevention program

Teach regarding avoidance of known gas-producing foods, such as cauliflower, cabbage, beans, cucumbers, onions, others

Teach calorie-count determination

Care Coordination/Case Management/ Discharge Planning

Assess need and initiate referral(s) for other agency/ community services, including aide, PT/OT/SLP, social worker, dietitian, pharmacist, wound specialist, and others

Physical Therapy

Evaluation

Therapeutic exercises for strengthening, balance, and endurance retraining as needed for functional mobility

Instruct patient/caregiver in safety in balance, gait/ambulation, and transfer training

Educate patient/caregiver on home programs for all instructions provided

Other interventions

Speech-Language Pathology

Evaluation, including swallowing assessment and determination of need for further testing to rule out swallowing disorder

Recommend appropriate liquid and food consistencies and progress diet as safe for patient

Instruct/perform techniques and exercise to stimulate or strengthen oral-motor function

Instruct in safe swallowing techniques/airway protection

Other interventions

Occupational Therapy

Evaluation

Instruct in safety and use of adaptive techniques and assistive devices for maximum independence in ADL

Training in compensatory techniques for ostomy/colostomy care and associated hygiene activities

Instruct in energy conservation for maximum functional activity level

Assess and instruct in home modification as needed for maximum safety and independence

Teach therapeutic exercise for strength, ROM and coordination of UE as needed for ADL and functional mobility

Educate patient/caregiver(s) on home programs for all instructions provided
Other interventions

Dietary Counseling
Nutritional evaluation of patient with feeding tube (ostomy, B-12 deficiency) for achievement of optimal nutrition and hydration
Other interventions

Other Considerations
Consult with wound specialist as needed
Other interventions, care management, etc. based on patient's unique condition and necds

8. Tips to Support Medical Necessity, Quality, and Reimbursement (see Care of Older Adults Template at the beginning of this Part)

Obtain prn orders for tube site dislodgement or other change related to a tube needing evaluation.
Obtain orders for enteral feeding formula, amount, frequency, and orders for water flush, amount, and frequency.
The manual removal of fecal impaction and bowel training are covered services by Medicare (see Part Six of this text). Document actual removal of the impaction and efforts related to teaching and bowel program management.

9. Evidence-Based and other Resources for Practice and Education

The Crohn's and Colitis Foundation of America (www.ccfa.org or 1-800-932-2423 or 1-800-343-3637) offer resources for professionals and patients.
The National Digestive Diseases Information Clearinghouse (www.digestive.niddk.nih.gov or 1-800-891-5389) has many resources in English and Spanish.

The Oley Foundation (www.oley.org or 1-800-776-OLEY or, outside the U.S. and Canada, 1-518-262-5079) has numerous support and information options available, including a Lifeline Letter bi-monthly newsletter for people living with home parenteral and/or enteral nutrition (HPEN) and fact sheets like "Questions New Tube Feeders Should Be Asking."

The Oral Cancer Foundation (www.oralcancerfoundation.org or 1-949-646-8000 has an information page which explains tube feeding, including a section on "Care of the Patient."

The United Ostomy Association of America (www.uoaa.org or 1-800-826-0826) offers information on ostomy care, frequently asked questions, and adjusting to an ostomy.

The Wound, Ostomy and Continence Nurses Society (www.wocn.org or 1-888-224-9626) offers fact sheets and patient guides including 'Basic Ostomy Skin Care, A Guide for Patients and Healthcare Providers."

GENITOURINARY/RENAL SYSTEM CARE

1. General Considerations

Patients in home care often have varying disease processes affecting the genitourinary (GU)/renal system, including urinary incontinence and other urinary problems (some necessitating indwelling catheters), prostate problems, and renal failure. According to the National Institutes of Health chronic renal failure and end-stage renal disease (ESRD) affect more than 19 million people in the United States. Diabetes and hypertension (high blood pressure) are the two most common causes and account for approximately two-thirds of the cases of chronic renal failure and ESRD. The National Kidney and Urologic Diseases Information Clearinghouse estimates that 4.5 percent of adults 20 years of age and older have physiological evidence of chronic kidney disease (8 million adults) determined as a moderately or severely reduced glomerular filtration rate.

Acute or chronic renal failure is treated by either peritoneal dialysis or hemodialysis. Dialysis is used to maintain life in patients when the kidneys have ceased to function adequately, and patients are either waiting for, or are not candidates for, a kidney transplant. Almost 400,000 people require dialysis or a transplant to survive, a number which has doubled in each of the last two decades, and experts project this number to increase as the population ages.

For Medicare patients, direct dialysis-related services are not covered under the Medicare home health benefit, as the ESRD program is its own benefit, and ESRD centers receive monies to care for all dialysis-related care. However, Medicare patients on hemodialysis or peritoneal dialysis (PD), or awaiting transplant, often have numerous other health problems that may necessitate home care. Document carefully those problems not related to the RF on the POC and throughout the clinical record.

Some GU cancer patients or those ending dialysis may be appropriate for palliative care, and readers are referred to the Oncology/Hematology System and Hospice and Palliative Care guidelines.

2. Potential Diagnoses and Codes

The diagnoses and codes listed here include some of the most common genitourinary/renal conditions in home care, and have been alphabetized for easy identification. The ICD-9-CM system requires a focused review of the patient's medical information in addition to the physician-assigned diagnoses. Should additional information be needed, refer to the coding books or a qualified coder.

Acute pyelonephritis	590.10
Acute renal failure	584.9
Admission for foley change	V53.6
Ascites	789.5
Attention to cystostomy	V55.5
Attention to nephrostomy	V55.6
Bacteremia	790.7
Benign prostatic hypertrophy	600.0X
Bladder atony	596.4
Bladder cancer	188.9
Calculus of kidney	592.0
Cancer of the kidney	189.0
Cancer of the prostate	185
Catheter, insertion, indwelling Foley	57.94
Chronic renal failure	585
Continuous ambulatory peritoneal dialysis (CAPD) (surgical)	54.98
Cystic kidney, congenital	753.10
Cystitis, unspecified	595.9
Glomerulonephritis	583.9
Hematuria	599.7
Hypercalcemia	275.42
Hyperosmolarity	276.0
Hyperparathyroidism	252.00

Continued

Hyperpotassemia	276.7
Hypertension, unspecified	401.9
Hypoglycemia	251.2
Hypoglycemia, in diabetic	250.8X
Hypopotassemia	276.8
Incontinence of urine, unspecified	788.30
Kidney, calculus of	592.0
Nephrosclerosis	403.90
Nephrotic syndrome	581.9
Nephrotic syndrome, due to diabetes	250.40 and 581.81
Neurogenic bladder	596.54
Obstructive uropathy	599.6
Peritonitis	567.9
Prolapse, uterovaginal	618.4
Prostate cancer	185
Prostatitis	601.X
Prostatitis, acute	601.0
Proteinuria	791.0
Pyelonephritis	590.80
Pyelonephritis, acute	590.10
Renal failure, acute	584.9
Renal failure, chronic	585
Renal failure, unspecified	586
Renal polycystic disease	753.12
Retention of urine	788.20
Septicemia	038.9
Stress, urinary incontinence, female	625.6
Surgical dressing change	V58.31
Suture removal	V58.32
Tubular necrosis, acute	584.5
Urinary incontinence	788.30
Urinary obstruction, unspecified	599.6
Urinary retention	788.20
Urinary tract infection (UTI)	599.0
Urosepsis	599.0
Uterine prolapse	618.1
Vaginal prolapse	618.0
Vaginitis	616.10
Others	

3. OASIS Considerations

The following are some of the OASIS items (referred to as *M0*) that specifically target or affect the system addressed in this guideline. Please keep in mind that this list is not all-inclusive, since patient comorbidities vary, as do other variables unique to the patient's situation. OASIS items that may be used in determining the case-mix index are highlighted.

M0420—Pain
M0430—Intractable Pain
M0510—Urinary tract infection
M0520—Urinary incontinence or urinary catheter
M0530—Urinary incontinence occurrence
M0650/M0660—Ability to dress upper/lower body
M0670/M0680/M0690—Bathing, toileting, transferring ability
M0700—Ambulation/locomotion
M0780—Management of oral medications
M0800—Management of injectable medications
M0826—Therapy Need

4. Associated Nursing Diagnoses (see Part Seven)

5. Supportive Factors for the Determination and Documentation of Homebound Status

Review the generic recommendations for documenting homebound status, and Medicare's definition of homebound in #5 of the template located at the beginning of this Part of this text. Other supportive factors for determining and documenting homebound status for patients with genitourinary/renal problems may include:

Taxing effort as evidenced by severe SOB (M0490), other (specify in functional terms)
Post-surgery, on activity restrictions

Infected postoperative site (specify); infection precautions and antibiotics
Need for walker and/or assistance to ambulate (M0700)
Pain (M0240/M0430) at level ____ (specify) when _____ (specify activity)
Severe fatigue with post-dialysis weakness
Indwelling urinary catheter (M0520)
Incontinent of urine (M0520)
Very frail, cannot walk unsupported (M0700)
Other reasons, including non-genitourinary/renal

6. Potential Interdisciplinary Goals and Outcomes

The template presented at the beginning of this Part lists patient-centered goals/outcomes that can be individualized according to the identified needs of the patient and family. The goals/outcomes listed below are specific examples related to genitourinary/renal system care, and each begins with the statement "By the end of the projected episode of care, the patient and/or family/caregiver will:"

Demonstrate ability to change appliance, no skin breakdown, verbalizes signs/symptoms necessitating follow-up, and who to contact
Maintain functional continence
Maintain patent catheter, no skin breakdown, infection-free
Demonstrate correct use of pessary
Choose foods congruent with renal diet regimen
Practice timed voiding
Verbalize signs/symptoms of UTI
Demonstrate proper care of catheter and drainage devices
Practice pelvic floor strengthening exercises
Verbalize and make long-term decisions related to care, including transplantation, kind of dialysis, or the stopping of treatment per patient choice
Other goals/outcomes as appropriate for patient

7. Skills, Interventions/Services, and Management

The template presented at the beginning of this Part lists generic skills, interventions, and management of the different home care services that can be individualized according to the identified needs of the patient and family. Skills and interventions utilized by home care clinicians specific to genitourinary/renal system care include:

Assessment

Observe external genitalia for abnormalities

Percuss over kidneys, noting tenderness

Palpate suprapubic area

Assess urine output; color, amount, frequency, signs of incontinence and/or retention

Assess for signs/symptoms of UTI; frequency, nocturia, hesitancy, retention, urgency, incontinence, dysuria, fever, hematuria, change in color, pain/fullness

If Foley catheter, determine:

- Catheter size, balloon size
- Frequency of change, when last changed
- Condition of catheter and drainage bag
- Determine how often bag emptied

Medication/Therapeutic Regimens

Comprehensive patient education protocol for catheter care initiated, including irrigation, signs/ symptoms of infection, need for hydration, changing the bag, cleaning the bag, need to keep the bag off the floor and below patient's waist or lower, and who should be called with questions

Instruct in ways to promote continence and decrease incontinent episodes

Teach care of ileal conduit, including skin care, appliance change, equipment ordering, infection control, and signs and symptoms to report

Teach patient/caregiver how to use flow sheet for tracking of intake and output, TPR, weight, BPs, BS, dietary, medication schedule(s), and other self-observational information

Administer EPO injection of _____ (specify dose and frequency) SQ (document reason that the patient is unable to self-inject; anxiety, arthritic hands, or other limitations)

Instruct care of suprapubic catheter, including cleansing of area, monitoring of temperatures qd, voids and post-void residuals, and their recordings

Insert/change indwelling catheter (specify, e.g., #16 Fr/5 cc) monthly/prn

Insert/change catheter q month and prn for catheter problems (specify number and reasons)

Insert pessary _____ (specify per orders) and assess for correct placement, effectiveness in older adult woman with arthritic hands who can no longer provide self-care

Nutrition/Hydration/Elimination

Teach regarding need to decrease renal workload to delay/prevent further kidney damage and way to do this

Initiate plan for renal diet and teach appropriate food/fluid choices

Teach regarding electrolyte and fluid restrictions

Monitor intake and output, patient to report weight loss/gain of ____ lbs. (specify parameters)

Care Coordination/Case Management/ Discharge Planning

Assess need and initiate referral(s) for other agency/ community services, including aide, PT/OT/SLP, social worker, dietitian, renal clinical specialist, pharmacist, wound specialist, and others

Physical Therapy

Evaluation

Therapeutic exercises for strengthening and endurance retraining as needed for daily functioning

Pelvic floor strengthening

Instruct patient/caregiver in safety in balance, ambulation, and transfer training

Educate patient/caregiver on home programs, including behavioral techniques for incontinence management

Assessment and instructions in wheelchair if needed

Other interventions

Occupational Therapy

Evaluation

Instruct in safety and use of adaptive techniques and assistive devices for maximum independence in ADL and personal hygiene associated with disease process

Training in therapeutic exercises

Instruct in energy conservation

Assess and instruct in home modification as needed for maximum safety and independence

Teach therapeutic exercise to improve UE strength and coordination as needed for self-care for ADL and functional mobility

Educate patient/caregiver(s) on home programs for all instructions provided

Other interventions

Dietary Counseling

Nutritional evaluation of patient with renal failure for achievement of optimal nutrition and hydration

Comprehensive nutritional assessment of patient with cancer of the prostate and weight loss

Other interventions

Other Considerations

Teach regarding need for infection control precautions and the specific steps/activities to support these precautions

Other interventions, care management, etc. based on the patient's condition and unique needs

8. Tips to Support Medical Necessity, Quality, and Reimbursement (see Care of Older Adults Template at the beginning of this Part)

The Medicare ESRD program is a special and separate Medicare benefit from that of home care. All dialysis-related care is to be provided by the dialysis center, which is paid directly for the provision of the ESRD care. For this reason and because the RHHI will NOT pay if the care is the same (e.g., duplicative and not medically necessary), clarify before and at admission the roles of the home care provider versus the role of the dialysis center. This should be done during the preadmission or admission process. Although home care organizations care for patients with renal disease, the care provided is usually directed toward another medical problem. This includes the patient's uncontrolled hypertension, dressing changes for abdominal sites, neurovascular ulcer sites, or other wound care, medication management, CVA, diabetes that is poorly controlled, and others. When completing the POC, ESRD is usually not listed as the primary diagnosis; the primary diagnosis/code should be the reason the home care organization will be seeing a particular patient (e.g., diabetes, hypertension, wound care), who also is an ESRD patient.

For EPO therapy, if the patient is not receiving dialysis, nursing visits to administer these injections are usually covered as long as the drug frequency and duration are reasonable and necessary, based on the patient's unique medical conditions and assuming that all other coverage criteria are met (e.g., homebound). The actual drug, epoetin (Epogen), is not covered under the Medicare home care program.

9. Evidence-Based and other Resources for Practice and Education

The American Urological Association (AUA) (www.auanet.org) has information on their website for both patients and professionals, and physician-created resources for both pediatric and adult conditions on their urology health site (www.urologyhealth.org).

The National Association for Continence (NAFC) (www.nafc.org or 1-800-BLADDER [1-800-252-3337]) has information on incontinence, including treatment options and explanations and how to find help.

The National Federation of the Blind (NFB) (www.nfb.org or 1-410-296-7760) publishes *Voice of the Diabetic* four times a year as a free service to diabetics and others, including health care programs and information related to kidney disease. It is available on the web or in standard print.

The National Kidney and Urologic Diseases Information Clearinghouse (www.kidney.niddk.nih.gov or 1-800-891-5390) offers information on treatment, booklets such as the "Kidney Failure Glossary," and other resources for patients and professionals. There is also a new Spanish website at www.nkdep.nih.gov/espanol. A brochure is offered that highlights the risk factors commonly associated with renal failure, diabetes and high blood pressure, specifically targeting Hispanic and Latino populations who are at high risk of diabetes and hypertension.

The National Kidney Foundation (NKF) (www.kidney.org or 1-800-622-9010) provides many services, including patient peer counseling, education, medication programs, transportation, and financial services. A very useful patient education resource is "What You Should Know About Infectious Disease: A Guide for Hemodialysis Patients and Their Families." This 13-page booklet reviews infection control, vaccines, and information about numerous infectious diseases. Also available is "It's Just

Part of My Life," a booklet for young adults living with kidney disease and dialysis, and a newsletter entitled "Family Focus."

The Simon Foundation for Continence (www.simonfoundation.org or 1-800-23SIMON [1-800-237-4666]) offers information for both patients and professionals defining incontinence, diagnosis, prevention in all age groups, and educational resources including books with titles such as *Managing Incontinence: A Guide to Living With Loss of Bladder Control.*

The Wound, Ostomy and Continence Nurses Society (www.wocn.org or 1-888-224-9626 offers fact sheets and patient guides for incontinence.

HEPATOBILIARY AND PANCREATIC SYSTEM CARE

1. General Considerations

Patients in home care often have varying disease processes affecting the liver, biliary tract, and/or pancreas. These are often considered together because of their anatomic proximity and their related functions and symptoms that result from pathological conditions. Problems include cystic fibrosis and varying types of hepatitis. Other problems necessitating home care include cancers and obstructions. Hepatitis can have many causes, such as viruses, alcohol use, drugs, toxins, and sepsis. There are new and emerging kinds of hepatitis, but the most common are hepatitis A, hepatitis B, and hepatitis C (C used to be called non-A/non-B). There are also hepatitis D and E, but these are rare in the United States. Please note that because the pancreas also has an endocrine function, this function, and diabetes mellitus specifically, is addressed in the Endocrine System care guideline.

Patients with cancer of the liver or pancreas may be appropriate candidates for palliative care. Readers are referred to the Oncology/Hematology System and Hospice and Palliative Care guidelines. There is also a specific Cystic Fibrosis Care guideline in the maternal and child care section of this handbook.

2. Potential Diagnoses and Codes

The diagnoses and codes listed here include some of the most common hepatobiliary and pancreatic conditions in home care, and have been alphabetized for easy identification. The ICD-9-CM system requires a focused review of the patient's medical information in addition to the physician-assigned diagnoses. Should additional information be needed, refer to the coding books or a qualified coder.

3

Aftercare following surgery to digestive system	V58.75
Aftercare following transplant	V58.44
Ascites	789.5
Cholangitis	576.1
Cholecystitis, unspecified	575.10
Cholelithiasis	574.20
Cirrhosis, biliary	571.6
Cirrhosis, liver	571.5
Cirrhosis, liver, alcoholic	571.2
Constipation	564.0
Cyst on liver	573.8
Cystic fibrosis	277.00
ETOH, abuse	305.00
ETOH, dependence	303.90
Hepatitis	573.3
Hepatitis A	070.1
Hepatitis B	070.30
Hepatitis C	070.51
Hepatitis, viral	070.9
Liver abscess	572.0
Malaise and fatigue	780.79
Malnutrition	263.9
Pancreatic insufficiency	577.8
Pancreatitis	577.0
Pancreatitis, recurrent	577.1
Postoperative wound infection	998.59
Status post transplant	V42.X
Surgical dressing change	V58.31
Suture removal	V58.32
Transplant, complications of	996.8X
Transplant organ rejection	996.80
Others	

3. OASIS Considerations

The following are some of the OASIS items (referred to as *M0*) that specifically target or affect the system addressed in this guideline. Please keep in mind that this list is not all-inclusive, since patient comorbidities vary, as do other variables unique to the patient's situation. OASIS items that may be used in determining the case-mix index are highlighted.

M0230/M0240/M0246—Diagnoses, Severity Index, and Payment Diagnoses
M0250—Therapies
M0420/M0430—Pain
M0430—Intractable Pain
M0482/M0484/M0486—Surgical Wound
M0488—Surgical Wound Status
M0650/M0660—Ability to dress upper/lower body
M0670/M0680/M0690—Bathing, toileting, transferring ability
M0700—Ambulation/locomotion
M0780—Management of oral
M0810/M0820—Management of equipment
M0826—Therapy need

4. Associated Nursing Diagnoses (see Part Seven)

5. Supportive Factors for the Determination and Documentation of Homebound Status

Review the generic recommendations for documenting homebound status, and Medicare's definition of homebound in #5 of the template located at the beginning of this Part of this text. Other supportive factors for determining and documenting homebound status for patients with hepatobiliary and pancreatic problems may include:

Taxing effort as evidenced by ascites causing severe SOB (M0490), other (specify in functional terms)
Post-surgery, on activity restrictions
Infected postoperative ______ site (M0488) (specify), on infection precautions with intravenous antibiotics
Need for walker and/or assistance to ambulate (M0700)
Inability to negotiate stairs inside/outside of home

High bilirubin level, low-grade fever, and up only with assistance
Distended abdomen, up only with maximum assistance
Pain (M0420) at level ____ (specify) when _____ (specify activity)
Other reasons, including non-hepatobiliary/pancreatic

6. Potential Interdisciplinary Goals and Outcomes

The template presented at the beginning of this Part lists patient-centered goals/outcomes that can be individualized according to the identified needs of the patient and family. The goals/outcomes listed below are specific examples related to hepatobiliary and pancreatic system care, and each begins with the statement "By the end of the projected episode of care, the patient and/or family/caregiver will:"

Achieve replacement of electrolytes lost secondary to medication therapies (or other reasons)
Demonstrate optimal liver function
Other goals/outcomes as appropriate for patient

7. Skills, Interventions/Services, and Management

The template presented at the beginning of this Part lists generic skills, interventions, and management of the different home care services that can be individualized according to the identified needs of the patient and family. Skills hepatobiliary and pancreatic system care include:

Assessment

Assess orientation
Assess color of sclera and skin; observe for jaundice
Assess color of urine and stools
Measure abdominal girth

Assess signs/symptoms of deterioration: fever, jaundice, abdominal pain/fullness, increased girth, etc.
Assess, monitor for presence of, fluid retention/edema and measure _____ (specify site)

Nutrition/Hydration/Elimination

Monitor intake and output, patient to report weight loss/gain of over __ lbs. (specify parameters)
Teach patient/caregiver record-keeping for daily weights and other aspects of self-observational care
Teaching related to decreasing liver workload to delay/ prevent further damage (e.g., no alcohol)
Teach regarding electrolyte and fluid restrictions
Assess for long-term ability of the patient and family to comply with therapeutic regimen (e.g., infection control, abstinence from alcohol, other drugs)

Physical Therapy

Evaluation
Therapeutic exercises for strengthening and endurance retraining as needed for mobility and daily functioning
Instruct patient/caregiver for safety in balance, ambulation and transfer training
Educate patient/caregiver on home programs for all instructions provided
Assessment and instructions in wheelchair and/or other assistive devices as needed
Other interventions

Occupational Therapy

Evaluation
Instruct in safety and use of adaptive techniques and assistive devices for maximum independence in ADL and associated personal hygiene as needed

Instruct in energy conservation and diaphragmatic breathing for maximum functional activity level and minimal SOB
Assess and instruct in home modification as needed for maximum safety and independence
Teach therapeutic exercise to improve UE strength and coordination as needed for ADL and functional mobility
Educate patient/caregiver(s) on home programs for all instructions provided
Other interventions

Other Considerations

Other interventions, care, management, etc. based on the patient's unique condition and needs

8. Tips to Support Medical Necessity, Quality, and Reimbursement (see Care of Older Adults Template at the beginning of this Part)

9. Evidence-Based and other Resources for Practice and Education

The American Cancer Society (ACS) (www.cancer.org or 1-800-ACS-2345) has professional and patient resources on liver and pancreatic cancer.
The Centers for Disease Control and Prevention (CDC) (www.cdc.gov or 1-800-311-3435 has up-to-date information and resources in English and Spanish on hepatitis.
The Cystic Fibrosis Foundation (www.cff.org or 1-800-344-4823 [1-800-FIGHT-CF]) offers many resources related to cystic fibrosis.
The National Digestive Diseases Information Clearinghouse (NDDIC) (www.digestive.niddk.nih.gov or 1-800-891-5389) offers information and resources for acute and chronic pancreatitis.
The National Cancer Institute (www.cancer.gov) has many resources available for both professionals and patients on liver and pancreatic cancer.

INFECTION AND IMMUNOLOGIC SYSTEM CARE

1. General Considerations

This Infection and Immunologic System Care guideline includes the most commonly seen infection and immunological problems in home care. The immune system comprises various mechanisms that recognize and eliminate or neutralize antigens that are recognized as foreign bodies. Similarly, infections are fought with various approaches by the body to destroy the infection. This care guideline addresses acquired immunodeficiency syndrome (AIDS), infected wounds, conditions that put patients at risk of infection (e.g., central lines, etc.), and numerous other infections resulting from various causes that are treated at home.

According to the Centers for Disease Control and Prevention (CDC), it is estimated that approximately 40,000 persons become infected with Human Immuno-Deficiency Virus (HIV) each year. It is also estimated that 27 percent of cases are women while 73 percent of the affected population are male. However, women make up nearly one-third of all new HIV infections and their risk is steadily increasing. Instances for young people are also rising and the CDC believes about half of all newly diagnosed HIV cases are in people less than 25 years of age. The number of people diagnosed with AIDS and living with AIDS has increased by 30 percent just from 2000 to 2004.

There has been much in the national media about the estimated 2 million nosocomial infections that occur annually in the United States. The costs are estimated to be $4 billion annually and infections are responsible for 88,000 deaths. Many of these patients come to home care for continued care (e.g., antibiotics and other interventions) after their catastrophic hospital stays. Unfortunately, experts predict that in the coming years, infectious disease caused by both new and re-emerging pathogens will grow in significance as a public health issue in the United States.

According to the Centers for Disease Control and Prevention (CDC), handwashing continues to be the single most important and least expensive means of infection prevention, yet studies demonstrate that compliance rarely exceeds 40 percent. This seemingly low-tech procedure is critical in all health care settings, as microbes become increasingly resistant to antibiotics. The emphasis for patients with infections and compromised immunological function is impeccable infection control, heightening the importance of the home care team who serve as role models for patient and caregivers.

For patients with tuberculosis (TB), readers are also referred to the Respiratory/Pulmonary Care guideline. For patients for whom palliative, supportive care is appropriate, readers are referred to the Hospice and Palliative Care guideline.

2. Potential Diagnoses and Codes

The diagnoses and codes listed here include some of the most common infection and immunologic conditions in home care, and have been alphabetized for easy identification. The ICD-9-CM system requires a focused review of the patient's medical information in addition to the physician-assigned diagnoses. Should additional information be needed, refer to the coding books or a qualified coder.

Acquired immunodeficiency syndrome (AIDS) (general)	042
AIDS and anemia	042 and 285.9
AIDS, recurrent bacterial infections	042
Abscess, abdominal wall	682.2
Abscess, chest wall	682.2
Amputation, infected site	997.62
Anorexia	783.0
Appendicitis, perforation with abscess	540.1

Appendicitis, with perforation	540.0
Appendix, abscess	540.1
Bacteremia	790.7
Bone, aseptic necrosis, unspecified site	733.40
Burkitt's lymphoma and AIDS	200.20 and 042
Candidiasis, unspecified site	112.9
Candidiasis, esophageal	112.84
Candidiasis, oral	112.0
Candidiasis, vaginal	112.1
Cellulitis	682.9
Cellulitis, arm	682.3
Cellulitis, foot	682.7
Cellulitis, trunk	682.2
Cellulitis, right or left lower leg	682.6
Chorioretinitis	363.20
Colitis	558.9
Cryptococcus	117.5
Cytomegalovirus	078.5
Cytomegalovirus, colitis	008.69 and 078.5
Cytomegalovirus, esophagitis	530.19 and 078.5
Cytomegalovirus, kidney	590.81 and 078.5
Cytomegalovirus, retinitis	363.20 and 078.5
Dehydration	276.5
Dementia, AIDS	042 and 294.10
Diarrhea, AIDS	042 and 787.91
Dysphagia	787.20
Encephalitis	323.9
Encephalopathy, AIDS	348.3 and 042
Endocarditis	424.90
Esophagitis	530.10
Fluid and electrolyte imbalance	276.9
Foot abscess	682.7
Herpes simplex	054.9
Herpes zoster	053.9
Hickman catheter insertion, venous (surgical)	38.93
Histoplasmosis	115.90

Continued

Hypovolemia	276.5
I and D, knee (surgical)	80.26
I and D, skin (surgical)	86.04
Immune deficiency disorder	279.3
Infected knee	686.9
Infection, postoperative wound	998.59
Influenza with pneumonia	487.0
Kaposi's sarcoma	176.9
Lupus, systemic erythematosus	710.0
Lyme disease	088.81
Lymphocytic interstitial pneumonia	516.8
Lymphoma	202.80
Lymphoma, non-Hodgkin's	202.80
Lymphoma, brain	202.81
Malaise and fatigue	780.79
Malnutrition	263.9
Meningitis	322.9
Meningitis, viral	047.9
Mycobacterium avium intracellulare or *intracellulare,* pulmonary	031.0
Mycobacterium tuberculosis	011.80
Myocarditis	429.0
Neuropathy, peripheral	356.9
Neutropenia	288.0
Osteomyelitis	730.20
Osteomyelitis, acute, site unspecified	730.20
Osteomyelitis, foot, ankle	730.27
Osteomyelitis, lower leg, knee	730.26
Osteomyelitis, pelvic region, thighs	730.25
Osteomyelitis, site unspecified, acute	730.00
Pelvic inflammatory disease, acute	614.3
Pericarditis, acute	420.90
Peritonitis, postoperative infection	998.59 and 567.2
Pneumocystosis carinii pneumonia	136.3
Pneumonia, aspiration	507.0
Pneumonia, bacterial	482.9
Pneumonia, nonspecific	486
Pneumonia, viral	480.9
Polymyositis	710.4
Polyradiculoneuropathy	357.0
Postoperative wound, infection	998.59
Rheumatoid arthritis	714.0

Salmonella infection, unspecified	003.9
Salmonella septicemia	038.8
Sepsis	038.9
Septicemia	038.9
Shigella	004.9
Shigella, dysentery	004.0
Sinusitis	473.9
Staphylococcal infection, unspecified	041.10
Syphilis, unspecified	097.9
Systemic lupus erythematosus (SLE)	710.0
Thrombocytopenia	287.5
Total parenteral nutrition (TPN) (surgical)	99.15
Toxoplasmosis	130.9
Tuberculosis, pulmonary	011.90
Upper respiratory infection	465.9
Urinary tract infection	599.0
Varicella	052.9
Vascular access device, insertion (VAD) (surgical)	86.07
Wasting syndrome	799.4
Wound infection, postoperative	998.59
Zoster virus	053.9
Others	

3. OASIS Considerations

The following are some of the OASIS items (referred to as *M0*) that specifically target or affect the system addressed in this guideline. Please keep in mind that this list is not all-inclusive, since patient comorbidities vary, as do other variables unique to the patient's situation. OASIS items that may be used in determining the case-mix index are highlighted.

M0230/M0240/M0246—Diagnoses, Severity Index, and Payment Diagnoses
M0250—Therapy at home
M0390—Vision
M0420—Pain

M0430—Intractable Pain
M0440—Wound/lesion
M0445/M0450/M0464—Pressure ulcer
M0450—Pressure ulcer status
M0468/M0470/M0474—Stasis Ulcer
M0476—Stasis Ulcer Status
M0482/M0484/M0486—Surgical Wound
M0488—Surgical Wound Status
M0490—Short of breath (SOB)
M0510—UTI
M0650/M0660—Ability to dress upper/lower body
M0670/M0680/M0690—Bathing, toileting, transferring ability
M0700—Ambulation/locomotion
M0780/M0790—Management of oral, inhalant medications
M0800—Injectable medications
M0810/M0820—Management of equipment
M0826—Therapy Need

4. Associated Nursing Diagnoses (see Part Seven)

5. Supportive Factors for the Determination and Documentation of Homebound Status

Review the generic recommendations for documenting homebound status, and Medicare's definition of homebound in #5 of the template located at the beginning of this Part of this text. Other supportive factors for determining and documenting homebound status for patients with infections and immunologic problems may include:

Taxing effort as evidenced by severe SOB (M0490), other (specify in functional terms)
Post-surgery, on activity restrictions
Unsteady gait, increased risk for falls
Severely immunosuppressed-medically prohibited from going outside
Terminal condition, unable to ambulate without assistance

Impaired mental status and needs supervision 24 hours a day
Reverse isolation due to _____ (specify)
Need for walker and/or assistance to ambulate (M0700)
Inability to negotiate stairs inside/outside of home
Infected wound (pressure ulcer, stasis ulcer, surgical wound)
Infected postoperative ____ site (M0488) (specify), on infection precautions with intravenous antibiotics
Incapacitating malaise related to infection
Pain (M0420) at level ____ (specify) when _____ (specify activity)
Other reasons, including non-infection/immunologic

6. Potential Interdisciplinary Goals and Outcomes

The template presented at the beginning of this Part lists patient-centered goals/outcomes that can be individualized according to the identified needs of the patient and family. The goals/outcomes listed below are specific examples related to infections and immunologic system care, and each begins with the statement "By the end of the projected episode of care, the patient and/or family/caregiver will:"

Demonstrate independent management of ordered therapy (TPN, G-tube, infusion, etc.) and all related site and line care
Verbalize potential complications related to infection and drug therapy
Verbalize understanding of reason and goal of infusion therapy for infection
Verbalize knowledge of potential adverse effects of infusion therapy and actions to take
Minimize symptoms of malnutrition; support optimal intake/nutrition
Achieve replacement of electrolytes lost secondary to medication therapies (or other reasons)
Other goals/outcomes as appropriate for patient

7. Skills, Interventions/Services, and Management

The template presented at the beginning of this Part lists generic skills, interventions, and management of the different home care services that can be individualized according to the identified needs of the patient and family. Skills and interventions utilized by home care clinicians specific to infections and immunologic system care include:

Assessment

Obtain temperature; oral, tympanic, axillary

Assess for signs/symptoms of inflammation/infection

- Neurological
  - Altered level of consciousness
  - Severe headache
  - Stiff neck
  - Pain or lesions along a nerve
- Respiratory
  - Swollen, tender tonsils with exudate
  - Productive cough with yellow/green sputum
  - Course crackles on lung auscultation
- Gastrointestinal
  - Nausea, vomiting, diarrhea
  - Hyperactive bowel sounds
- Urinary tract infection
  - Urgency, frequency, hematuria, pain on urination
  - Confusion in elderly
- Skin/wound infection
  - Warmth, redness, swelling, pain
  - Purulent drainage

Palpate for swollen lymph nodes: cervical, axillary, groin

Palpate abdomen for signs/symptoms of tenderness, especially right-sided tenderness

If intravenous line:

- Observe catheter for condition and that it is intact
- Measure and record length of central catheter, noting signs of migration

- Assess entry site of catheter for signs/symptoms of inflammation
- Palpate around entry site, determining if exudates present
- Determine flush, type, amount, frequency
- Determine IV med/solution, type, amount, frequency, duration of infusion
- Determine dressing change, type and frequency

Assess immunocompromised patient's skin and mucous membranes for problems, including bacterial infection, thrush, rash, or other changes

Teaching

Instruct regarding infection control and standard precautions at home

Teach patient/caregiver about water-borne illness, water to avoid, and water that is safe to drink (must drink water free of the parasite cryptosporidium)

Teach patient to call nurse for parenteral or central line problems such as leakage, blockage, swelling, pain, expulsion

Instruct immunocompromised patient/caregiver regarding pet care and infection control, cross contamination; check with physician about certain types of pets

Instruct patient/caregiver in all aspects of effective handwashing techniques, proper care and disposal of body fluids/excretions, soiled dressings, supplies, washing of linens, use of bleach solution, etc.

Medication/Therapeutic Regimens

Administer antibiotic _______(specify type and dose) over _____ (specify prescribed time line) via _____ (specify)

Heparin flush of _____ (specify) per organizational protocol/orders

Teach care of heparin lock for intermittent antibiotic medication

Change injection cap (weekly and prn) according to agency protocol
Teach patient/family signs and symptoms of phlebitis, occlusion, displacement, infection, other problems
Demonstrate/teach use of tools to manage medications (e.g., Medisets, etc.)
Where possible, integrate medication regimen times with other routine activities that occur the same time each day, such as meals or television shows
Establish/start peripheral line for infusion of _____ (specify)
Perform central/peripheral line dressing changes using aseptic technique or per prescribed plan

Nutrition/Hydration/Elimination

Teach immunosuppressed patient/caregiver regarding food preparation and handling, particularly hand washing, handling uncooked foods, and the need to cook all eggs, meat, fish, and/or poultry products
Evaluate for signs/symptoms of dehydration
Counsel patient with anorexia about diet and nutrition
Encourage intake and supplements to maintain lean body mass
Weigh patient every visit and report changes to physician
Monitor intake and output, patient to report weight loss of over __ lbs. (specify)

Safety

Evaluate patient for specialized support surfaces to avoid pressure ulcers
Disposal of biohazardous waste and sharps

Physical Therapy

Teach strengthening exercises/home exercise program
Implement progressive ambulation program
Teach endurance training/conditioning
Instruct/supervise caregiver in safe methods to assist patient

Teach therapeutic exercises to patient/caregiver
Instruct on bed mobility exercises
Assess and teach regarding safe balance, gait, and transfer training
Instruct patient/caregiver in pain management related to mobility
Other interventions

Speech-Language Pathology

Evaluation of swallow and speech, including assessment to determine the need for further swallowing tests to rule out aspiration
Educate patient/caregiver on safety precautions and prevention of swallowing dysfunction, including food textures and body positioning
Collaborate with nutritionist/dietitian for optimal nutrition
Teach exercises for maximum strength in articulation proficiency for verbal/vocal expression and for lip, tongue, and facial control for maximum swallowing skills
Teach alternative and effective communication program to enable the patient to express his/her needs, even if only for periods of fatigue
Educate patient/caregiver on each home program for all instructions provided
Other interventions

Occupational Therapy

Instruct in safety and use of adaptive techniques and assistive devices for maximum independence in ADL and related functional mobility, within the patient's tolerance
Instruct in energy conservation and diaphragmatic breathing for maximum functional activity level and minimal SOB
Assess and instruct in home modification as needed for maximum safety and independence
Teach therapeutic exercise for maximum UE strength, ROM and coordination as needed for ADL and functional mobility

Assess and address the patient's needs to improve body image and other psychological effects of the disease process
Educate patient/caregiver(s) on home programs for all instructions provided
Other interventions

Other Considerations

Address/teach regarding sexuality concerns and implications for safer sexual expression, including the use of latex condoms, abstinence, the use of dental dams during oral sex, and other methods
Address need for guardianship or power of attorney
Assess spiritual needs and plan
Assist with planning funeral, other plans, if appropriate
Implement nonpharmacologic interventions—may include therapeutic massage, distraction therapy, imagery, progressive muscle relaxation, humor, biofeedback, music therapies, and others
Other interventions, care, management, based on the patient's condition and unique needs

8. Tips to Support Medical Necessity, Quality, and Reimbursement (see Care of Older Adults Template at the beginning of this Part)

9. Evidence-Based and other Resources for Practice and Education

AIDS Info (a service of DHHS) (www.aidsinfo.nih.gov or 1-800-HIV-0440 [1-800-448-0440]) offers resources and a hot line for educational/other information, clinical trial information, and telephone consultation.
The Centers for Disease Control and Prevention's (CDC) National Prevention Information Network (formerly the AIDS Clearinghouse) (www.cdcnpin.org or 1-800-458-5231) offers information and publications, including a 35-page booklet entitled "Caring for Someone with AIDS at Home."

The CDC also offers a National AIDS Hotline: 1-800-342-AIDS (1-800-342-2437).

The Health Resources and Services Administration (HRSA) (www.hab.hrsa.gov or 1-800-ASK-HRSA [1-800-275-4772]) has HIV/AIDS information including a resource "A Clinical Guide on Supportive and Palliative Care for People with HIV/AIDS" (2003).

McGoldrick, M. (2007). Infection Prevention and Control Program. Saint Simons Island, GA: Home Health Systems. (www.homecareandhospice.com)

Rhinehart, E. and McGoldrick, M. (2006). Infection Control in Home Care and Hospice. Sudbury, MA: Jones and Bartlett. (www.homecareandhospice.com)

The Substance Abuse and Mental Health Services Administration (SAMHSA) (www.kap.samhsa.gov) offers many resources. One brochure entitled "Drugs, Alcohol, and HIV/AIDS: A Consumer Guide," offers information on drugs and the spread of HIV/AIDS as well as an entire page of resources both for those suffering from AIDS and those with substance abuse problems.

The Test Positive Aware Network (TPAN) (www.tpan.com or 1-773-989-9400) provides information on AIDS/HIV medical developments, drug interactions, and more. Test Positive also offers a journal, "Positively Aware," which can be ordered.

INTEGUMENTARY SYSTEM CARE

1. General Considerations

This Integumentary System Care guideline encompasses varying aspects of skin and wound care-related problems, including pressure ulcers, cellulitis, acute and postoperative wounds, infusion sites, and parenteral therapy sites.
It has been estimated that three to five million Americans suffer from chronic wounds that resist healing despite months and even years of traditional treatment. Readers are referred to the Gastrointestinal System Care guideline for patients who have ostomies or other GI-related wound conditions.

2. Potential Diagnoses and Codes

The diagnoses and codes listed here include some of the most common integumentary conditions in home care, and have been alphabetized for easy identification. The ICD-9-CM system requires a focused review of the patient's medical information in addition to the physician-assigned diagnoses. Should additional information be needed, refer to the coding books or a qualified coder.

Diagnosis	Code
Acute wound, postoperative infection	998.59
Aftercare following surgery	V58.7X
Amputation status, with infected stump AKA	997.62, V49.76
Appendicitis, perforation with abscess	540.1
Bacteremia	790.7
Bullous pemphigoid	694.5
Cellulitis	682.9
Cellulitis, toe	681.10
Chronic ulcer, lower limb, unspecified	707.10
Chronic ulcer, unspecified site	707.9
Decubitus ulcer (pressure ulcer)	707.0X

Dehydration	276.51
Fluid and electrolyte imbalance	276.9
Gangrene, toe	785.4
Gangrene, upper or lower extremity	785.4
Heel ulcer, right or left	707.14
Hernia	553.9
Infection, postoperative wound	998.59
Intestinal obstruction	560.9
Leg ulcer	707.10
Leg varicosity with ulcer	454.0
Lymphedema	457.1
Malnutrition	263.9
Non-surgical dressing change	V58.30
Osteomyelitis, acute	730.0X
Pain in limb	729.5
Paraplegia	344.1
Peripheral vascular disease	443.9
Peristomal rash	782.1
Peritonitis, postoperative infection	998.59 and 567.2
Posthemorrhage anemia	285.1
Postoperative wound, infection	998.59
Pressure ulcer	707.0X
Pressure (decubitus) ulcer	707.0X
Septicemia	038.9
Skin eruption	782.1
Skin, excoriation	919.8
Staphylococcal infection, unspecified	041.10
Stasis ulcer	454.0
Surgical dressing change	V58.31
Surgical wound, dehiscence or rupture	998.3
Suture removal	V58.32
Thrombophlebitis	451.9
Ulcer, heel with cellulitis	707.14 and 682.7
Ulcer, right or left heel	707.14
Varicose leg ulcer	454.0
Venous insufficiency	459.81
Venous thrombosis	453.9
Venous varicose, with ulcer	454.0
Wound infection, postoperative	998.59
Wound, surgical, non-healing	998.83
Others	

3

3. OASIS Considerations

The following are some of the OASIS items (referred to as *M0*) that specifically target or affect the system addressed in this guideline. Please keep in mind that this list is not all-inclusive, since patient comorbidities vary, as do other variables unique to the patient's situation. OASIS items that may be used in determining the case-mix index are highlighted.

M0230/M0240/M0246—Diagnoses, Severity Index, and Payment Diagnoses
M0250—Therapy at home
M0350/M0360/M0370/M0380—Caregiver availability/ assistance (for dressing changes)
M0420—Pain
M0430—Intractable Pain
M0440—Wound/lesion
M0445/M0450/M0464—Pressure ulcer
M0450—Pressure ulcer status
M0468/M0470/M0474—Stasis Ulcer
M0476—Stasis Ulcer Status
M0482/M0484/M0486—Surgical Wound
M0488—Surgical Wound Status
M0520—Urinary incontinence
M0540—Bowel incontinence
M0650/M0660—Ability to dress upper/lower body
M0670/M0680/M0690—Bathing, toileting, transferring ability
M0700—Ambulation/locomotion
M0780—Management of oral medications
M0810/M0820—Equipment Management
M0826—Therapy Need

4. Associated Nursing Diagnoses (see Part Seven)

5. Supportive Factors for the Determination and Documentation of Homebound Status

Review the generic recommendations for documenting homebound status, and Medicare's definition of homebound in #5 of the template located at the beginning of this Part of this text. Other supportive factors for determining and documenting homebound status for patients with integumentary problems may include:

Taxing effort as evidenced by severe SOB (M0490), other (specify in functional terms)
Need for walker and/or assistance to ambulate (M0700)
Inability to negotiate stairs inside/outside of home
Restricted activity, legs elevated due to _____ (specify)
Large (specify site, etc.) open wound(s)
Open draining _____ lesions with pain (M0420) on any activity
No weight-bearing per physician's orders
Surgically restricted after abdominal surgery
Open infected wound with weakness
Continual oozing liquid drainage from wound site (specify)
Unsteady gait
Multiple functional limitations due to severe pain (symptoms, burns on thigh)
Foot wound with poor balance and painful ambulation
Patient not to bear weight on leg with open wound sites
Morbid obesity (specify height and weight)
Reverse isolation
Infected postoperative site (M0488) (specify), on infection precautions with intravenous antibiotics
Pain (M0420) at level ____ (specify) when _____ (specify activity)
Activity restricted due to _____ (specify)
Other reasons, including non-integumentary

6. Potential Interdisciplinary Goals and Outcomes

The template presented at the beginning of this Part lists patient-centered goals/outcomes that can be individualized according to the identified needs of the patient and family. The goals/outcomes listed below are specific examples related to integumentary system care, and each begins with the statement "By the end of the projected episode of care, the patient and/or family/caregiver will:"

_____ percent of tissue regeneration within _____ (specify weeks)
Optimal circulation and nutrition for patient to support healing
Implement measures to prevent wound deterioration
Demonstrate optimal nutrition/hydration needs maintained/addressed as evidenced by patient's weight maintained/decreased by/increased by _____ lbs
Demonstrate ability to change dressings and provide ordered wound care
Maintain infection control standards maintained as taught

7. Skills, Interventions/Services, and Management

The template presented at the beginning of this Part lists generic skills, interventions, and management of the different home care services that can be individualized according to the identified needs of the patient and family. Skills and interventions utilized by home care clinicians specific to integumentary system care include:

Assessment

Observe skin for any lesions (skin abnormalities) or wounds, especially over bony prominences and lower extremities; note rashes, bruises, burns, pustules, and broken skin integrity
Assess skin color, condition, texture, temperature, turgor, edema
If wounds, describe:

- Measurements: length, width, depth, tunneling, undermining

- Assess condition of wound bed using colors (red-pink-yellow-black) and tissue type (granulation, slough, necrotic tissue)
- Assess periwound area
- Assess drainage (color, consistency, amount, odor)

Assess for need of special support surfaces to enhance healing or prevent skin breakdown

Monitor patient for evidence of infection, metabolic problems, or other complications in patient on TPN

Evaluate healing process and progress toward outcome

Check _____ pulses for equality, strength, rate

Assess peripheral circulation

Administer Braden/other standardized tool/scale to identify/determine risk for skin breakdown

Medication/Therapeutic Regimens

Instruct on use of/care of special support surfaces (air mattress, Clinitron bed, etc.) _____ (specify)

Teach patient/caregiver effective hand-washing techniques and infection control techniques

Teach patient/caregiver ordered wound care and dressing change, including dressing disposal

Teach self-observational and record-keeping skills to patient and caregiver for documenting response to _____ therapy

Teach operation and troubleshooting of access device and pump (e.g., alarms, 800 numbers, who to call, etc.)

Provide wound care to site-specify supplies, frequency, and specific wound orders must include each step specifically and may include:

1. Cleanse with _____ (specify)
2. Apply _____ (specify) to wound bed
3. Apply _____ (specify) to periwound area
4. Dress wound with _____ (specify)
5. Secure wound with _____ (specify)

Teach patient correct application of compression stockings
Medicate patient with pain medication before dressing change
Teach signs/symptoms of infection

Safety

Teach about the need for safe, clean storage of supplies
Teach wound inspection, care, infection control, adhering to standard precautions, etc.
Teach patient/caregiver protocol for disposal of biohazardous waste (e.g., sharps, saturated dressings, etc.)
Initiate plan for high protein/vitamin/mineral diet and food choices available

Care Coordination/Case Management/ Discharge Planning

Assess need and initiate referral(s) for other agency/community services, including aide, PT/OT/SLP, social worker, pharmacist, wound specialist, but especially dietitian
Contact wound specialist for assessment of wound and recommend plan to discuss with physician for possible change in POC
Manage and identify risk factors to the healing or development of (further) pressure ulcers/other wounds (e.g., activity level, incontinence, diabetes history, immobility)

Physical Therapy

Assessment

Nutritional status
Wound characteristics (size, depth, drainage, color, pain, odor, location, healing phase)
Activities, positions, and postures that produce trauma or aggravate the wound
Circulatory and sensory status of wound site

Interventions/Teaching

Therapeutic exercises for maximum strengthening and endurance training for mobility and daily functioning

Instruct patient/caregiver in safety in balance, ambulation, and transfers

Instruct regarding wheelchair, prosthetic and/or other assistive devices for functional mobility such as ambulation, bed mobility, transfers, etc.

Teach pain management related to mobility, with use of modality agents as appropriate

Instruct in LE prosthetics and functional positioning for prevention of pressure ulcers

Educate patient/caregiver on each home program for all instructions provided

Provide strengthening exercises/home exercise program

Teach bed mobility and transfers

Other interventions

Occupational Therapy

Instruct in safety and use of adaptive techniques and assistive devices for maximum independence in ADL; coordinate w/nurse for bowel and bladder training program

Instruct in energy conservation

Assess and instruct in home modification as needed for maximum safety and independence

Instruct on use of splints, prosthetics, and/or other supports for functional positioning, to prevent pressure ulcers

Teach therapeutic exercise for maximum UE strength, ROM, and coordination as needed for ADL and functional mobility

Educate patient/caregiver(s) on home programs for all instructions provided

Other interventions

Medical Social Services

Evaluation of emotional and social factors affecting POC implementation

Evaluation/assessment as patient's problems adversely impact the POC and impede progress toward identified goals (e.g., cannot afford nutritional supplements, supplies; depressed and noncompliant)

Home assessment

Financial counseling

Identification and resolution of problems with treatment plan implementation

Other interventions

Dietary Counseling

Comprehensive nutritional assessment and plan

Nutritional evaluation of patient with wound and recommendations for achievement of optimal body weight and to promote wound healing

Other interventions

Other Considerations

Dietitian consult

Wound specialist consult

Other considerations, based on the patient's condition/unique needs

8. Tips to Support Medical Necessity, Quality, and Reimbursement (see Care of Older Adults Template at the beginning of this Part)

Document the specific wound(s): exact location, size (length, width, depth, tunneling, undermining), drainage (color, amount, consistency), wound bed (color, type of tissue), periwound area condition.

Document all steps of wound care provided, not just "wound care as ordered."

Document progress or deterioration in wound healing; take measurements at least once a week or per agency protocol.

If wound culture is obtained, document the results in the clinical record.

Specify and document the specific teaching accomplished, to whom it was directed, and the behavioral outcomes of that teaching.

Document the patient/caregiver's level of participation in care, if any.

Document your supplies needed on the POC and obtain the specific orders.

When appropriate, take photograph(s) to substantiate documentation at onset and every 3 weeks, have patients sign release; place one photograph in clinical records.

Document if patient or family member unable/unwilling to change dressing and reason (retinopathy, location of wound, family only able to provide evening care, severity of wound, etc.).

If you are providing daily care, seven days a week, there must be a realistic and projected endpoint (specific date) to the daily care.

Obtain prn visit orders (1 to 2) for wound care necessitating a home visit for assessment (e.g., excessive drainage requiring dressing change, pain, etc.). Similarly, for infusion patients also obtain 1 to 2 prn visits for problems necessitating a home visit to assess/identify/troubleshoot.

Wound care is an area in which some managed-care companies and other payers are attempting to reduce the number of visits. It is the clinician's responsibility to remember that effective wound care is not just the dressing change that is performed, but also includes: (1) observation and assessment of the wound; (2) teaching and training activities related to the wound and associated care; and (3) the actual hands-on care provided. Observation and assessment of the wound, in addition to a focus on the importance of infection control should occur at every visit, and the documentation should address the healing or deterioration of the wound. In your documentation, clearly stress these three skills that contribute to safe, effective wound care.

For wound care and all care regimens needing supplies or equipment, a physician's order must be obtained and filed in the clinical record. If the care specifies Opsite, 4 × 4s, Adaptic gauze, Kerlix, specific solutions or ointments, Montgomery straps, DuoDerm, or others, an order is needed for these supplies. These are only examples and the supplies vary as much as the patient's needs. Remember, all care provided is under the physician's POC, and, as such, all need orders.

Wound dressing or care orders should always include the specific treatment instructions, such as the use of aseptic or clean technique, the wound location, frequency of change, and any special supplies needed to safely and effectively follow the POC.

Daily Care

Remember that for Medicare patients, the term *"daily"* is defined as 7 days a week. If your patient needs daily or BID dressing changes, obtain an order from the physician with an estimate for the "finite and predictable endpoint." This needs to be a date, for example, 10/10/08, **NOT** "when the pressure ulcer heals." *If a patient needs daily care with no reasonable finite projected endpoint in sight, the services do not meet the intermittent definition and will not be covered by Medicare.* An example would be a patient who has had a wound for years and the physician agrees it may not ever heal. Daily, indefinite, long-term care is generally not covered by the Medicare home care program. If you have a question as to whether a patient meets the criteria, speak with your manager, who may ask your RHHI representative for guidance or input. In addition, remember that daily insulin injections (and only in those rare cases where the patient is unable or unwilling to self-inject) is the only exception to daily visits/care. Please review the *HHA Manual* or information from your manager or from the home health intermediary representative should further information be needed. The *HHA Manual* is located in Part Seven of this handbook for your review of Medicare coverage.

9. Evidence-Based and other Resources for Practice and Education

The Agency for Healthcare Research and Quality (AHRQ) (www.ahrq.gov or 1-800-358-9295) offers many resources, including "Clinical Practice Guideline Number 3: Preventing Pressure Ulcers: Patient Guide" and "Pressure Ulcers in Adults: Prediction and Prevention." Consumer versions of each are available in English and Spanish.

Baranoski, S., & Ayello, E. (2008). *Wound care essentials: Practice principles.* Philadelphia: Lippincott Williams & Wilkins.

Hess, C.T. (2004). *Clinical guide: Wound care (5th Ed.).* Philadelphia: Lippincott Williams & Wilkins.

The Mayo Clinic (www.mayoclinic.com) offers information on their website about the causes, risk factors, symptoms, complications, and more of pressure ulcers. There is also an "Anatomy of Your Skin" diagram showing the layers of your skin so you can see what effects a pressure ulcer has.

The National Pressure Ulcer Advisory Panel (NPUAP) (www.npuap.org or 1-202-521-6789) displays examples of extensive pressure ulcers. They offer a "Frequently Asked Questions" page, an archive of past newsletters, and a site where one can sign up for the newsletter.

The Paralyzed Veterans of America (PVA) at (www.pva.org or 1-800-424-8200) offers numerous publications, including "Pressure Ulcer Prevention and Treatment

Following Spinal Cord Injury" and "Pressure Ulcers: What You Should Know," available in both English and Spanish.

3

The Wound, Ostomy and Continence Nurses Society (www.wocn.org or 1-888-224-9626) offers educational resources and programs, including the "WOCN Guidance on OASIS Skin & Wound".

MUSCULOSKELETAL SYSTEM CARE

1. General Considerations

Musculoskeletal (MS) problems are commonly seen in home care. This MS System Care guideline addresses problems that most frequently necessitate home care and therapy services, and is directed toward optimizing function and comfort while minimizing disability. This section includes patients with amputations, fractures, arthritis, and joint replacements and those who have a history of falls, and/or osteoporosis. Because of functional and mobility considerations, multiple sclerosis is also included in this section.

Rheumatic diseases are the leading cause of disability among older adults. According to the National Institutes of Health Senior Health, more than 40 million people in the United States have some form of arthritis, and many have chronic pain that limits daily activity. Osteoarthritis (OA) is by far the most common form of arthritis, affecting more than 20 million people. Rheumatoid arthritis (RA) is the most disabling form of arthritis. More than 2 million people have this disease. Gout occurs in approximately 840 out of every 100,000 people.

The Centers for Disease Control and Prevention (CDC) report that more than 95 percent of hip fractures among adults ages 65 and older are caused by falls. These injuries can cause severe health problems and lead to reduced quality of life and premature death. In 2003, there were more than 309,500 hospital admissions for hip fractures. As many as 20 percent of hip fracture patients die within a year of their injury. Women sustain about 80 percent of all hip fractures. Knees, hips, and shoulders are the most common joint replacement surgeries, although elbows and ankles can be replaced as well.

For patients with a CVA, please refer to the Neurologic System Care guideline. For patients who require supportive care, readers are referred to the Hospice and Palliative Care guideline.

2. Potential Diagnoses and Codes

The diagnoses and codes listed here include some of the most common musculoskeletal conditions in home care, and have been alphabetized for easy identification. The ICD-9-CM system requires a focused review of the patient's medical information in addition to the physician-assigned diagnoses. For Medicare, it is not appropriate to use codes for acute fractures as primary diagnoses in home care. Should additional information be needed, refer to the coding books or a qualified coder.

Abnormality of gait	781.2
Aftercare following joint replacement	V54.81
Aftercare for healing pathologic fracture	V54.2X
Aftercare for healing traumatic fracture	V54.1X
Ankle fracture, left or right	824.8
Ankle, fracture, closed reduction with internal fixation (surgical)	79.16
Ankylosing spondylitis (AS)	720.0
Aphasia	784.3
Arthritis	716.9X
Arthritis, degenerative	715.9X
Arthritis, juvenile	714.3X
Arthritis, traumatic	716.1X
Arthritis, rheumatoid	714.0
Arthritis, spine	721.9X
Arthropathy, general	716.90
Arthropathy, pelvis	716.95
Aseptic necrosis, femur	733.42
Ataxia	781.3
Backache	724.5
Cerebral vascular accident (CVA)	434.91
Congenital hip deformity	755.63
Contracture, joint	718.4X
Debility	799.3
Deconditioning, muscle	728.9
Degenerative joint disease (DJD)	715.9X
Degenerative joint disease, hip, thigh	715.95
Degenerative joint disease, lower leg, knee	715.96
Difficulty walking	719.7X

Disc displacement	722.2
Dislocated hip	835.00
Dislocation, right or left hip prosthesis	996.4X
Disuse, atrophy, muscle	728.2
Dysarthria	784.5
Dysphagia	787.2
Fibromyalgia	729.1
Gait, abnormality of (unsteady)	781.2
Generalized weakness	780.79
Gout	274.9
Hemiplegia	342.90
Hemiplegia/hemiparesis	342.90
Hypercalcemia	275.42
Hypotension	458.9
Infected right or left AKA stump	997.62, V49.76
Infected right or left BKA stump	997.62, V94.75
Intervertebral disc disorders, unspecified	722.9
Joint contracture	718.40
Joint crepitus	719.60
Joint effusion	719.00
Juvenile arthritis	714.30
Knee, degenerative arthritis	715.96
Knee, internal derangement	717.9
Laminectomy syndrome	722.80
Long-term (current) antibiotic therapy	V58.62
Long-term (current) use of anticoagulants	V58.61
Lower limb amputation status	V49.7X
Lumbago	724.2
Lumbar stenosis	724.02
Lyme disease	088.81
Meniscus tear	836.2
Multiple sclerosis	340
Muscle atrophy (disuse)	728.2
Muscle spasm	728.85
Muscle spasm, back	724.8
Muscle weakness	728.9
Muscular dystrophy	359.1
Muscular scoliosis	737.39
Myasthenia gravis	358.0
Myositis	729.1

Continued

Neuropathy	355.9
Occupational therapy	V57.21
Osteoarthritis, acute exacerbation	715.90
Osteoarthritis, hip, thigh, pelvis	715.95
Osteoarthritis, leg, knee	715.96
Osteoarthritis, spine	721.90
Osteomyelitis	730.2X
Osteoporosis	733.00
Paget's disease	731.0
Pain, cervical	723.1
Pain, generalized	780.96
Pain, limb	729.5
Pain, low back (lumbar)	724.2
Pain, radicular	729.2
Pain, sacroiliac	724.6
Pain, sciatic	724.3
Pain, trigeminal	350.1
Paralysis	344.9
Paralysis agitans (Parkinson's)	332.0
Paraplegia	344.1
Parkinson's disease	332.0
Pathological fracture, unspecified	733.10
Pathological fracture, vertebrae	733.13
Pelvic fracture	808.8
Physical therapy	V57.1
Pulmonary embolism	415.19
Quadriplegia	344.00
Reflex sympathetic dystrophy, unspecified	337.20
Rheumatoid arthritis	714.0
Rheumatoid arthritis, spine	720.0
Rib(s), fracture	807.00
Rotator cuff, tear	840.4
Sciatica	724.3
Site of joint replaced	V43.60-V43.69
Spinal cord compression	336.9
Spinal stenosis	724.00
Sprain, lumbar, acute	847.2
Sprain, lumbosacral, acute	846.0
Sprain, sacral, acute	847.3
Sprain (strain)	848.8
Stenosis, spinal	724.00

Surgical dressing changes	V58.31
Suture removal	V58.32
Syncope	780.2
Tear, rotator cuff	840.4
Therapeutic drug monitoring	V58.83
Thrombophlebitis, deep vein, leg	451.19
Thrombosis	453.9
Thrombosis, deep vein, leg	453.8
Torn rotator cuff	840.4
TKR, failed	996.77
Walking, difficulty	719.70
Others	

3. OASIS Considerations

The following are some of the OASIS items (referred to as *M0*) that specifically target or affect the system addressed in this guideline. Please keep in mind that this list is not all-inclusive, since patient comorbidities vary, as do other variables unique to the patient's situation. OASIS items that may be used in determining the case-mix index are highlighted.

M0230/M0240/M0246—Diagnoses, Severity Index, and Payment Diagnoses
M0420—Pain
M0430—Intractable Pain
M0482/M0484/M0486—Surgical Wound
M0488—Surgical Wound Status
M0520/M0530—Urinary incontinence
M0540—Bowel incontinence
M0650/M0660—Ability to dress upper/lower body
M0670/M0680/M0690—Bathing, toileting, transferring ability
M0700—Ambulation/locomotion

M0780—Management of oral medications
M0826—Therapy Need

4. Associated Nursing Diagnoses (see Part Seven)

5. Supportive Factors for the Determination and Documentation of Homebound Status

Review the generic recommendations for documenting homebound status, and Medicare's definition of homebound in #5 of the template located at the beginning of this Part of this text. Other supportive factors for determining and documenting homebound status for patients with musculoskeletal problems may include:

Post-surgery, on activity restrictions
Need for walker and/or assistance to ambulate (M0700)
Inability to negotiate stairs inside/outside of home
Pain (M0420/M0430) at level ____ (specify) when _____ (specify activity)
Patient is chair-bound (M0700) and needs assistance with activities due to an exacerbation of _______ (specify)
Patient is a new AKA due to diabetes or _____ (specify), and cannot bear weight, wound site not healing
Chair-bound due to recent exacerbation of joint disease symptoms (e.g., pain, swelling)
Patient's home is on third floor with no elevator, unable to use/negotiate stairs
Post-amputation after motorcycle accident; residual site to be wrapped and leg elevated
Paralysis, endurance, and poor ambulation postoperatively
No weight bearing, s/p revision surgery due to _____ (specify)
S/P femoral fracture with no bending, no reaching, no stairs
Patient cannot stand or bear weight per protocol

Knee safety precautions with no weight bearing for _____ (specify)
Unsteady gait, increased risk for falls after hip replacement
Decreased ROM and strength after surgery for joint replacement
Other reasons, including non-musculoskeletal

6. Potential Interdisciplinary Goals and Outcomes

The template presented at the beginning of this Part lists patient-centered goals/outcomes that can be individualized according to the identified needs of the patient and family. The goals/outcomes listed below are specific examples related to musculoskeletal system care, and each begins with the statement "By the end of the projected episode of care, the patient and/or family/caregiver will:"

Demonstrate decreased spasticity/normalized muscle tone with increased coordination
Demonstrate decreased risk for falls through balance/strengthening fall prevention program
Verbalize how to protect the residual limb from further injury to avoid higher-level amputation
Demonstrate return to stable MS status as with decreased or controlled symptoms, etc.
List self-care behaviors that support optimal health maintenance with MS (e.g., avoiding fatigue, extreme weather, exposure to illness/infection)
Demonstrate optimal nutrition/hydration in patient prone to constipation
Demonstrate hip, knee, or other precautions
Achieve an increased level of function and safety
Demonstrates ability to perform home exercise program (HEP) safely

Demonstrate incision-site care
Demonstrate independence in bed mobility and ability to self-position for comfort and safety
Verbalize signs/symptoms of infection (wounds)
Verbalize potential complications related to decreased mobility/immobility
Achieve maximum functional restoration of limb lost due to _____ (specify)
Demonstrate improved ROM from _____ percent to _____ percent (specify)
Demonstrate improved ambulation/locomotion as demonstrated by _____
Demonstrate stabilization in transferring
Demonstrate conditioning, strengthening, and functional, comfortable use of prosthesis
Demonstrate increased endurance, comfort, balance
Demonstrate increased functional use of affected limb
Other goals/outcomes as appropriate for patient

7. Skills, Interventions/Services, and Management

The template presented at the beginning of this Part lists generic skills, interventions, and management of the different home care services that can be individualized according to the identified needs of the patient and family. Skills and interventions utilized by home care clinicians specific to musculoskeletal system care include:

Assessment

Observe skeletal structure, body alignment, and musculature; note obvious abnormalities such as amputations or joint deformities/deviations
Ask patient to move muscles and joints assessing range of motion and strength:

- Facial muscles: raise eyebrows, puff cheeks, smile, show teeth

- Torso: shrug shoulders, bend over and take off shoes/socks
- Extremities: raise hands above head, squeeze hands, raise legs, flex and dorsiflex foot

Palpate painful joints while patient puts joint through range of motion, listen and feel for crepitus

Observe patient get out of chair, walk 10 feet, turn around and sit down

Ask patient to "walk through" ADLs

- Does the patient have the manual dexterity and range of motion to perform grooming and dressing?
- How does the patient bathe and toilet? Ask patient to demonstrate getting in and out of tub/shower and on/off toilet

Observe for and note any assistive devices the patient uses during ambulation or ADLs

Assess for need of special adaptive equipment (e.g., trapeze, grab bars, elevated toilet seat, etc.)

Assess muscle weakness and swallowing problems in patients with myasthenia gravis

Assess/evaluate patient for specialized support surfaces to avoid pressure ulcers

Assess ____ wound site (specify)

Medication/Therapeutic Regimens

Teach family and caregiver proper, safe body alignment and positions, including hip safety precautions

Teach patient/caregiver ordered wound care, what to observe and report (increased pain, swelling, tenderness, drainage, and other signs of infection) and who to notify

Teach/initiate home safety program/fall protocol

Teach patient/caregiver about anticoagulation therapy, including schedule, need for blood tests, side effects to observe for, interactions with foods/medications, and missed dose management

Teach safety/bleeding precautions of patient on anticoagulant therapy

Teach patient about and observe for adverse side effects of nonsteroidal anti-inflammatory drugs (NSAIDs)
Provide wound care
Comfort measures of patient's choice provided to patient who is essentially bed-bound/chair-bound and alert, including back rub, hand massage, music of choice, and supportive interventions
Teach regarding anticoagulant medication interactions with foods

Safety

Provide safety management related to transfers and mobility and function after amputation
Initiate fall protocol in patient with history of falls
Emergency response system

Physical Therapy

Assessment

Prior level of function
Specific strength (on 0–5 scale) and ROM (in degrees of movement) deficits
Functional impact of deficits
Standardized functional tests for assessment of gait (e.g., Tinetti, Dynamic Gait Index, Timed Get Up and Go)

Interventions/Teaching

Strengthening exercises/home exercise program
Assessment of wheelchair and seating
Assessment of upper body strength for trapeze or other methods to maintain function/bed mobility
Progressive ambulation
Establish and/or revise home exercise program
Provide heat or cold therapy as specified per orders

Teach CPM immobilizer use
Teach safe use of crutches or other ambulatory devices
Endurance training/conditioning
Instruct/supervise caregiver in safe methods to assist patient
Therapeutic exercises
Bed mobility exercises
Balance, gait, and transfer training
Stair climbing
Pain management
Instruct patient/caregiver in home safety, potential complications, precautions, edema
Initiate prosthetic training in collaboration with prosthetic supplier
Teach home exercise program with progressive ambulation to walker
Teach patient/caregiver safe ambulation, transfer, and site care
Other interventions

Speech-Language Pathology

Evaluation of swallow and speech skills
Educate patient/caregiver on safety precautions and prevention of swallowing dysfunction, including food textures and body positioning to reduce risk of aspiration
Collaborate with dietitian for optimal nutrition
Teach exercises for maximum articulation proficiency for verbal/vocal expression and/or for lip, tongue, and facial control for optimum swallowing skills
Teach alternative and effective communication program to enable expression of needs
Educate patient/caregiver for all instructions provided
Initiate dysphagia and speech program

Word fluency exercises
Other interventions

Occupational Therapy

Instruct in safety and use of adaptive techniques and assistive devices for maximum independence in ADL, stump wrapping, and doffing/donning of prosthesis
Instruct in energy conservation and work simplification for maximum functional activity level and pain prevention
Assess and instruct in home modification as needed for maximum safety and independence
Instruct on use of splints, prosthetics, and/or other support devices for functional positioning, joint protection, and precautions for preventing skin breakdown
Teach therapeutic exercise for maximum UE strength, ROM and coordination, with minimal inflammation, for ADL and functional mobility
Assess and address the need to improve body image and other psychological effects of the disease process
Educate patient/caregiver(s) on home programs for all instructions provided
Residual site wrapping/shrinkage
Teach preprosthetic training and exercise program
Assess for adaptive equipment for independent ADLs
Other interventions

Dietary Counseling

Nutritional evaluation of patient for achievement of optimal nutrition and hydration to facilitate healing
Comprehensive nutritional assessment and plan
Nutritional assessment of patient with MS on high protein with increased roughage diet for constipation management
Other interventions

Other Considerations

Joint (other, specify) rehabilitation program (per physician order)
Other interventions, care management, etc. based on patient's unique condition and needs

8. Tips to Support Medical Necessity, Quality, and Reimbursement (see Care of Older Adults Template at the beginning of this Part)

Keep in mind that some of these patients may have Medicare as their secondary payer (MSP) or insurer because the musculoskeletal problem may have occurred from trauma or a fall. For example, if your patient fell at a grocery store, it may be an attorney to whom the bills are directed, not Medicare. If the patient is known to have had trauma, check with your manager so that billing gets directed from the beginning of the POC to the correct payer.

9. Evidence-Based and other Resources for Practice and Education

The American Academy of Neurology (www.neurolog.org or 1-800-879-1960) offers practice parameter and evidence-based review of assessing patients for risk of falls.
The American Academy of Orthopedic Surgeons (www.aaos.org) offers an Orthopedic Connection page specifically for patients (www.orthoinfo.org) with information about patient-centered care for arthritis, osteoporosis, and joint replacement, including the articles "Activities After a Hip Replacement" and "Keep Moving for Life."
The American Geriatrics Society (www.americangeriatrics.org or 1-212-308-1414) offers information and a clinical practice guideline on the prevention of falls in older persons.

The Amputee Coalition of America (ACA) (www.amputee-coalition.org or 1-888-267-5669) offers information about prosthetics, rehabilitation, and peer support group, as well as a Spanish section with information about the ACA and its programs and many of the organizations most popular and informative articles all translated. The ACA also publishes *In Motion*, a bimonthly publication with news, resources, and support for those with amputated limbs.

The Arthritis Foundation (www.arthritis.org or 1-800-568-4045 or 1-404-872-7100) has free brochures available, including "Meet Your Arthritis Health Care Team." They also publish the *Arthritis Today* magazine which you can subscribe to through their website.

The Myasthenia Gravis Foundation (www.myasthenia.org or 1-800-541-5454) supplies information and offers patient support groups.

The National Institute of Arthritis and Musculoskeletal and Skin Diseases Information Clearinghouse (www.niams.nih.gov or 1-877-22-NIAMS [1-800-22-64267]) offers numerous Q&A publications and other resources, including "Questions and Answers About Arthritis and Rheumatic Diseases."

The National Institutes of Health Osteoporosis and Related Bone Diseases National Resource Center (www.niams.nih.gov/Health_Info/Bone/ or 1-800-624-BONE [800-624-2663]) offers information on health topics including "Bone Health (General)," "Paget's Disease," and more.

The National Multiple Sclerosis Society (www.nationalmssociety.org or 1-800-FIGHT-MS [800-344-4867]) offers clinical bulletins on topics such as "Aging with MS," "Overview of Multiple Sclerosis," and "Swallowing Disorders and Their Management," as well as brochures, including "Managing Specific Issues," "Staying Well," and "Newly Diagnosed."

The National Osteoporosis Foundation (www.nof.org or 1-202-223-2226) offers patient information, including "Fall Prevention" and "Medications and Osteoporosis," as well as fact sheets like "Bone Density" and "Bone Basics." They also offer professional resources, clinical guideline information, and more.

The Parkinson's Disease Foundation (www.pdf.org or 1-800-457-6676) supplies information and offers patient support groups.

NEUROLOGIC SYSTEM CARE

1. General Considerations

This care guideline incorporates primarily neurologic conditions and addresses amyotropic lateral sclerosis (ALS), brain tumors, cerebral vascular accidents (CVAs), Parkinson's and trauma resulting in neurologic impairment/ pathology. According to the National Institutes of Health, more than 700,000 people in the United States have strokes for the first time each year. Nearly three-quarters of all strokes occur in people over the age of 65, and the risk of having a stroke more than doubles each decade after the age of 55. The National Institute of Neurological Disorders and Stroke reports that stroke is the third leading cause of death in the country. And stroke causes more serious long-term disabilities than any other disease. Though men have a higher risk of stroke (by about 1.25 times), women are more likely to die from a stroke.

According to the National Institute on Aging Alzheimer's Disease (AD) is the most common dementia in older adults, and affects an estimated 4.5 million Americans. AD usually begins after age sixty and risk increases with age. About 5 percent of men and women ages 65 to 74 have AD, and nearly half of those age 85 and older may have the disease. More than 100,000 people a year die from AD. The major difference between AD and other dementias is that AD is progressive. Brain tumors are abnormal growths of primary, metastatic, or developmental origin where the clinical manifestations are determined by the area of the brain involved and the extent of the disease.

The emphasis in home care for all of these patients is directed toward safety and optimal function. Trauma and head injury are a growing part of home care practice where efforts are directed toward rehabilitation and optimal function. Some patients with end-stage neurologic disease need skilled, compassionate hospice or palliative care through death, with support also provided to their family/caregivers—readers are referred to the Hospice and Palliative Care guideline for further information.

2. Potential Diagnosis and Codes

The diagnoses and codes listed here include some of the most common neurologic conditions in home care, and have been alphabetized for easy identification. The ICD-9-CM system requires a focused review of the patient's medical information in addition to the physician-assigned diagnoses. For Medicare, it is not appropriate to use acute cerebrovascular accident (CVA) as the primary diagnosis in home care. Should additional information be needed, refer to the coding books or a qualified coder.

Diagnosis	Code
Abnormal gait	781.2
Acoustic neuroma	225.1
Aftercare following pathologic fracture	V54.2X
Aftercare following traumatic fracture	V54.1X
AIDS	042
AIDS, with dementia	042 and 294.10
Alzheimer's disease (AD)	331.0
Alzheimer's disease, with dementia	331.0, 294.10
Amyotropic lateral sclerosis (ALS, Lou Gehrig's disease)	335.20
Aphasia	784.3
Arthritis, traumatic	716.1X
Attention to indwelling urinary catheter	V53.6
Bladder incontinence	788.30
Cancer of the brain, primary	191.9
Cancer of the brain, secondary	198.3
Carotid artery occlusion	433.10
Cerebrovascular disease (CVD), with late effect, aphasia	438.11
Cerebrovascular disease (CVD), with late effect, dysphagia	438.82 and 787.20

Continued

Cerebrovascular disease (CVD), with late effect, hemiplegia	438.20
Cerebrovascular disease (CVD), with late effect, unspecified	438.9
Combined therapies	V57.89
Contusions, multiple	924.8
Creutzfeldt-Jakob disease and dementia	046.1 and 294.10
Dementia, Alzheimer's	331.0 and 294.10
Diabetes mellitus with neurological manifestations	250.60
Disc displacement	722.2
Dysarthria	784.5
Dysphagia	787.20
Encephalopathy, unspecified	348.3
Falls, history of	V15.88
Gait abnormality	781.2
Glioma, unspecified site	191.9
Head injury	959.01
Hemiplegia or hemiparesis	342.90
History of falls	V15.88
Huntington's chorea	333.4
Incontinence of feces	787.6
Incontinence of urine	788.30
Intractable spasticity	781.0
Joint contracture	718.4X
Korsakoff's disease	294.0
Lou Gehrig's disease (ALS)	335.20
Meniere's disease	386.00
Meningitis, unspecified	322.9
Metastases (general)	199.1
Metastatic brain tumor	198.3
Multiple sclerosis	340
Muscle disuse/atrophy	728.2
Muscular dystrophy	359.1
Nonpsychotic brain syndrome	310.9
Occupational therapy	V57.21
Organic brain syndrome (OBS)	310.9
Paralysis	344.9
Paralysis agitans (Parkinson's disease)	332.0
Paraplegia	344.1
Parkinson's disease	332.0
Physical therapy	V57.1

Pneumonia	486
Pneumonia, aspiration	507.0
Presenile dementia	290.10
Pressure (decubitus) ulcer	707.0X
Quadriplegia, unspecified	344.00
Reflex sympathetic dystrophy	337.20
Respiratory failure	518.81
Sciatica	724.3
Seizure disorder	780.39
Senile dementia	290.0
Spasticity, intractable	781.0
Speech therapy	V57.3
Spinal cord compression	336.9
Spinal cord disease	336.9
Spinal cord disease, congenital	742.9
Spinal cord injury, traumatic, unspecified	952.9
Spinal cord tumor	239.7
Spinal stenosis	724.00
Subdural hematoma	852.20
Subdural hematoma, nontraumatic	432.1
Subdural hematoma, traumatic	852.20
TIA/Transient ischemic attacks	435.9
Unipolar affective disorder	296.99
Urinary incontinence	788.30
Urinary retention	788.20
Urinary tract infection	599.0
Vertigo	780.4
Others	

3. OASIS Considerations

The following are some of the OASIS items (referred to as *M0*) that specifically target or affect the system addressed in this guideline. Please keep in mind that this list is not all-inclusive, since patient comorbidities vary, as do other variables unique to the patient's situation. OASIS items that may be used in determining the case-mix index are highlighted.

M0230/M0240/M0246—Diagnoses, Severity Index, and Payment Diagnoses

3

M0250—Therapy at home
M0350/M0360/M0370/M0380—Caregiver availability/ assistance
M0420—Pain
M0430—Intractable Pain
M0520/M0530—Urinary incontinence/Catheter
M0540—Bowel incontinence
M0560/M0570/M0580/M0590/M0610/M0620/M0630—Cognitive/emotional functioning
M0650/M0660—Ability to dress upper/lower body
M0670/M0680/M0690—Bathing, toileting, transferring ability
M0700—Ambulation/locomotion
M0780—Management of oral medications
M0810/M0820—Equipment management
M082—Therapy Need

4. Associated Nursing Diagnoses (see Part Seven)

5. Supportive Factors for the Determination and Documentation of Homebound Status

Review the generic recommendations for documenting homebound status, and Medicare's definition of homebound in #5 of the template located at the beginning of this Part of this text. Other supportive factors for determining and documenting homebound status for patients with neurologic problems may include:

Ventilator-dependent
Needs assistance for any activity
Bedbound with ALS except up with maximum assistance
Unsafe, unsteady gait with maximum assistance
S/P brain surgery—too weak to leave home without maximum assistance
Diagnosis of malignant lesion and too weak to safely leave home alone

On large doses of steroids, meningitis postop—not safe to leave home
Limited mobility due to headache pain and unsafe ataxic gait
Pain, weakness
Medically restricted because of risk of infection postoperatively
Diagnosis of dementia, cannot leave home unattended
Unsafe for patient without supervision
Confusion level precludes safe leaving of home without supervision
Needs 24-hour supervision due to mental status or confusion
Other medical problems (specify) making patient homebound
Impaired neurologic status, cannot ambulate
Paralysis left side S/P CVA
Unsteady ambulation
Frail, needs assistance to ambulate
Bedridden with severe SOB
Cannot safely leave home without assistance
S/P CVA, has significant sided weakness
Lesion causing mental status changes, homebound for safety reasons
Comatose, S/P trauma
Aphasia and lethargy due to progression of tumor malignancy
Residual weakness S/P CVA, AMI
Feeding tube and Foley catheter—primarily bed-bound/chair-bound
Right or left hemiplegia or hemiparesis
Requires maximum assistance to ambulate (M0700)
Quadriplegia
Pressure ulcer right buttock, feeding tube, needs total care

6. Potential Interdisciplinary Goals and Outcomes

The template presented at the beginning of this Part lists patient-centered goals/outcomes that can be individualized according to the identified needs of the patient and family. The goals/outcomes listed below are specific examples related to neurologic system care, and each begins with the statement "By the end of the projected episode of care, the patient and/or family/ caregiver will:"

Demonstrate safe, consistent, and nurturing physical environment
Demonstrate ability to communicate effectively through speech or some alternative form of communication
Actively participate in decisions about care and daily activities
Demonstrate proper positioning and care for bedbound patient
Demonstrate seizure care regimen and other care for optimal control
Demonstrate safe, effective use of energy conservation techniques for maximum functional activity level
Demonstrate home exercise program for neuromuscular re-education
Demonstrate proper use of splints and/or other positioning devices
Achieve maximum independence in home program for cognitive and/or perceptual motor retraining
Report optimal function s/p CVA
Demonstrate seizure control, symptomatic relief, and pain management in patient with brain tumor
Other goals/outcomes as appropriate for patient

7. Skills, Interventions/Services, and Management

The template presented at the beginning of this Part lists generic skills, interventions, and management of the different home care services that can be individualized according to the identified needs of the patient and family. Skills and interventions utilized by home care clinicians specific to neurologic system care include:

Assessment

Assess patient's level of consciousness, orientation, memory

Assess ability to see near (if literate, ask patient to read medication labels) and far (including seeing well enough to walk safely)

Assess ability to hear and understand; to speak and be understood

Assess pupils equal and reactive to light (PERLA)

Perform simple cranial nerve assessment:

- Ask patient to look up, down, side to side, and diagonally up and down
- Ask patient to raise eyebrows, squeeze eyes shut, puff cheeks, smile, show teeth

Assess ability to move muscle groups:

- Raise arms above head, squeeze your hands
- Raise legs, flex and dorsiflex foot

Observe patient get out of chair, walk 10 feet, turn around and sit down; note gait, balance and coordination

If pain, perform complete pain assessment for each pain site:

- Location
- Quality
- Intensity (1–10 scale)
- Timing: onset, frequency, duration
- What makes it better or worse?
- Effect of pain medication

Assess skin at risk for pressure ulcer (chair-bound/bedbound, limited activity, limited mobility, incontinence, etc.)

Offer spiritual counseling/support to patient/caregiver verbalizing concern over the reason or meaning of suffering

Support patient/caregiver through radiation/chemotherapy/ modalities for tumor reduction

Assist patient/family through grieving process

Medication/Therapeutic Regimens

Teach proper, safe body alignment and positions

Teach regarding skin care needs, including the need for frequent position changes, pressure pads and mattresses available, and the importance of prevention in skin breakdown

Assess/teach symptoms/interventions if patient has autonomic dysreflexia

Teach patient/caregiver ordered wound care; what to observe for (increased pain, swelling, tenderness, drainage, and other signs of infection), and when/who to report

Teaching and training of family caregivers related to skin care, positioning, and feeding regimens and/or feeding pumps

Teach caregiver to observe for increased secretions and teach safe suctioning when needed

Teach patient radiation therapy regimen, schedule, and which effects to monitor

Teach patient/caregiver regarding steroid therapy and side effects

Teach caregiver daily care of catheter (e.g., indwelling, suprapubic, etc.)

Teach family care of the immobilized or bedridden patient

Teach/initiate home safety program/fall protocol

Care and management of the patient with gastrostomy, jejunostomy, percutaneous endoscopic gastrotomy (PEG), or other (specify) feeding tube

Teach patient/caregiver administration of _____ and safe disposal of sharps

Instruct the patient about the need to have prescriptions filled before the last dose(s) of medications

Provide wound care as ordered
Comfort measures of patient's choice provided to patient who is essentially bed-bound/chair-bound and alert, including back rub, hand massage, music of choice, and supportive interventions

Nutrition/Hydration/Elimination
Monitor patient who has nutritional supplements and water via feeding tube daily
Maintain nutrition/hydration by offering patient high-protein diet and foods of choice as tolerated

Physical Therapy
Assessment
Movement and postural control
Prior level of function
Level of cognitive impairment/functioning
Sensory/perceptual integrity

Interventions/Teaching
Teach therapeutic exercises for muscle re-education to increase strength and ROM for mobility, e.g. ambulation, transfers and bed mobility, and for prevention of joint contractures
Instruct patient/caregiver in safety with balance, ambulation, and transfers
Instruct regarding walker, wheelchair and/or other assistive devices for functional mobility (e.g., ambulation, bed mobility, and/or transfers)
Assess and instruct in home modification for safety and independence in mobility
Provide use of physical agents/modalities to facilitate muscle retraining
Instruct in LE positioning for prevention of pressure ulcers
Educate patient/caregiver on each home program for all instructions provided
Other interventions

Speech-Language Pathology

Evaluation of swallow, speech, and cognitive function, with ongoing re-assessment

Educate patient/caregiver on safety precautions and prevention of swallowing dysfunction, including food textures and body positioning to reduce risk of aspiration

Collaborate with nutritionist/dietitian for optimal nutrition

Teach program for articulation proficiency for verbal skills, both expressive and receptive (dysphasia)

Teach program for lip, tongue, and facial control for optimum swallowing skills (dysphagia)

Assess and establish program for memory and other cognitive functions as needed; coordinate with OT

Teach alternative and effective communication program to enable expression of needs

Educate patient/caregiver on each home program for all instructions provided

Other interventions

Occupational Therapy

Instruct in safety and use of adaptive techniques and assistive devices for maximum independence in ADL, including hygiene

Instruct in energy conservation for maximum functional activity level

Assess and establish cognitive retraining program and compensatory system, coordinate with SLP

Assess and instruct in home modification as needed for maximum safety and independence

Instruct on use of splints and/or other support devices for functional positioning, reduction and/or prevention of contractures, including precautions for preventing skin breakdown

Teach therapeutic exercise for maximum UE strength, ROM and coordination
Assess and address the needs to improve body image and other psychological effects of the disease process
Educate patient/caregiver(s) on home programs for all instructions provided
Others interventions

Medical Social Services
Evaluate patient adjustment to health problems
Assess emotional/financial factors impacting POC implementation
Provide financial counseling related to loss of job because of illness and spouse being full-time primary caretaker
Identify community supports/services
Assess social and emotional factors
Provide counseling
Provide community resource referral(s)
Evaluate home, family/caregiver ability and availability
Evaluate patient for nursing home placement
Other interventions

Dietary Counseling
Nutritional evaluation of patient with neurological disease for achievement of optimal nutrition/hydration
Comprehensive nutritional assessment and plan
Assessment of diet history, calculation of nutrient intake
Other interventions

Other Considerations
Stroke (other, specify) rehabilitation program (per physician order)
Other interventions, care management, etc. based on patient's unique condition and needs

8. Tips to Support Medical Necessity, Quality, and Reimbursement (see Care of Older Adults Template at the beginning of this Part)

9. Evidence-Based and other Resources for Practice and Education

The Alzheimer's Association (www.alz.org or their 24/7 helpline 1-800-272-3900) offers brochures and other resources for professionals and families, including information on getting the right diagnosis.

The American Stroke Association (www.strokeassociation.org or 1888-4-STROKE [1-888-478-7653]) offers a free subscription to *Stroke CONNECTION Magazine* and other resources for patients and professionals related to strokes.

The Amyotrophic Lateral Sclerosis Association (ALSA) (www.alsa.org or 1-818-880-9007) offers information on the symptoms, forms, genetics, and other facts about ALS, also called Lou Gehrig's Disease. Information is also available specifically for the patient, family, and caregiver including pages on "Facts About Family Caregivers" and "Caregiving Tips and Hints" for caring for an ALS patient.

Mace, N.L., & Rabins, P.V. *The 36-Hour Day: A Family Guide to Caring for Persons with Alzheimer's Disease, Related Dementing Illnesses, and Memory Loss in Later Life*. Baltimore: Johns Hopkins Press (www.press.jhu.edu or 1-800-537-5487). This is a practical book providing a day-by-day look at the difficulties of caring for loved ones with Alzheimer's disease and other dementia illnesses.

McLay, E., & Young, E. P. (2007). *Mom's OK, She Just Forgets: The Alzheimer's Journey from Denial to Acceptance, A Handbook for Families*. Amherst: Prometheus Books.

The National Institute of Health National Institute on Aging's (NIA) Alzheimer's Disease Education and Referral (ADEAR) Center (www.nia.nih.gov/Alzheimers or 1-800-438-4380) has information and booklets available to professionals as well as patients and families including an Alzheimer's Disease fact sheet which can be accessed from their website. Through ADEAR, two booklets from Duke University's Family Support Program for caregivers and families outlining the struggles and solutions when dealing with anger in dementia patients are available. "Hit Pause—Helping Dementia Families Deal With Anger," which is $3.00, and "Wait A Minute," for $2.00, are both available at the ADEAR website. NIA's ADEAR also offers the *Connections* newsletter which provides information about Alzheimer's disease and about caregiving, both professionally and at home or with family.

The National Institute of Neurological Disorders and Stroke (www.ninds.nih.gov 1-301-496-5751 or 1-800-352-9424) offers information pages on stroke treatment, prognosis, research, and more including "Stroke Rehabilitation Information" and "What You Need to Know About Stroke."

ONCOLOGIC/HEMATOLOGIC SYSTEM CARE

1. General Considerations

This Oncologic/Hematologic System Care guideline encompasses numerous kinds of cancers, including solid tumors and malignant blood dyscrasias. Health problems related to cancers, such as pathologic fractures, treatment modalities, and symptom management, are also addressed in this guideline.

Cancer is the second leading cause of death in the United States. According to the National Cancer Institute, millions of Americans are living with a diagnosis of cancer. Breast cancer is the most common non-skin cancer and the second leading cause of cancer-related death in women. It is estimated that 12.7 percent of women will be diagnosed with breast cancer sometime in their lives. Risk increases with age and it is estimated that each year there are about 213,000 new cases in women and 1,800 new cases in men.

Most cancers occur in people over the age of 65. Death rates for the four most common cancers (breast, prostate, lung, and colorectal), as well as for all cancers combined, continue to decline as survival rates rise. The National Brain Tumor Association estimates that more than 190,000 people in the United States will be diagnosed with a brain tumor each year. Of those, about 43,000 are primary brain tumors and about 150,000 are metastasis brain tumors.

Because many cancers are now considered chronic diseases, the home care clinician's role varies and includes impeccable assessment skills, expertise in technical, hand-on care, and ongoing case management and care coordination to optimize patient comfort. Home care efforts are directed toward support of the patient through surgery, chemotherapy, radiation, and other treatment modalities. Management of the disease and its symptoms, self-care knowledge and reporting, and cure or the arresting of the disease, when possible, is the goal.

Not all cancers are curable—patients sometimes present with a recurrence after years of remission. Many of these patients and their families choose hospice for their end-of-life care. For patients with life-limiting cancers who require supportive care, readers are also referred to the Hospice and Palliative Care guideline for information on the provision and care planning for these patients and their families.

2. Potential Diagnoses and Codes

The diagnoses and codes listed here include some of the most common oncologic/hematologic conditions in home care, and have been alphabetized for easy identification. The ICD-9-CM system requires a focused review of the patient's medical information in addition to the physician-assigned diagnoses. Should additional information be needed, refer to the coding books or a qualified coder.

Diagnosis	Code
Acoustic neuroma	225.1
Acquired immunodeficiency syndrome (AIDS)	042
Adenocarcinoma, lung	162.9
Adenocarcinoma, metastatic	199.1
Adrenal cancer	194.0
Aftercare following surgery for neoplasm	V58.42
Airway obstruction, chronic	496
Anemia	285.9
Aplastic anemia	284.9
Ascites, malignant	197.6
Astrocytoma, unspecified site	191.9
Attention to colostomy	V55.3
Attention to ileostomy	V55.2
Attention to nephrostomy	V55.6
Attention to tracheostomy	V55.0
Bladder cancer	188.9
Bladder metastases	198.1
Bone metastasis	198.5
Bowel obstruction	560.9
Brain cancer, primary	191.9

Continued

Brain cancer, secondary	198.3
Brain, tumor, recurrent	239.6
Breast, cancer	174.9
Cachexia	799.4
Cancer, brain, primary	191.9
Cancer, brain, secondary	198.3
Cancer, breast	174.9
Cancer pain	338.3
Cervix, cancer	180.9
Colon cancer	153.9
Colon lymphoma	202.83
Dehydration	276.51
Depression, reactive (situational)	300.4
Dysphagia	787.2
Electrolyte and fluid imbalance	276.9
Endometrial cancer	182.0
Esophagus, cancer of the	150.9
Ewing's sarcoma	170.9
Fracture, pathological, unspecified	733.10
Fracture, pathological, vertebrae	733.13
Gastric cancer, metastatic	197.8
Glioma, unspecified site	191.9
Head or neck, cancer of the	195.0
Hickman venous catheter, insertion (surgical)	38.93
Hodgkin's disease	201.90
Intestinal obstruction	560.9
Kaposi's sarcoma	176.9
Kidney (renal) cancer	189.0
Larynx, cancer of the	161.9
Leukemia, acute	208.00
Leukopenia	288.0
Liver cancer	155.2
Liver, metastatic cancer of	197.7
Lung, adenocarcinoma	162.9
Lung cancer, squamous cell	162.9
Lymphedema (postmastectomy)	457.0
Lymphoma (non-Hodgkin's)	202.80
Malaise and fatigue	780.79
Malignant neoplasm of the breast	174.9
Melanoma, malignant	172.9

Metastasis, general	199.1
Metastatic brain tumor	198.3
Metastatic lung cancer	197.0
Metastatic pleural cancer	197.2
Multiple myeloma	203.00
Nasopharyngeal cancer	147.9
Nausea with vomiting	787.01
Neuroblastoma, unspecified site	194.0
Neutropenia	288.0
Obstruction, intestinal	560.9
Oropharyngeal cancer	146.9
Osteosarcoma	170.9
Ovarian cancer	183.0
Pancreatic cancer	157.9
Pathological fracture, unspecified site	733.10
Pathological fracture, vertebra	733.13
Pharynx cancer	149.0
Prostate cancer	185
Radiation enteritis	558.1
Radiation myelitis	323.8 and 990
Rectosigmoid cancer	154.0
Rectum, cancer of the	154.1
Renal cancer (kidney)	189.0
Renal cell cancer, metastatic	198.0
Sarcoma, unspecified site	171.9
Secondary malignant neoplasm, breast	198.81
Seizures	780.39
Septicemia	038.9
Skin carcinoma	173.9
Spinal cord compression	336.9
Spinal cord tumor	239.7
Stomach, cancer of the	151.9
Testis, cancer of the	186.9
Tongue, cancer of the	141.9
Trachea, cancer of the	162.0
Uterine sarcoma, metastatic	198.82
Uterus, cancer of the	179
Vulvar cancer	184.4
Others	

3

3

3. OASIS Considerations

The following are some of the OASIS items (referred to as *M0*) that specifically target or affect the system addressed in this guideline. Please keep in mind that this list is not all-inclusive, since patient comorbidities vary, as do other variables unique to the patient's situation. OASIS items that may be used in determining the case-mix index are highlighted.

M0230/M0240/M0246—Diagnoses, Severity Index, and Payment Diagnoses
M0250—Therapies
M0270—Rehabilitative prognosis
M0280—Life expectancy
M0350/M0360/M0370/M0380—Caregiver availability/assistance
M0420—Pain
M0430—Intractable pain
M0490—Dyspnea
M0500—Respiratory treatments
M0650/M0660—Ability to dress upper/lower body
M0670/M0680/M0690—Bathing, toileting, transferring ability
M0700—Ambulation/locomotion
M0780/M0790—Management of oral, inhalant medications
M0800—Management of Injectable Medications
M0810/M0820—Equipment management
M0826—Therapy Need

4. Associated Nursing Diagnoses (see Part Seven)

5. Supportive Factors for the Determination and Documentation of Homebound Status

Review the generic recommendations for documenting homebound status, and Medicare's definition of homebound in #5 of the template located at the beginning of this Part of this text. Other supportive factors for determining and documenting homebound status for patients with oncologic/ hematologic problems may include:

Taxing effort as evidenced by severe SOB (M0490), other (specify in functional terms)
Post-surgery, on activity restrictions
Need for walker and/or assistance to ambulate
Inability to negotiate stairs inside/outside of home
Pain (M0420/M0430) at level ____ (specify) when _____ (specify activity)
Infected postoperative site (M0488), on infection precautions while being treated with intravenous antibiotics
Diagnosis of metastatic cancer; needs assistance with all activities
Bone marrow transplant patient severely immunosuppressed
Paralysis secondary to brain surgery for tumor
Activity restricted-lung cancer patient with SOB, coughing, bronchitis; outside temperature is 90 degrees, heat and humidity present with a smog alert
On immunosuppressive medications (specific) and physician-ordered wound care at home for infection control
On medically ordered protective isolation
Medically restricted to home per physician due to extensive reconstructive therapy for head and neck cancer
Severe weakness and SOB due to chemotherapy and radiation
Diagnosis of metastatic cancer with bone pain
Severe SOB on all activity, receiving oxygen
S/P brain surgery, too weak to leave home without assistance
Cancer causing mental status changes, patient cannot leave home unattended for safety reasons
Comatose patient with metastatic cancer
Aphasia and lethargy due to progression of malignancy
Other reasons, including non-oncologic/hematologic

6. Potential Interdisciplinary Goals and Outcomes

The template presented at the beginning of this Part lists patient-centered goals/outcomes that can be individualized

according to the identified needs of the patient and family. The goals/outcomes listed below are specific examples related to oncologic/hematologic system care, and each begins with the statement "By the end of the projected episode of care, the patient and/or family/caregiver will:"

Implement plan for home modifications for safety and optimal function
Demonstrate management of complications or side effects of chemotherapy/radiation, including decreased resistance, increased fatigue and SOB, nausea and vomiting
Maintain skin integrity in bedridden cancer patient as evidenced by problem-free skin
Demonstrate control of pain and other symptoms
Demonstrate ability to administer oxygen as ordered and manage equipment safely
Be supported with skilled and compassionate palliative care for end-stage disease through death
Other goals/outcomes as appropriate for patient

7. Skills, Interventions/Services, and Management

The template presented at the beginning of this Part lists generic skills, interventions, and management of the different home care services that can be individualized according to the identified needs of the patient and family. Skills and interventions utilized by home care clinicians specific to oncologic/hematologic system care include:

Assessment

Assess conjunctiva of eyes and skin color, noting pallor
Assess cardiopulmonary system for signs/symptoms of anemia or impaired function
Assess for signs/symptoms of infection using immunologic system assessment techniques
Assess skin for signs/symptoms of bruising or bleeding
Assess urine and stools for signs/symptoms of bleeding

Perform complete pain assessment for each pain site:

- Location
- Quality
- Intensity (1–10 scale)
- Timing: onset, frequency, duration
- What makes it better or worse?
- Effect of enlarged lymph nodes: cervical chain, axillary, groin

Observation of side effects of chemotherapy, including anemia, fatigue, stomatitis, others

Assess/evaluate patient for specialized support surfaces to avoid pressure ulcers

Assessment and observation of patient status after ______ surgery (specify) for signs/symptoms of infection, other complications

Ongoing management and assessment of the effectiveness of the plan/program for pain and other symptom control/relief

Assess patient/caregiver anxiety level and coping skills and support use of positive coping skills

Medication/Therapeutic Regimens

Teach about skin care and care of sites receiving radiation

Teach regarding the care and safety of the affected arm postmastectomy; increased risk of infection and signs, symptoms of cellulitis, no BPs, venipunctures in that arm

Teach patient/caregiver importance of round-the-clock and regularly scheduled analgesia

Teach importance of meticulous mouth care and comfort measures for side effects that affect the mouth/throat (sore gums, tender mouth areas, etc.)

Teach all aspects of tracheostomy, colostomy care

Teach caregiver skin care, including the need for position changes, pressure pads and mattresses for comfort, and the prevention of skin breakdown

Teach patient/caregiver ordered wound care, what to observe for (increased pain, swelling, tenderness, drainage, and other signs of infection), and when/who to report

Teach patient/caregiver about radiation/chemo therapy, including schedule, need for blood tests, side effects to observe for, interactions with foods/medications, others

Provide wound care as ordered

Comfort measures of patient's choice provided to patient who is essentially bed-bound/chair-bound and alert, including back rub, hand massage, music of choice, and supportive interventions

Nutrition/Hydration/Elimination

Assess for changes in appetite and intake either due to the disease or the antineoplastic therapies to identify patients at risk for malnutrition and implement plan to optimize nutrition

Teach the patient/caregiver to offer small, frequent snacks

Maintain optimal nutrition and hydration by offering patient high-protein diets with snacks/foods, supplements of patient's choice

Safety

Teach safe and correct use of home oxygen therapy, and provide written information on safe use of oxygen

Physical Therapy

Teach therapeutic exercises for maximum strength, function, ROM

Instruct patient/caregiver adaptive techniques for maximum independence and safety with balance, ambulation, and transfers

Assessment and instructions for use of walker, wheelchair and/or other assistive devices for functional mobility, including bed mobility; assist in arrangements to obtain necessary equipment

Assess and instruct in home modification for safety and independence in mobility
Provide use of physical agents/modalities for pain management
Assess and instruct in functional positioning for prevention of pressure ulcers and joint contractures
Educate patient/caregiver on each home program for all instructions provided
Other interventions

Speech-Language Pathology

Evaluation of swallow, speech and cognitive function, with ongoing re-assessment
Educate patient/caregiver on safety precautions and prevention of swallowing dysfunction, including food textures and body positioning to reduce risk of aspiration
Collaborate with dietitian, recommend appropriate food texture and diet modification
Teach program for lip, tongue, and facial control for optimum swallowing skills (dysphagia)
Instruction in voice training with prosthesis
Teach program for articulation proficiency for verbal skills, both expressive and receptive (dysphasia)
Assess and establish program for memory and other cognitive dysfunction and coordinate with OT
Teach alternative and effective communication program
Educate patient/caregiver on each home program for all instructions provided other interventions
Other interventions

Occupational Therapy

Instruct in safety and use of adaptive techniques and assistive devices for maximum independence in ADL, including hygiene
Instruct in energy conservation and diaphragmatic breathing techniques for maximum functional activity level and minimal SOB

Assess and instruct in home modification for maximum safety and independence

Instruct on use of splints and/or other support devices for functional positioning, reduction and/or prevention of contractures, maximum comfort, and teach precautions to prevent skin breakdown

Teach therapeutic exercise for maximum UE strength, ROM, and coordination

Assess and establish cognitive retraining program and compensatory system, coordinate with SLP

Assess and address the need to improve body image and other psychological effects of the disease process

Educate patient/caregiver(s) on home programs for all instructions provided

Other interventions

Medical Social Services

Evaluation/assessment as patient's problems adversely impact the POC and impede progress toward identified goals (e.g., cannot afford medications or ordered nutritional supplements, depressed and noncompliant)

Assess the patient's adjustment to cancer diagnosis (or recurrence) and associated problems

Identify eligibility for services and benefits

Psychosocial assessment of patient regarding disease, prognosis, and implications

Consideration of hospice services, other palliative care

Other interventions

Dietary Counseling

Nutritional evaluation of patient with cancer for optimal nutrition/hydration

Comprehensive nutritional assessment and plan

Assessment of diet history, calculation of nutrient intake, others

Collaborate with SLP on care for patient with head and neck resection

Provide information on safest diet consistency
Evaluation of patient with anorexia, weight loss
Plan for improved nutrition/hydration
Evaluation of patient on tube feedings
Monitoring/managing to support optimal nutrition/ hydration
Teach caregiver aspects of nutritional care
Other interventions

Other Considerations

Pain management program
Nonpharmacological interventions of progressive muscle relaxation, imagery, positive visualization, music, and humor therapy of patient's choice
Other interventions, care management, etc. based on patient's unique condition and needs

8. Tips to Support Medical Necessity, Quality, and Reimbursement (see Care of Older Adults Template at the beginning of this Part)

There are many facets of cancer that demand supportive, skillful, and compassionate care. For an in-depth text about hospice and palliative care, readers are referred to the *Hospice and Palliative Care Handbook: Quality, Compliance and Reimbursement* (Mosby, 1999).

9. Evidence-Based and other Resources for Practice and Education

The American Cancer Society (www.cancer.org or 1-800-ACS-2335 or 1-800-395-LOOK [1-800-395-5665]) has support groups like "I Can Cope" and "Look Good … Feel Better" for women undergoing chemotherapy or radiation. They also offer numerous resources and information related to various cancers for patients, families, and professionals.

Cancer Care (www.cancercare.org or 1-800-813-HOPE [1-800-813-4673]) offers information for anyone dealing with cancer, whether you are a patient, family member, friend, or health professional providing care. They provide online support groups, fact sheets with titles including "Prevention and Early Detection" and "Young Adults with Cancer," as well as fact sheets and publications in Spanish.

The City of Hope National Medical Center (www.cityofhope.org 1-626-256-HOPE [1-626-256-4673]) offers information on adult and pediatric cancers of all sorts for patients and caregivers, families, and professionals. Information pages on each type of cancer include what the cancer is, what parts of the body the cancer effects and how, and what each stage of the cancer involves. They also have information on treatment and patient referral options and what trials and research is going on now.

Cope, D.G., & Reb, A.M. (Eds.) (2006). *An Evidence-Based Approach to the Treatment of Care of the Older Adult with Cancer.* (www.ons.org or 1-866-257-4667). This book details commonly occurring cancers in aging patients, palliative care considerations, symptom management, alternative therapies, and other issues specifically for older adult patients.

The Intercultural Cancer Council (www.iccnetwork.org) provides fact sheets and information about minorities and cancer, underserved population, as well as news, statistics, and links to other resources for health care professionals and patients alike. They also publish a newsletter entitled *The Voice* which can be viewed or subscribed to through their website.

The National Cancer Institute (NCI) (www.cancer.gov or 1-800-4-CANCER [1-800-422-6237]) produces a newsletter entitled the *NCI Cancer Bulletin* with articles on research and training to help reduce the suffering caused by cancer.

The National Coalition for Cancer Survivorship (NCCS) (www.canceradvocacy.org or 1-301-650-9127) offers a free educational resource called the *Cancer Survivor Toolbox*. This includes topics on communication, negotiating, concerns for the older adult, and more.

The Oncology Nursing Society (www.ons.org or 1-866-257-4ONS [1-866-257-4667]) has a "Breast Cancer Patient Resource Area" on their website, as well as links to organizations and journals to help patients.

Cancer. Net (www.cancer.net/portal/site/patient or 1-703-797-1914) offers many other patient and clinician education materials.

PSYCHIATRIC/PSYCHOSOCIAL SYSTEM CARE

1. General Considerations

This Psychiatric and Psychosocial System Care guideline includes the most common psychiatric problems seen in home care. According to the National Institute of Mental Illness, it is reported that of the nearly 35 million Americans age 65 and older, an estimated 2 million have a depressive illness (e.g. major depressive disorder, dysthymic disorder, or bipolar disorder) and another 5 million may have "subsyndromal depression," or depressive symptoms that fall short of meeting full diagnostic criteria for a disorder. Research has shown that in the United States about 19 million people—one in ten adults—experience depression each year, and *nearly two-thirds do not get the help they need.* Major depression and dysthymia affect twice as many women as men. This two-to-one ratio exists regardless of racial and ethnic background or economic status. In America alone, more than 6 million men have depression each year and about 1 woman in 5 has depression.

Depression in the older adult population is of particular concern as an under-reported and under-treated health problem. Considering the multiple problems and losses many older adults experience, home care clinicians have an important role in identifying these problems and intervening appropriately. Many of these patients are also caregivers for adult children, grandchildren or their aging spouses, which only adds to their burdens. Psychotherapy, medications, or a combination of both, often relieve the symptoms for these at-risk patients.

2. Potential Diagnoses and Codes

The diagnoses and codes listed here include some of the most common psychiatric/psychosocial conditions in home care, and have been alphabetized for easy identification. The ICD-9-CM system requires a focused review of the patient's medical information in addition to the physician-assigned diagnoses. Should additional information be needed, refer to the coding books or a qualified coder.

Diagnosis	Code
Agoraphobia without panic attacks	300.22
AIDS, with dementia	042 and 294.10
Alcoholism	303.9X
Alzheimer's disease (AD)	331.0
Anorexia nervosa	307.1
Anxiety state	300.00
Bipolar disorder	296.7
Bulimia	307.51
Constipation	564.0
Creutzfeldt-Jakob disease/dementia	046.1 and 294.10
Dementia	294.8
Depression, reactive	300.4
Depressive disorder	311
Depressive psychosis	296.20
Drug addiction	304.XX
Hypochondriasis	300.7
Korsakoff's dementia	294.0
Mania	296.00
Nonpsychotic brain syndrome	310.9
Obesity	278.00
Obesity, morbid	278.01
Obsessive-compulsive disorder	300.3
Organic brain syndrome	310.9
Panic disorder	300.01
Panic disorder with agoraphobia	300.21
Personality disorder, unspecified	301.9
Polyaddiction	304.8X
Post-traumatic stress disorder	309.81
Presenile dementia	290.10
Psychosis, unspecified	298.9
Schizophrenia, simple	295.0X
Schizophrenia, undifferentiated	295.9X
Senile dementia	290.0
Traumatic stress disorder	308.3
Unipolar affective disorder	296.99
Others	

3. OASIS Considerations

The following are some of the OASIS items (referred to as *M0*) that specifically target or affect the system addressed in this guideline. Please keep in mind that this list is not all-inclusive, since patient comorbidities vary, as do other variables unique to the patient's situation. OASIS items that may be used in determining the case-mix index are highlighted.

M0230/M0240/M0246—Diagnoses, Severity Index, and Payment Diagnoses
M0350/M0360/M0370/M0380—Caregiver availability/assistance
M0560/M0570/M0580/M0590/M0610/M0620/M0630—Cognitive, emotional, behavioral functioning
M0650/M0660—Ability to dress upper/lower body
M0670/M0680/M0690—Bathing, toileting, transferring
M0700—Ambulation/locomotion
M0710/M0770—IADLs
M0780—Management of oral medications
M0800—Management of injectable medications
M0826—Therapy Need

4. Associated Nursing Diagnoses (see Part Seven)

5. Supportive Factors for the Determination and Documentation of Homebound Status

Review the generic recommendations for documenting homebound status, and Medicare's definition of homebound in #5 of the template located at the beginning of this Part of this text. Other supportive factors for determining and documenting homebound status for patients with psychiatric/psychosocial problems may include:

Needs supervision due to psychiatric condition
Phobias, refuses to leave home or go outside

Delusional (M0610/M0620), must be accompanied when leaving home
High level of depression (M0590), leaves home only for visits with psychiatrist and needs to be driven
Agoraphobic, does not leave home
Acute anxiety (M0580), cannot safely leave home
Due to psychiatric condition, unsafe to leave home unattended
Acute depression (M0590) with vegetative symptoms
Paranoid (M0610/M0620), says everyone is "out to get" her/him—will not leave home
Needs walker and assistance to ambulate (M0700)
Very frail, cannot walk unsupported (M0700)
Disoriented with impaired thoughts/confusion/agitation (M0560/M0570)
Psychiatric problem (specify), demonstrated in part by a refusal to leave home
Paralysis, endurance, and poor ambulation (M0700)
Severely immunosuppressed and depressed (M0590)—does not go outside
Confusion levels (M0560/M0570) preclude patient from leaving home safely for needed psychotherapy
Cannot safely leave home unattended (not oriented to place, person) (M0560/M0570)
Mental status deterioration, cannot leave home (hallucinations, outbursts) (M0610/M0620)
Behaviors pose risk to self/others, cannot leave home unattended (M0610/M0620)
Other reasons, including non-psychiatric/psychosocial

6. Potential Interdisciplinary Goals and Outcomes

The template presented at the beginning of this Part lists patient-centered goals/outcomes that can be individualized according to the identified needs of the patient and family. The goals/outcomes listed below are specific examples related to psychiatric/psychosocial system care, and each begins with the statement "By the end of the projected episode of care, the patient and/or family/caregiver will:"

Demonstrate improvement/stabilization in anxiety level
Demonstrate improvement/stabilization in cognitive functioning
Demonstrate behavioral stabilization and increased coping skills related to appropriate functioning and depression
Demonstrate appropriate grief/bereavement expression and support
Verbalize decreased episodes of panic and ability to leave home with assistance of _____ (specify)
Demonstrate increased independence with home program for reality orientation and/or cognitive skills by _____ (specify date)
Other goals/outcomes as appropriate for patient

7. Skills, Interventions/Services, and Management

The template presented at the beginning of this Part lists generic skills, interventions, and management of the different home care services that can be individualized according to the identified needs of the patient and family. Skills and interventions utilized by home care clinicians specific to psychiatric/psychosocial system care include:

Assessment

Assess orientation, memory, and mood
If memory is of concern, perform mini-mental status exam
If anxiety is of concern, ask about intensity, frequency, effect of the anxiety to perform ADLs, including sleeping, and what makes it better or worse

If depression is of concern, ask patient about:

- Intensity, frequency, duration, and effect on ability to perform normal ADLs, including eating, sleeping
- What makes it better or worse?
- Thoughts or plans to harm oneself

Assess patient's caregiver for ability to cope and manage:

- Is the caregiver able to get enough sleep?
- Is the caregiver showing signs/symptoms of stress and/or depression?

Determine patient's support system, including family, neighbors, faith-based community members and available community resources

Does the patient's illness/condition provoke feelings of spiritual distress or concern?

Are there particular cultural beliefs, values, or practices that the home health staff should know about to promote the most respectful and helpful care?

Is the patient/family having problems affording the things needed for health and well-being—medications, food, shelter, needed care?

Observation and assessment of cognitive/affective behaviors

Observation and assessment of patient's hygiene, personal care, independence, safety, home setting, other parameters

Assess patient and provide/plan for psychotherapy

Assess mental status and any changes, including hallucinations, delusions, history of hospitalizations, depression, chemical dependency, anxiety disorder, sleep disturbances

Assess patient for suicidal ideation

Observation and assessment of patient for neuropsychiatric complications of illness, including confusion, depression, anxiety, hostility, paranoia

Assess patient's/caregiver's emotional status/coping ability, capability

Assess patient for side effects/drug interactions of psychotropic medications with other medication therapy for numerous medical diseases

Assess/evaluate behavior modification plan, including support, teaching, evaluation of compliance/adherence

Assess patient behavior, including anxiety, cooperation, ability to communicate, eye contact, other behaviors

Assess for the long-term ability of patient and family to comply with therapeutic regimens

Observation and assessment of patient on tricyclic antidepressants to assist in pain relief/management of neuropathic origin

Assess patient/caregiver anxiety level and coping skills and support use of positive coping skills

Provide support and intervention to patient too withdrawn to leave bed or home with severe grief reaction

Provide active, nonjudgmental listening to patient expression of a desire to "end it all" and initiate referral(s) to other team members for counseling and interventions

Teaching

Teach patient/family about depression and signs/symptoms of exacerbation that require additional intervention

Teach patient/family about bipolar disease and symptoms and signs/symptoms of escalation that necessitate calling the doctor and/or being re-evaluated

Instruct patient/caregiver on the risks/problems associated with using illicit or other drugs and alcohol with prescribed drugs

Medication/Therapeutic Regimens

Monitor medication regimen and compliance with lithium therapy

Administer _____ (specify psychotropic medication, dose, route) injection per physician order

Therapeutic intervention/support to address patient's symptoms and behaviors

Provide/set-up patient with medication box to facilitate medication planning and adherence

Review/coordinate blood-level monitoring of antidepressants for effectiveness
Assess effectiveness and manage the patient's response to therapeutic treatments and interventions, and report any changes or unfavorable responses to the physician (i.e., extrapyramidal symptoms)
Monitor/assess effectiveness of new antipsychotic drug(s) (specify) for severe agitation, psychotic behavior, and suicidal thoughts or planning
Encourage family/caregiver to give the patient medications on the designated written schedule and around the clock
Evaluate behaviors related to medication plan, including support, teaching, and evaluation of compliance/adherence
Assess whether the patient is taking the prescribed medications correctly (e.g., status of supply, hoarding, running out of medication "quickly")

Nutrition/Hydration/Elimination

Assess hydration and nutrition status and provide nutritional information/education
Instruct patient regarding bowel movement, the need to prevent constipation, and avoiding constipation or straining
Teach patient about the stool softeners, dietary recommendations, and need for adequate hydration for optimal bowel function
Teach regarding psychotropic medication interactions with foods
Implement bowel management/constipation prevention program

Care Coordination/Case Management/ Discharge Planning

Assess need and initiate referral(s) for other agency/ community services, including aide, PT/OT/SLP, social worker, psychiatrist/psychologist, community mental health services, dietitian, pharmacist, and others

Physical Therapy

Physical therapy is usually not indicated for this care system unless patient has another problem. If the patient also has mobility or ADL deficits in functioning, please refer to the Musculoskeletal Care guideline.

Occupational Therapy

Assess safety of home and patient awareness

Instruct patient/caregiver of adaptive techniques and use of assistive devices for maximum independence in ADLs

Provide cognitive retraining and reality orientation with home program of therapeutic activities

Instruct in effective functional communication skills for expressing needs

Plan, implement, and supervise therapeutic activity program

Other interventions

Medical Social Services

Evaluate/assess patient's problems that adversely impact the POC and impede progress toward identified goals (e.g., cannot afford medications, problematic living situation)

Assess and identify optimal coping strategies

Assess financial situation and concerns, provide counseling regarding food acquisition, ability to prepare, and costs of needed medications

Provide crisis intervention and counseling for planning and decision making

Psychosocial assessment of patient's mental status and safety

Provide therapeutic interventions/counseling directed toward patient's symptoms, identified problems

Assess health and mental status factors impacting on the POC not being able to be implemented

Provide emotional/spiritual support to patient in crisis

Assess depression, fear, anxiety in patient with numerous health concerns and poor supports

Provide grief counseling and intervention/support related to loss/illness/grief
Identify caregiver role strain necessitating relief measures, alternative caregivers for POC implementation
Identify suicidal ideation and plan for safety and resolution
Provide referral/linkage to community services and resources
Other interventions

Dietary Counseling
Nutritional evaluation of patient for achievement of optimal nutrition and hydration in depressed patient with anorexia
Comprehensive nutritional assessment and plan

Other Considerations
Observe for sleeping, eating, and other changes in lifestyle patterns
Psychotherapeutic interventions, including crisis intervention, reality orientation, others (specify)
Other interventions, care management, etc. based on patient's unique condition and needs

8. Tips to Support Medical Necessity, Quality, and Reimbursement (see Care of Older Adults Template at the beginning of this Part)

Psychiatric evaluation, therapy, and training are listed as one of the 15 coverable skilled nursing services by Medicare. Readers are referred to Part Six for the full text of the Medicare "Coverage of Services" section, which lists three psychiatric patient examples. Psychiatrically trained nurses are nurses who have special training and/or experience beyond the standard curriculum required for a registered nurse. It is also important to note that Medicare law precludes agencies that primarily provide care and treatment of mental disease from participating as home health agencies; this means the psychiatric nursing services must be furnished by an agency that does not provide care and treatment of mental diseases.

9. Evidence-Based and other Resources for Practice and Education

The Agency for Healthcare Research and Quality (AHRQ) (www.ahrq.gov or 1-800-358-9295) has a patient guide entitled "Depression is a Treatable Illness" (AHCPR Pub. No. 93-0053).

The American Psychiatric Nurses Association's website is www.apna.org.

The American Psychiatric Association (www.psych.org or 1-202-682-6220) provides information and resources for patients and family on symptoms and treatment of depression. They also sponsor a mental health website (www.healthyminds.org) that offers numerous mental health resources for professionals and consumers.

The Centers for Disease Control and Prevention (CDC) (www.cdc.gov) offers information on depression, including "Preventing Suicide: Program Activities Guide," a booklet with information on the causes and risks related to suicide as well as prevention.

The Depression and Bipolar Support Alliance (www.dbsalliance.org or 1-800-826-3632) offers information about depression, anxiety, bipolar disorder, and other mood altering disorders including causes, signs, and treatment options.

The National Institute of Mental Health (www.nimh.nih.gov or 1-866-615-6464) has many resources available.

The Paralyzed Veterans of America (PVA) (www.pva.org or 1-800-424-8200) offers many publications including "Depression Following Spinal Cord Injury" and a consumer guide entitled "Depression: What You Should Know" for mood disorders, including depression with information on signs, treatments, and more.

PULMONARY/RESPIRATORY SYSTEM CARE

1. General Considerations

This care guideline addresses the most common pulmonary/respiratory conditions seen in home care. This includes chronic obstructive pulmonary disease (COPD), pneumonia, and tuberculosis (TB), as well as patients with tracheostomies and other related respiratory or lung conditions. According to the Centers for Disease Control and Prevention (CDC), COPD is a leading cause of death, illness, and disability in the United States. COPD takes many forms, including asthma, emphysema, and chronic bronchitis. More than 12 million people are diagnosed with COPD and an additional 12 million who likely have COPD but are not yet diagnosed. COPD is a common reason why older adults are hospitalized and is the fourth leading cause of death in the United States, costing more than $14.5 billion annually. Likewise, approximately 12 million people in the U.S. suffer from asthma, and 5000 die each year from severe asthma.

Noncompliance, episodic care, the home environment, no caregiver, or a lack of competent caregivers all contribute to this cycle. Malnutrition has been estimated to occur in 70 percent of patients with COPD. Air swallowing or physiologic changes to the diaphragm contribute to patients feeling very full early in meals and often too tired to prepare or eat meals. These patients expend increased energy in labored breathing. Because of these factors, COPD patients require more calories to prevent weight loss.

TB is a contagious disease of the lung that continues its resurgence and now infects one-third of the world's population. This is particularly problematic because there are drug-resistant strains that are becoming more common. Because TB is spread by airborne droplets, everyone exposed is susceptible. Treatment must continue for the entire course of care, even though the patient may feel better and be tempted to quit taking the medications.

Should your patient have end-stage lung disease, such as lung cancer or severe COPD, refer to the Hospice and Palliative Care guideline. Should your patient have cystic fibrosis, there is a Cystic Fibrosis Care guideline in the Maternal-Child section of this book.

2. Potential Diagnoses and Codes

The diagnoses and codes listed here include some of the most common pulmonary/respiratory conditions in home care, and have been alphabetized for easy identification. The ICD-9-CM system requires a focused review of the patient's medical information in addition to the physician-assigned diagnoses. Should additional information be needed, refer to the coding books or a qualified coder.

Diagnosis	Code
Aftercare following organ transplant	V58.44
Airway obstruction, chronic	496
Asphyxia	799.0
Asthma	493.90
Asthma, with status asthmaticus	493.91
Asthma, with acute exacerbation	493.92
Attention to tracheostomy	V55.0
Bronchiolitis	466.19
Bronchitis	490
Bronchitis, acute	466.0
Bronchitis, acute, with COPD	491.21
Bronchopneumonia	485
Cancer of the esophagus	150.9
Cancer of the larynx	161.9
Cancer of the pharynx	149.0
Cancer of the tongue	141.9
Cancer of the trachea	162.0
Congestive heart failure	428.0
Chronic obstructive pulmonary disease (COPD)	496
Chronic obstructive pulmonary disease (COPD), exacerbation	491.21
Cor pulmonale	416.9
Cystic fibrosis	277.00

Dehydration	276.51
Dysphagia	787.2
Emphysema	492.8
Heart failure	428.9
Hemoptysis	786.3
Influenza with pneumonia	487.0
Interstitial emphysema	518.1
Laryngeal cancer	161.9
Left heart failure	428.1
Long-term oxygen use	V46.2
Lung cancer	162.9
Lung disease	518.89
Pleural effusion	511.9
Pneumonia	486
Pneumonia, aspiration	507.0
Pneumonia, *Pneumocystis carinii*	136.3
Pneumonia, viral	480.9
Pneumonia with influenza	487.0
Protein-calorie malnutrition	263.9
Pulmonary edema	514
Pulmonary embolism	415.19
Pulmonary fibrosis	515
Respiratory failure	518.81
Trachea or bronchi, disease	519.1
Tracheitis, acute	464.10
Transplant, lung, rejection (failure)	996.84
Tuberculosis, bronchial	011.30
Tuberculosis, bronchus	011.30
Tuberculosis, lung (pulmonary)	011.90
Upper respiratory infection	465.9
Others	

3. OASIS Considerations

The following are some of the OASIS items (referred to as *M0*) that specifically target or affect the system addressed in this guideline. Please keep in mind that this list is not all-inclusive, since patient comorbidities vary, as do other variables unique to the patient's situation. OASIS items that may be used in determining the case-mix index are highlighted.

M0230/M0240/M0246—Diagnoses, Severity Index, and Payment Diagnoses
M0350/M0360/M0370/M0380—Caregiver availability/ assistance
M0420—Pain
M0430—Intractable Pain
M0482/M0484/M0486—Surgical Wound
M0488—Surgical Wound Status
M0490—Dyspnea
M0500—Respiratory treatments
M0580—Anxiety
M0650/M0660—Ability to dress upper/lower body
M0670/M0680/M0690—Bathing, toileting, transferring
M0700—Ambulation/locomotion
M0780/M0790—Management of oral, inhalant medications
M0810/M0820—Management of equipment
M0826—Therapy Need

4. Associated Nursing Diagnoses (see Part Seven)

5. Supportive Factors for the Determination And Documentation of Homebound Status

Review the generic recommendations for documenting homebound status, and Medicare's definition of homebound in #5 of the template located at the beginning of this Part of this text. Other supportive factors for determining and documenting homebound status for patients with pulmonary/ respiratory problems may include:

Taxing effort as evidenced by severe SOB (M0490), other (specify in functional terms)
Post-surgery, on activity restrictions
Need for walker and/or assistance to ambulate (M0700)
Inability to negotiate stairs inside/outside of home
Infected postoperative chest site (M0488), on infection precautions with intravenous antibiotics post surgery

Pain (M0420/M0430) at level ____ (specify) when _____ (specify activity)
Chest pain (M0420) caused by minimal exertion
Unsteady gait, increased risk for falls (M0700)
Respiratory distress (M0490) with talking and standing, oxygen dependent at all times
Activity restricted due to COPD, other (specify)—patient SOB (M0490) and temperature outside is 90 degrees with humidity and smog alert
Other reasons, including non-pulmonary/respiratory

6. Potential Interdisciplinary Goals and Outcomes

The template presented at the beginning of this Part lists patient-centered goals/outcomes that can be individualized according to the identified needs of the patient and family. The goals/outcomes listed below are specific examples related to pulmonary/respiratory system care, and each begins with the statement "By the end of the projected episode of care, the patient and/or family/caregiver will:"

Demonstrate ability to administer oxygen as ordered and manage equipment safely
Demonstrate improvement in dyspnea (as evidenced by _____ (specify)
Demonstrate adequate oxygenation as evidenced by _____ (specify) (e.g., decreased dyspnea)
Achieve replacement of electrolytes lost secondary to medication therapies (or other reasons)
Demonstrate pulse measurement and signs/symptoms which require physician notification
Maintain patent airway and mobilization of secretions by use of respiratory treatments, medications, and effective cough
Verbalize factors (e.g., environmental allergies, smoking) that trigger exacerbation of respiratory problem

Demonstrate resolution of pneumonia with improved lung sounds, decreased SOB, improved CBC
Demonstrate improved respiratory status (cough, sputum production, oximetry, anxiety)
Verbalize understanding of respiratory isolation and demonstrate compliance
Demonstrate safe and effective secretion removal
Optimize functional capacity while minimizing hospital admissions/readmissions within the limits of the disease process
Participate in respiratory care plan as appropriate (e.g., suctioning, oxygen delivery)
Demonstrate smoking cessation
Demonstrate independence in trach care
Demonstrate effective diaphragmatic breathing techniques, purse-lipped breathing to decrease SOB for maximum functional activity level
Demonstrate improved muscle tone, relaxation, and/or sleep patterns
Be supported with skilled and compassionate palliative care for end-stage disease through death
Other goals/outcomes as appropriate for patient

7. Skills, Interventions/Services, and Management

The template presented at the beginning of this Part lists generic skills, interventions, and management of the different home care services that can be individualized according to the identified needs of the patient and family. Skills and interventions utilized by home care clinicians specific to pulmonary/respiratory system care include:

Assessment

Observe patient breathing; note signs/symptoms of SOB, DOE, orthopnea, use of accessory muscles and posture assumed to breathe

Observe skin color, oral mucosa, and nail beds
Obtain respiratory rate; note rhythm and depth of respirations
Palpate sinuses, noting pain or tenderness
Assess nose, checking for signs/symptoms of congestion or discharge
Assess oral cavity and throat, looking for signs/symptoms of URI (e.g., enlarged tonsils, exudates on tonsils)
Observe thorax for deformities and for respiratory excursion
Auscultate lung fields, upper and lower, anterior and posterior, during inspiratory and expiratory phases; note especially fine crackles, course crackles, and wheezes
Obtain pulse oximetry reading
Assess capillary refill of nail beds
If cough, note:

- Productive or non-productive, timing, what makes it better or worse
- Productive cough; note color, consistency, amount

If oxygen, note:

- Liters/minute, used intermittently/constantly, how delivered
- Back-up plans for power emergency (for concentrator), and for travel
- Knowledge of safe use

If tracheostomy, note:

- Type and size of trach tube, cuffed/not cuffed
- Integrity of skin around trach site
- Frequency of suctioning
- Color, consistency of mucous suctioned

Assess oxygen decompensation at rest and with activity using O_2 saturation pulse oximetry
Assess need for chest physiotherapy, other pulmonary treatment
Assess wound site (specify), change dressings (specify orders and frequency), and teach patient/caregiver wound care, infection control, and symptoms that necessitate additional care

3

Medication/Therapeutic Regimens

Measure pulse oximetry q _____ for signs/symptoms cardiorespiratory distress (specify frequency per doctor's order)

Teach use, care, and management of respiratory treatments/rx (e.g., Pulmonaide, IPPB), nebulizers, aerosol inhalers, etc. and care/cleaning of supplies/ equipment

Teach patient effective coughing, deep breathing, and pursed lip or diaphragmatic breathing

Teach patient/caregiver to identify and avoid specific factors that precipitate an exacerbation (asthma)

Teach and train family/caregivers about disease and importance of infection control procedures

Patient/family cautioned to avoid use of aerosol sprays, powders, and other particles that could be aspirated

Teach home use of peak flow meter, incentive spirometer

Teach patient/family about pneumonia and symptomatology and signs/symptoms that necessitate calling the doctor

Teach care of tracheostomy, site care, and related infection control measures

Teach CPR with tracheostomy

Teach about and observe for side effects of steroids

Provide/teach chest PT

Teach patient/caregiver ordered wound care and dressing changes

Safety

Review backup ventilator support system and emergency backup procedure(s)

Teach patient about the safe disposal of copious secretions

Teach safe and correct use of home oxygen therapy, and provide written information on safe use of oxygen

Care Coordination/Case Management/ Discharge Planning

Assess need and initiate referral(s) for other agency/ community services, including aide, PT/OT/SLP, social worker, dietitian, pharmacist, wound specialist, especially respiratory therapist

Physical Therapy

Assessment

Vital signs at rest, during and after activity or exercise
Perceived exertion or dyspnea scale during activities or exercise
Breathing patterns at rest and with activity
Pulmonary signs/symptoms in response to increased oxygen demand of activity/exercise

Interventions/Teaching

Teach therapeutic exercises for maximum strength, balance
Teach adaptive techniques and diaphragmatic breathing for ambulation and transfers, for minimal SOB, and maximum safety and independence
Teach patient/caregiver(s) home programs for all instructions provided
Other interventions

Speech-Language Pathology

Comprehensive speech and swallowing evaluation
Evaluation of speech/communication options (e.g., artificial larynx, esophageal speech, voice prosthesis)
Dysphagia and speech program
Teach care of voice prosthesis, including removal, cleaning, and safe site maintenance
Develop and teach communication system
Establish home maintenance program and teach patient/ caregiver
Laryngeal speech program
Assess and teach regarding new Electrolarynx
Teach swallowing/safe swallowing skills

Coach patient in adaptive activities to trach (e.g., eating, speaking)
Food texture recommendations for safety and optimal nutrition
Collaborate with dietitian/nutritionist
Other interventions

Occupational Therapy
Teach home modification for safety with ADL and functional mobility
Teach adaptive techniques and use of assistive devices for maximum safety and independence in ADL
Teach energy conservation, diaphragmatic breathing, and relaxation techniques for SOB
Teach therapeutic UE exercise for strength, ROM, and coordination for ADL
Teach patient/caregiver(s) home programs for all instructions provided
Other interventions

Dietary Counseling
Nutrition and hydration in patient with severe SOB, anorexia, and weight loss
Provide adequate nutrition to prevent malnutrition and loss of respiratory muscle mass
Achieve and maintain desired weight
Comprehensive nutritional assessment and plan
Nutritional assessment of patient with TB and significant weight loss
Coordinate/collaborate with SLP
Other interventions

Pharmacy Services
Evaluation of patient taking multiple medications (e.g., nebulizers, inhalers, antibiotics, steroids, aminophylline) for possible interactions

Medication monitoring regarding therapeutic levels and dosages in patient with complex respiratory care regimen
Assessment of medication regimen and plan for safety and compliance
Other interventions

Respiratory Therapy
Assess patient on oxygen with tracheostomy
Manage oxygen therapy and monitor oxygenation status
Provide respiratory treatments per orders (e.g., suction, nebulizer, incentive spirometry)
Other interventions

Other Considerations
Pulmonary rehabilitation program (per physician order)
Engage patient and support comfort, choice, enjoyment, and dignity
Support patient experiencing grieving process (e.g., "normal" eating, breathing, loss of spit/saliva and ability to smell, change in speaking)
Emotional support for patient and caregiver during radiation and chemotherapy for cancer of the larynx, other (specify)
Other interventions, care management, etc. based on patient's unique condition and needs

8. Tips to Support Medical Necessity, Quality, and Reimbursement (see Care of Older Adults Template at the beginning of this Part)

9. Evidence-Based and other Resources for Practice and Education

The Agency for Healthcare Research and Quality (AHRQ) (www.ahrq.gov or 1-800-358-9295) offers resources and clinical guidelines related to respiratory and pulmonary problems. In conjunction with the AHRQ, the National

Quit Line (www.smokefree.gov or 1-800-QUIT-NOW [1-800-784-8669]) offers help and support for smokers who want to quit.

The American Association of Respiratory Care (www.aarc.org or 1-972-243-2272) offers conferences, clinical practice guidelines, and other resources.

The American Lung Association (www.lungusa.org or 1-800-232-5864) has information available on treatment and support both for patients and healthcare professionals.

The Centers for Disease Control (CDC) (www.cdc.gov) has a TB site with up-to-date information and research resources for patients and healthcare professionals.

The Francis J. Curry National Tuberculosis Center (www.nationaltbcenter.edu) offers information, an e-newsletter one can sign up for, web-based workshops and more related to TB.

The National Heart Lung and Blood Institute (www.learnaboutcopd.org or 1-301-592-8573) offers information, research, and news about COPD.

The World Health Organization (www.who.org) offers TB fact sheets, handouts and other information. If you click on "products" there are numerous TB-related topics, information and presentations.

PART FOUR

HOSPICE AND PALLIATIVE CARE

Clinical Guidelines for Assessment, Care Planning, and Documentation

HOSPICE AND PALLIATIVE CARE

1. General Considerations

Palliative care encompasses care when "cure" is not (or no longer) possible; it is care directed toward comfort and works to control symptoms (e.g., pain, nausea, etc.) and improve the quality of life for the patient and family. There is no one diagnosis that comprises who may need hospice, palliative, or end-of-life care. All kinds of patients can need this specialized and compassionate care. According to the Centers for Disease Control and Prevention (CDC), the leading causes of death are heart disease, cancers, stroke and other cerebrovascular diseases, respiratory diseases, accidents, diabetes, and Alzheimer's disease. All of these patients can be appropriate for compassionate palliative, end-of-life care.

Hospice is a kind of palliative care. According to the Centers for Disease Control and Prevention (CDC), expectations about quality of life throughout the lifespan, including at its very end, are increasing. Unfortunately, death itself is ultimately not preventable, and most people will die as a result of chronic disease. The end of life is associated with a substantial burden of suffering among dying individuals and also has health and financial consequences that extend to family members and society.

The data indicates that as many as 50% of dying persons with cancer or other chronic illnesses experience unrelieved symptoms during their final days. Because most deaths occur within hospitals, end-of-life care has been recognized as an important clinical issue needing improvement. The medicalization of disease processes, the denial of the psychosocial and spiritual components in health and disease, and the historical treatment through death (whether appropriate or what the patient wishes) have made people with end-stage disease demand an alternative; hospice and palliative care offer that option. According to the National Hospice and Palliative Care Organization (NHPCO),

1.2 million patients received services through hospice programs in 2005, and approximately one-third of all deaths in 2005 in the U.S. were under the care of a hospice program.

Although cancer is the second leading cause of death in the U.S., NHPCO reports that in 2005 it only accounted for 46% of all hospice admissions. The top non-cancer diagnoses included heart disease (12%), dementia (9.8%), debility (9.2%), and lung disease (7.5%). Regardless of the diagnosis, pain and symptom management form the foundation for the best hospice and palliative care. Pain is one of the most frequent symptoms reported by patients, is highly subjective, and can only be defined by the one experiencing the pain. The patient is always the expert on his or her pain, history, and often the measures that help bring relief.

A thorough patient assessment includes rating pain using one of several varied methods, which should be performed at the time of the initial evaluation and at intervals thereafter if a positive response to the experience of pain is elicited. There are numerous pain therapy choices and emerging, improving oral delivery systems (immediate-release, controlled-release, sustained-release drugs).

Hospice and palliative care are specialty practices directed toward making each day the best it can be for patients with a life-limiting illness and their families as the focus changes from cure to care. This care includes a specialized team approach, called the *interdisciplinary team (IDT)* or *group (IDG)*. In addition to meeting the patient's medical needs, hospice care addresses the physical, psychosocial, and spiritual needs of the patient as well as the family and/or caregiver. Spiritual care, bereavement support, and volunteer assistance are hallmarks of this growing specialty. Readers are referred to the Oncology Care guideline or other care guidelines should they also be appropriate.

2. Potential Diagnoses and Codes

This list contains some of the most common reasons patients are referred to hospice or palliative care services. It is by no means an all-inclusive or exhaustive list. It is important to note that there is no particular diagnosis or group of diagnoses that make a patient "appropriate" for hospice. Generally it is the presentation of the patient, the prognosis by the physician of a life-limiting illness (when the disease runs its natural course), and the patient's (and family's) wishes for skillful and compassionate hospice or palliative care as their option for end-of-life care. It may be appropriate to refer a patient to hospice care when any of the following are present: early stage cancer has progressed to metastatic disease; functional status has declined and the patient requires increased assistance for ADLs; weight loss; recurrent intractable infections with or without hospitalization; treatment is negatively impacting quality of life or there is a lack of response to treatment for the disease; worsening or difficult to control symptoms. The documentation should support the decrease in functional status, weight loss, etc.

These codes have been alphabetized to assist in easy identification. Keep in mind that the ICD-9-CM system requires a focused review of the medical information in addition to the physician-assigned diagnosis. Should additional information be needed, refer to the coding books or a qualified coder. Keep in mind that some diagnoses may be secondary diagnoses.

Adenocarcinoma, metastatic, unspecified site	199.1
Adrenal cancer	194.0
Aftercare following surgery for neoplasm	V58.42
Airway obstruction, chronic	496
Alzheimer's disease	331.0
(ALS) Amyotrophic lateral sclerosis	335.20
Anorexia	783.0
Aplastic anemia	284.9
Astrocytoma, unspecified site	191.9
Bladder cancer	188.9
Bone metastasis	198.5
Brain, cancer of the (primary)	191.9
Brain cancer, metastatic	198.3
Brain tumor, recurrent	239.6

Breast cancer	174.9
Cancer of the brain (primary)	191.9
Cancer of the breast	174.9
Cancer of the cervix	180.9
Cancer of the colon	153.9
Cancer of the esophagus	150.9
Cancer of the head and neck	195.0
Cancer of the larynx	161.9
Cancer of the pharynx	149.0
Cancer of the tongue	141.9
Cancer of the trachea	162.0
Cardiomyopathy	425.4
Cerebrovascular accident (CVA)	436
Cervix, cancer of the	180.9
Chronic obstructive pulmonary disease (COPD)	496
Chronic obstructive pulmonary disease (COPD), with exacerbation	491.21
Cirrhosis of the liver	571.5
Colon cancer	153.9
Dysphagia	787.2
Dysphagia and CVA, late effect	438.82 and 787.20
Emphysema	492.8
Esophagus, cancer of the	150.9
Fracture, pathological	733.1X
Gastric cancer, metastatic	197.8
Glioma, unspecified site	191.9
Heart failure	428.9
Huntington's disease	333.4
Kaposi's sarcoma	176.9
Kaposi's sarcoma with acquired immunodeficiency syndrome (AIDS)	042 and 176.9
Kidney, cancer of the (renal)	189.0
Laryngeal cancer	161.9
Larynx, cancer of the	161.9
Leukemia, acute	208.00
Leukemia, acute lymphocytic (ALL)	204.00
Leukemia, acute myelogenous (AML)	205.00
Leukemia, chronic	208.10
Leukemia, chronic myelogenous (CML)	205.10
Leukopenia	288.0
Liver, malignant neoplasm	155.2
Lou Gehrig's disease (ALS)	335.20
Lung cancer	162.9

Continued

4

4

Lupus	710.0
Lymphoma with bone metastasis	202.80 and 198.5
Metastasis, general	199.1
Multiple myeloma	203.00
Nasopharyngeal cancer	147.9
Oropharyngeal cancer	146.9
Ovarian cancer	183.0
Pain, cancer associated	338.3
Palliative care	V66.7
Pancreas, cancer of the	157.9
Parkinson's disease	332.0
Pharynx, cancer of the	149.0
Pleural effusion	511.9
Pneumonia	486
Pneumonla, aspiration	507.0
Pneumonia, viral	480.9
Pneumonia, *Pneumocystosis carinii*	136.3
Pressure ulcer	707.0X
Prostate cancer	185
Pulmonary edema	514
Pulmonary edema, acute with cardiac disease	428.1
Pulmonary embolism	415.19
Pulmonary fibrosis	515
Radiation enteritis	558.1
Radiation myelitis	323.8 and 990
Rectosigmoid cancer	154.0
Rectum, cancer of the	154.1
Renal cell cancer, metastatic	198.0
Renal failure, chronic	585
Respiratory failure, acute	518.81
Respiratory insufficiency, acute	518.82
Seizure disorder	780.39
Skin cancer	173.9
Stomach, cancer of the	151.9
Tongue, cancer of the	141.9
Transplant, lung, rejection (failure)	996.84
Uterine sarcoma, metastatic	198.82
Uterus, cancer of the	179
Wilms' tumor	189.0
Others	

3. Potential Interdisciplinary Goals and Outcomes

Patient/caregiver expresses satisfaction with care as verbalized

Compliance/adherence to care regimen as demonstrated and verbalized by patient/caregiver by ___ (specify date)

Patient's wishes, dignity, and privacy are respected

Dyspnea, chest pain, and other symptoms controlled

Patient/caregiver is knowledgeable about pain, other symptom regimen, relief measures, and care for optimal relief/control

Patient will experience increased comfort and pain control through self-report and ___ (specify parameters)

Patient maintains functional mobility and ambulation as long as possible

Pain and other symptoms managed in setting of patient's choice

Planned and effective bowel program, as evidenced by regular bowel movements and patient/family report of comfort

Enhanced quality of life as verbalized by patient/family (e.g., alert, pain-free, able to putter in garden)

Patient cared for and family supported through death, with physical, psychosocial, spiritual, and other dimensions, needs, acknowledged/addressed

Effective infection control and palliation

Grief/bereavement expression and support provided

Comfort and individualized interventions of patient with immobility/bedbound status (e.g., skin, urinary, muscular, vascular)

Patient and family supported through death

Patient and family receives hospice support and care, and family members and friends are able to spend quality time together

Patient supported through and receives the maximum benefit from palliative chemotherapy/radiation with minimal complications

Patient/caregiver states dosages of medications, verbalizes rationale for ongoing monitoring (steroids, analgesics)
Patient maintains patent airway and mobilization of secretions and verbalizes decreased dyspnea
Patient states pain will be at ___ on 0–10 scale by ___ (specify)
Patient's/caregiver's anxiety improved by ___ (specify)
Patient/caregiver will verbalize potential complications related to oxygen therapy
Patient demonstrates compliance to therapeutic, preventative, and maintenance care regimens
Patient can communicate effectively through speech or some alternative form of communication
Patient has safe nutritional intake without risk of aspiration
Improved safe swallowing skills, speech, and strength of oral-motor movements
Patient eating foods and using supplements of recommended texture/consistency
Secretion removal is safe and effective as taught by nurse
Optimize functional capacity while minimizing hospital (re)admissions within the limits of the disease process
Patient/caregiver actively participates in all aspects of care plan and wishes/choices are respected/honored
Symptoms managed to patient's satisfaction on current plan of care
Respect for patient's beliefs and knowledge about disease and self
Understanding of disease process with maximum level of functioning
Caregiver able to care for patient by ___ (specify)
Patient/caregiver verbalize knowledge of potential adverse effects of medication therapy and actions to take
Patient achieves and agency supports self-determined life closure
Patient performs self-observational aspects of care (specify)
Patient experiences a sense of control over decisions about life situations

Patient adapts to changed body and body image
Patient experiences adaptive adjustment to diagnosis and illness
Caregiver system assessed and development of stable caregiver plan facilitated
Patient/caregivers supported with skillful and compassionate care through death
Comfort, companionship, and friendship extended to patient and family
Volunteer and other support provided as defined by the patient/family
Spiritual support provided
Patient will have palliative care and maintain comfort through death as desired at home
Educational tools/plan incorporated into daily care and patient/caregiver verbalizes understanding of needed care
Patient/caregiver demonstrates ADL program for maximum safety and independence
Patient demonstrates effective energy conservation techniques for maximum functional activity level by ___ (specify)
Patient demonstrates effective diaphragmatic breathing techniques to decrease shortness of breath (SOB) for maximum functional activity level by ___ (specify)
Patient/caregiver demonstrates safe use of adaptive techniques and assistive devices for maximum independence in ADL by ___ (specify)
Home modifications for safety and independence arranged for completion by ___ (specify)
Patient/caregiver will be independent in upper extremity exercise program for maximum functional skills by ___ (specify)
Improvement in pain interfering with activity per patient self-report
Improvement in dyspnea as evidenced by ___ (specify) or patient self-report

4

Family feels safe and comfortable managing patient's care at home (between home visits)
Improvement in anxiety level per patient self-report
Patient and family execute advance directives/health power of attorney decisions
Patient participates in diversional activities of choice
Patient and family are supported in acceptance of diagnosis
Patient and family discuss issues of death and dying (per culture)
Patient/family progresses through stage of grief
Patient/family feels spiritually supported
Patient offered nutrition of choice
Patient/caregiver copes adaptively with body image change, stress, and illness
Optimal strength, mobility, and function achieved by ___ (specify)
Financial problems addressed with patient able to access medications as ordered on plan of care (POC)
Safety and stability in complex medication regimen
Laboratory reports reviewed for therapeutic dosages and effective patient response
Improved muscle tone, relaxation, and/or sleep patterns
POC successfully implemented because of resolution of identified problems that were impeding progress
Patient able to access community resources
Successful linkage(s) with community resources established
Survivors receive follow-up bereavement counseling after patient's death
Others

4. Associated Nursing Diagnoses (see Part Seven)

5. Supportive Factors for the Determination and Documentation of Homebound Status

The homebound requirement is only for patients admitted to a Medicare-certified home health agency. Homebound is not a requirement for admission to a Medicare-certified or other hospice. However, the following statements help support hospice appropriateness and functional decline and should be stated in the clinical documentation.

Patient becomes exhausted after 50 feet with a walker and must sit down to catch his/her breath
Patient has severe COPD and SOB; 100 degrees heat and humidity outside with a high pollen count; patient does not leave air conditioning on during high pollen/heat/humidity days
Patient needs walker and assistance of one to ambulate
Patient very frail, cannot walk unsupported
Unable to leave home without ambulance due to condition/weight and walking is a considerable and taxing effort
Paralysis, endurance, and poor ambulation
Unsteady gait, increased risk for falls
Respiratory distress with talking and standing—oxygen dependence at all times
Stairs outside home—must be carried in and out
Exit of building approximately 800 to 1000 feet from home door; severe SOB, inability to safely negotiate/use stairs
Patient on opioid sedatives around the clock due to cancer and is unsafe to leave home unattended
Others

6. Skills, Interventions/Services, and Management

Clinicians who provide hospice and palliative care must exercise acute and effective critical thinking, observation, technical, teaching and evaluation skills when performing clinical assessments, interventions, and management of their patients. The *major focus* for many of these patients and caregivers will be assessment and intervention for *pain relief and other symptom management* and *support/respite* for the caregiver(s).

Nursing

Critical Thinking/Assessment Components

Observation and complete systems assessment of patient with ___ (specify problem necessitating hospice/palliative care)

Present hospice/palliative care philosophy and information to patient/family

Assess patient, family, caregiver resources available for care and support

Discuss/clarify expectations of hospice care

Identify primary caregiver, if appropriate

Observation and assessment of patient with known end-stage lung disease admitted with dyspnea, complaint of dyspnea, poor activity tolerance, orthopnea, weight loss, and on oxygen therapy

Assessment of educational needs using standardized organizational protocol (e.g., home oxygen safety, pain management)

Evaluate lung sounds; assess amount, site(s) of wheezing, rhonchi, other findings

Offer/initiate volunteer support to patient and family

Assess the need for and collaborate with other interdisciplinary team (IDT) members (e.g., physician, aide, social worker, nutritionist/dietitian, spiritual counselor, pharmacist, volunteer[s], therapists, others)

Assess for need of continuous care or other appropriate/changed level of care

Perform psychosocial, spiritual, pain, other status assessment

Skilled observation and assessment of all systems

Assess patient response to care and interventions and report changes and undesirable responses to physician

Observation and assessment of/for wheezing, cough, dyspnea, use of accessory muscles, shortness of breath, weights, and other findings/symptoms/changes

Assess pain and evaluate pain management program's effectiveness

Assess all aspects of pain, including site(s), character, description, relation to activity or position, type (constant, spontaneous, chronic, episodic, sharp, bony, etc.), and other factors patient identifies

Evaluate pain in relation to other symptoms, including fatigue, confusion, nausea, constipation, depression, dyspnea

Evaluate need for noninvasive methods of pain control, including heat or cold applications and a transcutaneous electrical nerve stimulator (TENS) unit

Others

Case Management

Management and evaluation of the patient's POC

Implement organizational telehealth protocol

Initiate appropriate pathway/clinical path per organizational protocol (e.g., hospice, palliative pulmonary care)

Provide/teach with corresponding educational tools/information on admission

Teach and manage medication schedules for patient to optimize adherence and symptom relief and effective management

Consider telephone reminder mechanisms for patients with difficulty remembering medication schedule/management

Observe and assess for signs and symptoms of continuing decompensation and increased symptoms (specify) and measures to alleviate and control/relieve

Prevent secondary symptoms (e.g., all patients on opioids have a thorough bowel history and are initiated on a bowel management program to prevent constipation)

Assess and manage pain each visit, including source/type of pain (e.g., cancer pain, infection, arthritis, pathologic fracture, neurogenic, others), and identify need for change, addition, or other plan (e.g., dose adjustment, titration)

Provide/teach effective oral care and related comfort measures

Others

Teaching and Training

Assess learning patient/caregiver readiness, learning barriers, specific educational needs, how the patient may best learn (reading, pictures, listening, etc.) and the desired/assessed ability to learn

Teach patient oxygen care: cannula care, oxygen use, use of inhaler, and safety considerations (NO SMOKING and signs posted, no candles, no petroleum products on or near face, etc.)

Teach family or caregiver physical care of patient

Teach patient and family use of pain assessment tool/scale and reporting mechanisms

Teach patient and family realistic expectations of the disease

Teach care of the dying and signs/symptoms of impending/approaching death

Instruct patient/caregiver about medications, including route, schedule, desired effects/actions, possible side effects, and to immediately report untoward reactions/effects

Teach caregiver care of the weak, bedridden patient

Teach patient/caregiver about the importance of and the rationale for around-the-clock analgesia

Teach patient how to use/measure pain on the organization's standardized pain scale (e.g., 0–10, or other scale specific to the patient's ability and agency protocol)

Instruct patient/caregiver on specific symptoms (including those of imminent death) that necessitate calling the hospice nurse or physician

Teach patient/family use of standardized form/tool to use between hospice team members' visits (and for care coordination among the interdisciplinary team [IDT])

Teach patient/caregiver gentle care of irradiated skin sites and care of severely cracked, dry feet due to palliative chemotherapy

Teach patient/family about patient-controlled analgesia (PCA)

Teach patient/family fundamental principles of effective pain management (e.g. administering medications as prescribed rather than waiting for PRN dose or a crisis)
Instruct patient/caregiver about the need to have prescriptions, such as opioids, antidepressants, steroids, filled before the last dose(s) of medication
Teach patient (with trach from head/neck cancer)/caregiver infection control measures regarding cleaning cannula, storing supplies, etc.
Others.

Hydration and Nutrition

Assess hydration and nutrition statuses and provide nutritional information/education to patient at risk for poor nutritional status with end-stage lung disease
Teach patient and family to expect decreased nutritional and fluid intakes as disease progresses
Initiate bowel assessment and management program per physician
Assess and manage/expect family concerns related to anorexia, cachexia, such as dry mouth, painful chewing, difficulty speaking, and denture fit/size changes after radiation and therapy
Develop and implement bowel management program to prevent constipation
Teach patient, family, and aide the importance of noting/documenting bowel movements between scheduled nursing visits
Consider stool softeners, and offer laxative(s) of choice, and other methods per patient wishes and physician's orders
Evaluate the patient's bowel patterns and need for stool softeners, laxatives, dietary adjustments (where possible)
Teach and assess regarding prevention and early identification of constipation and its correction/resolution
Other interventions

Comfort, Safety, and Mobility

Teach disposal of sharps

Evaluate patient for specialized support services to avoid pressure ulcers

Patient/caregiver provided with information about oxygen and home safety

Assess relationship of pain to increased safety risks, such as history of falls in the home; counsel regarding safety precautions

Evaluate patient's need for equipment, including supplies to decrease pressure, alternating pressure mattress, gel foam seat cushion, patient lifts and heel and elbow protectors

Teach patient/family about proper body alignment and positioning in bed to prevent skin tears from shearing skin

Observe and assess skin areas for possible breakdown, including heels, hips, elbows, ankles, and other pressure-prone areas

Evaluate home safety and plan to support safety

Offer and provide presence and support

Provide comfort measures of backrub, hand massage, other comfort measures/therapeutic massage

Review backup ventilator support system and emergency backup procedure(s) for patient with ALS on ventilator

Confirm the community emergency preparedness plan for patient

Assess patient for a personal emergency response system (PERS) or other community safety resource(s)

Pain assessment and management each visit

Teach energy conservation techniques

Teach patient about the safe disposal of secretions

Engage patient and support comfort, choice, enjoyment, and dignity

Other interventions

Therapeutic/Medication Regimens

Implement nonpharmacologic interventions with medication schedule, including therapeutic massage, hypnosis, distraction imagery, progressive muscle relaxation, humor, music therapies, biofeedback, others of patient choice

Titrate the dose to achieve pain relief with minimal side effects (per the range specified in the physician's orders)
Teach patient and caregiver use of patient-controlled analgesia (PCA) pump
Teach about and observe for side effects of palliative chemotherapy, including constipation, anemia, fatigue, mouth sores, dry/cracking skin
Medication teaching and management
Provide/set-up patient/caregiver with medication box to facilitate medication planning and adherence
Instruct patient/caregiver about multiple medications, including schedule, functions, routes, rationales for the need for compliance, possible side effects, and what to report
Coordinate/collaborate teaching complex medication schedule with pharmacist, other members of the IDT
Medications changed using equianalgesic conversion tables/ physician orders (e.g., from oral morphine to an equianalgesic dose of transdermal fentanyl)
Instruct in the use of "breakthrough" or "rescue" dosing of pain medications
Others

Emotional/Spiritual Considerations

Provide a psychosocial assessment of the patient and family regarding disease and prognosis
Provide emotional support to patient and family
Evaluate patient for emotional/spiritual distress and other factors impacting pain
Assess mental status and sleep disturbance changes
Assess for and manage plans for psychosocial and/or spiritual pain (e.g., all pain, anxiety, interpersonal distress)
Assess and provide care/support related to depression, changed body image concerns, fever, mouth sores/ulcers, complaints of extreme fatigue, and dry/cracking skin in patient receiving palliative chemotherapy and questioning the meaning of it all

Ongoing acknowledgement of spirituality and related concerns of patient/family
Assess and acknowledge psychosocial aspects of pain and its control (e.g., depression, anxiety) with team support/ interventions
Others

Other Considerations

Assess progression of disease process
Support patient experiencing grieving process (e.g., "normal" eating, breathing, [loss of] spit and ability to smell, change in speaking) with head and neck cancer
Emotional support of patient and caregiver during palliative radiation and chemotherapy
Teach patient and caregiver role in an emergency and what to do, where to go
Other interventions, care, management, based on the patient's condition and unique needs

Home Health Aide

Assist with activities/exercises per case manager and prescribed plan
Safe ADL assistance and support
Observation, record-keeping, and reporting
Report patient complaints of unrelieved, new, or changed pain
Personal care
Meal preparation
Active listening skills
Other activities, tasks as delegated

Physical Therapy

Evaluation
Assess for equipment needs (e.g., Hoyer lift, grab bars, ramp, etc.)
Safety assessment of patient's environment

Teach home exercise program for strengthening and improved ambulation
Teach safe transfer training or bed mobility for patient with pain
Wheelchair and seating assessment
Pain management through various modalities and manual therapy techniques
Provide conditioning exercises
Instruct/supervise caregiver in home exercise program
Teach safe use of assistive devices
Teach fall precautions/protocol
Other interventions

Volunteer Support

Support, friendship, companionship, and presence
Comfort and dignity maintained
Errands and transportation
Advocacy and respite
Other services, based on the IDT recommendations and patient/caregiver needs

Spiritual Counseling

Provide spiritual assessment and care
Provide counseling, intervention, and support related to dimension of life's meaning (consistent with patient's beliefs)
Support, listening, presence
Participation in sacred or spiritual rituals or practices
Other spiritual care, based on the patient's/family's needs and belief systems
Other interventions

Speech-Language Pathology

Evaluate speech and swallowing
Evaluate speech/communication options (e.g., artificial larynx, esophageal speech, voice prosthesis)

Teach care of voice prosthesis, including removal, cleaning, and safe site maintenance
Develop and teach communication system
Establish safe home maintenance program and teach patient/caregiver
Food texture recommendations for safety and optimal nutrition
Collaborate with dietitian/nutritionist, other IDT members
Other interventions

Occupational Therapy

Evaluation
Assess for home modifications as needed for safety and maximum functional independence
Instruct in safety and use of adaptive equipment and assistive devices for maximum independence in ADL
Instruct in energy conservation for maximum independent functioning
Teach home exercise program for maximum functional activity level
Instruct and establish home program for functional positioning and/or use of splints/other supports to prevent skin problems
Other interventions

Medical Social Services

Evaluate/assess as patient's financial/other problems adversely impact the POC and impede progress toward identified goals (e.g., cannot afford nutritional supplements, medications, supplies)
Initiate linkage with community services and resources
Psychosocial assessment of patient, including understanding of/adjustment to illness and its implications
Assess psychosocial factors impacting patient/caregiver, including adjustment to illness, changed roles, and implications

Identify optimal coping strategies and strengths
Assess finances/resources and provide counseling regarding food acquisition, patient's ability to prepare meals, and costs of needed medications
Provide patient and family emotional/spiritual support
Assess fear, depression, anxiety
Facilitate communications among patient, family, and hospice team
Provide grief counseling and intervention related to illness/loss
Identify caregiver role strain necessitating respite/relief measures, additional support for family
Identify illness-related psychiatric conditions necessitating support, care, and intervention(s)
Other interventions

Bereavement Counseling

Assess needs of the bereaved family and friends
Provide presence and counseling
Initiate supportive bereavement visits, follow-up, and other interventions (e.g., mailings, telephone calls)
Other interventions

Dietary Counseling

Nutritional evaluation of patient for achievement of optimal nutrition and hydration in patient with severe SOB, anorexia, and weight loss
Comprehensive nutritional assessment and plan
Supportive counseling with patient/family indicating that patient will have a decreased appetite and possible inability to eat/drink
Assess/recommendations for swallowing difficulties, nausea, vomiting, and constipation associated with pain medications
Support and care with food and nourishment as desired by patient
Coordinate/collaborate with speech-language pathologist and other IDT members

Food and dietary recommendations incorporate patient choice and wishes
Other interventions

Pharmacy Services

Assess complex medication regimen and plan for team and patient education related to medication(s)/drug therapy
Monitor medications for therapeutic levels and dosages
Perform pain consult and provide input into interdisciplinary plan of care related to pain control, palliation, and optimal symptom management
Assess medication regimen for safety, efficacy, and drug/drug, drug/food interactions
Assess medication regimen and plan for safety and compliance
Other interventions

Music, Massage Art, and Other Therapies or Services

Evaluate/intervene based on patient and caregiver's unique wishes and needs that support care, comfort, and death in the setting of the patient's choice
Assess plan to engage patient and support comfort, quality of life, enjoyment, dignity, and pain/symptom relief
Provide pet therapy per patient choice, including patient's pet(s) if patient is in an inpatient facility
Other interventions

7. Patient, Family, and Caregiver Educational Needs

Educational needs are the daily and ongoing care regimens that contribute to safe and effective care between the hospice team's home visits. These include:

The basic tenets of hospice and the availability of care 24 hours a day, 7 days a week
How to reach/access the on-call system and what to say

The patient's specific daily self-care activities
The patient/caregiver's role in emergency preparedness
The importance of follow-up with health care providers
The specific signs, symptoms, and problems that necessitate calling health care providers or emergency services
Effective hand washing and other aspects of infection control
Information about the disease process and what to expect
Support groups and community resources
Other information and education, specific to the patient/caregiver

8. Tips to Support Medical Necessity, Quality, and Reimbursement

The patient should meet all the criteria of the hospice before admission (e.g., caregiver, prognosis) and throughout service. Specifically describe your assessments and interventions. Since pain management is such an integral part of hospice and palliative care, document especially the description (e.g., aching, sharp, bony, radiating), the location, the duration, the onset, the intensity, where it ranks on the organization's standardized pain tool, and other information. Keep in mind that this detail assists in painting a picture for any reviewer or payer as they make determinations on a particular patient's care.

- Document the specific care provided, the plan for the next visit, and the patient's response to the care.
- The clinical documentation (e.g., visit notes, POC) must be congruent and show the same clinical information.
- Document the specific reason(s) the patient is homebound in functional terms if patient is admitted to home care. (Medicare-certified hospices do not have homebound as admission criteria).
- Specify in the documentation any learning barriers.

- Document laboratory and other objective test findings that assist in painting a picture of the progress toward goal achievement (or deterioration).
- Document any identified barriers to learning-remember there is no requirement that the patient learn if he or she does not wish to learn.
- Document care coordination; communications with other team members, the physician, family members, etc.
- For emergency preparedness as well as numerous other reasons patients must assume responsibility for their own care long-term. It is always prudent to teach someone else in the home the patient's care regimen or, if the patient lives alone, a friend in the neighborhood or someone else of the patient's choosing.
- Document the specific supplies used as directed by your manager.
- Remember that many supplies are included as a part of the per day Medicare reimbursement rate.

For an interdisciplinary/care planning source for hospice, readers are referred to the *Hospice and Palliative Care Handbook: Quality, Documentation, and Reimbursement* (Mosby). For a flyer or more information, call 1-800-997-6397.

9. Evidence-Based and other Resources for Practice and Education

The Agency for Healthcare Research and Quality (AHRQ) (www.ahrq.gov) (1-800-335-9100) offers clinical practice guidelines on pain management.

The American Academy of Hospice and Palliative Medicine (www.aahpm.org) provides position statements and other resources regarding important issues related to hospice and palliative care.

The American Hospice Foundation (www.americanhospice.org) offers free publications, including "Talking About Hospice: Tips for Nurses," "Providing Care at Home: Can I Do It?" as well as select publications translated in Spanish.

Americans for Better Care of the Dying (www.abcd-caring.org) (1-703-647-8505) provides resources concerning public policy and hospice, and has useful links to other hospice resources.

The Center to Advance Palliative Care (www.getpalliativecare.org) has a new website which provides information for patients and families about what palliative care consists of, options for palliative care, and a page to help the patient/family decide if palliative care is the right choice. There are also other handouts, including "What should you know about palliative care."

Children's Hospice International (www.chionline.org) (1-800-242-4453) offers information about children's hospice, palliative care, and end-of-life care services and how to locate a program near you. There are also publications available both for families and professionals.

City of Hope Pain/Palliative Care Resource Center (*www.cityofhope.org/prc*) disseminates information and resources to assist others in improving the quality of pain management and end-of-life care. The site contains a variety of materials, including pain assessment tools, patient education materials, and end-of-life resources.

The Commission on Aging With Dignity (www.agingwithdignity.org) (1-800-594-7437 or 850-681-2010) offers a living will, "Five Wishes," for $5.00 a copy. Five Wishes is a living will and a durable power of attorney for health care, valid in most states, and addresses an individual's medical wishes, and also personal, emotional, and spiritual needs. The project was supported by a grant from The Robert Wood Johnson Foundation.

Compassionate Friends (www.compassionatefriends.org) (1-877-969-0010) is an organization which offers grief support for families after the death of a child. Chapters across the country hope to offer families an opportunity to work towards a positive resolution after the loss of a child of any age.

The Dougy Center for Grieving Children and Families (www.dougy.org) (1-866-775-5683) offers support for children, teenagers, and their families when dealing with the death of a loved one. Sections are specifically tailored for adults who want to help a grieving child, children, teens, and those working with students. This information is available through their website and centers across the country.

Dying Well (www.dyingwell.org) provides resources for people facing life-limiting illness, their families, and their professional caregivers.

The Hospice and Palliative Nurses Association (www.hpna.org) (1-412-787-9301) offers news and information on their site for caregivers, including tip sheets on skin care, dementia, and recognizing pain, and patient teaching sheets on "Hospice and Palliative Care," "Managing Pain," "Managing Anxiety" and more.

The Hospice Foundation of America (www.hospicefoundation.org) (1-800-854-3402) has information on hospice goals and care, grieving, and publications and videos for families and professionals. Also available on their website is their Hospice Foundation of America E-Newsletter which features updates on news and events regarding hospice care in the U.S.

The National Consensus Project (www.nationalconsensusproject.org) is an initiative to improve the delivery of palliative care in the U.S. Clinical Practice Guidelines describe core components of clinical palliative care programs, and are available for download.

The National Hospice and Palliative Care Organization at (www.nhpco.org) (1-703-243-5900) offers information for professionals, patients and caregivers.

www.Pain-Topics.org website provides free access to evidence-based clinical news, information, research, and education on the causes and effective treatment of the many types of pain.

Palliative Care Matters (www.pallcare.info) is designed for professionals working in hospice.

Booklet Resources:

Barbara Karnes Books, Inc. offers informational booklets on their website including: "Gone From My Sight—The Dying Experience," "My Friend, I Care," and "A Time to Live." All are available in English and Spanish and "Gone From My Sight" is also offered in Russian, French and Italian. They are $2.00 plus shipping and handling. This booklet and others are available on their site, *http://www.bkbooks.com*, or by writing to B.K. Books, P.O. Box 822139, Vancouver, WA 98682.

Palliative Care: Complete Care Everyone Deserves. This 16-page booklet is produced by the National Alliance for Caregiving (NAC) and Friends and Relatives of Institutionalized Aged (FRIA) of New York. A free copy of the booklet may be obtained by sending an e-mail to *info@caregiving.org*. The booklet may also be downloaded NAC's website, *www.caregiving.org/care.pdf* and FRIA's website at *www.fria.org*.

Book Resources:

Heffner, J.E., & Byock, I. (2002) Palliative and end-of-life pearls. Hanley & Belfus.

Kuebler, K.K., Berry, P.H., & Heidrich, D.E. (2007) Palliative & end-of-life care: Clinical practice guidelines (2nd ed.). Saunders.

Marrelli, T.M. (2007) Hospice and palliative care handbook: Quality, compliance and reimbursement (2nd ed.). Mosby: www.marrelli.com

Marrelli, T.M. (2008) Home health aide: Guidelines for care. Marrelli. (Aide Handbook and Instructor Manual) www.marrelli.com

Matzo, M.L., & Sherman, D.W. (2003) Gerontologic palliative care nursing. Mosby.

PART FIVE

MATERNAL/CHILD CARE

Clinical Guidelines for Assessment, Care Planning, and Documentation

5

ACQUIRED IMMUNE DEFICIENCY SYNDROME (AIDS) (CARE OF THE CHILD WITH)

1. General Considerations

AIDS affects three primary groups in the pediatric population: (1) infants who were exposed in utero or in the birth process; (2) children and adolescents who received blood or blood products before the blood supply was adequately tested (e.g., hemophiliacs); and (3) adolescents who acquired the disease primarily through sexual contact or injection drug use, including steroids. Since the beginning of the epidemic, 9441 children have been reported with AIDS. In 2005, 93 children with AIDS were reported to CDC, and most of these children (91 percent) were infected perinatally. Another 4 percent acquired HIV from a transfusion of blood or blood products, and another 2 percent acquired HIV from transfusion because of hemophilia.

Home care efforts in the care of these children are ultimately directed toward supportive care, infection control, and disease prevention.

2. Potential Diagnoses and Codes

The diagnoses and codes listed here include some of the most common conditions seen in children with AIDS, and have been alphabetized for easy identification. Check your state regulations related to AID/HIV coding as primary. If there are no restrictions, code HIV first followed by the associated complication. Keep in mind that the ICD-9-CM system requires a focused review of the patient's medical information in addition to the physician-assigned diagnoses. Should additional information be needed, refer to the coding books or a qualified coder.

AIDS (general)	042
Anemia	042 and 285.9
Candidiasis	042 and 112.XX
Cervical cancer, unspecified	042 and 180.9
Chorioretinitis, unspecified	042 and 363.20
Cytomegalovirus	042 and 078.5
Cytomegalovirus retinitis	042, 078.5, 363.20
Diarrhea	042 and 787.91
Encephalitis	042 and 323.9
Encephalopathy, due to AIDS	042 and 348.3X
Endocarditis	042 and 424.90
Esophagitis	042 and 530.10
Failure to thrive	042 and 783.41
Herpes simplex	042 and 054.9
Herpes zoster	042 and 053.9
Histoplasmosis	042 and 115.90
Kaposi's sarcoma	042 and 176.9
Lymphocytic interstitial pneumonia	042 and 516.8
Meningitis	042 and 322.9
Mycobacterium avium intracellulare, pulmonary	042 and 031.0
Neurological developmental delays, unspecified	042 and 315.9
Neuropathy, peripheral	042 and 357.4
Neutropenia	042 and 288.0
Peripheral neuropathy	042 and 357.4
Pneumocystosis carinii pneumonia	042 and 136.3
Pneumonia (bacterial)	042 and 482.9
Pneumonia (NOS)	042 and 486
Pneumonia (viral)	042 and 480.9
Polymyositis	042 and 710.4
Polyradiculoneuropathy	042 and 357.0
Quadriplegia	042 and 344.0X
Retinal detachment, unspecified	042 and 361.9
Retinal hemorrhage	042 and 362.81
Seizures	042 and 780.39
Sepsis	042 and 038.9
Shigella	042 and 004.9
Shigella, dysentery	042 and 004.0
Thrombocytopenia	042 and 287.5
Toxoplasmosis	042 and 130.9
Tuberculosis (pulmonary)	042 and 011.90
Wasting syndrome	042 and 799.4
Others	

5

5

3. Associated Nursing Diagnoses (see Part Seven)

4. Supportive Factors for the Determination and Documentation of Homebound Status

The homebound factor may or may not be a criterion for admission, based on the managed care program or third-party payer involved. However, the following are reasons the child with AIDs might be homebound:

Oxygen therapy
Fatigue
Dyspnea
Infection control, protecting child from further infection
Pain or other symptoms necessitating care at home
Medically weak and fragile
Severe immune suppression
Weakness
Others

5. Potential Goals and Outcomes

The following patient-centered goals/outcomes can be individualized according to the identified needs of the patient and family.

Nursing

Parent/child verbalizes satisfaction with care
Support growth and developmental tasks of childhood through illness
Successful pain and symptom management as verbalized by patient/caregiver
Patient will demonstrate adequate breathing patterns as evidenced by a lack of respiratory distress symptoms
Patient will be comfortable through illness
Patient/caregiver will demonstrate ____ percent compliance with instructions related to care

Patient and caregiver demonstrate and practice effective hand washing and other infection-control measures (specify, e.g., disposal of waste, cleaning linens, other aspects of care at home)
Adherence to POC by patient and caregivers and able to demonstrate safe and supportive care of child
Nutritional needs maintained/addressed as evidenced by patient's weight maintained/increased by ____ lbs.
Patient's pulmonary status will be maintained/improved
Patient/partner/caregiver integrating information and care regarding implications of disease and chronic/terminal nature
Laboratory values (specify) will be improved/within normal limits (WNL) for child
Patient's catheter will remain patent and infection free
Patient/caregiver adheres to/demonstrates compliance with multiple medication regimens (e.g., times, storage, refrigeration)
Patient's and family's educational and support needs met as verbalized by caregiver and adherence to plan
Palliative, curative, and symptomatic interventions to ensure optimal level of functioning in child
Other

Home Health Aide
Effective personal care and hygiene
ADL assistance
Safe home environment maintained
Other

Medical Social Services
Financial/access problems addressed, resources identified as demonstrated by food in the refrigerator and medication availability to patient
Plan of care implementation as validated by parent/other team members

Linkage with community services, support groups, and other resources
Other

Occupational Therapy

Home modifications for safety will be arranged for completion by ____ (date)
Patient/caregiver achieves maximum independence and safety with ADL within pain tolerance through instructions in use of assistive techniques and assistive devices by ____ (date)
Patient/caregiver demonstrates effective use of energy conservation and diaphragmatic breathing by ____ (date)
Patient/caregiver will be independent with program for positioning patient effectively to minimize pain
Optional function maintained
Other

Physical Therapy

Patient using home exercise program taught and has _____ percent increase in mobility/strength
Increased function and mobility; patient/caregiver able to perform exercise program by _____ (date)
Increased endurance as verbalized by patient/caregiver
Other

Speech-Language Pathology

Safe swallowing with decreased pain
Swallowing improved with decreased problems, verbalized by patient/caregiver
Recommended food list/textures for safety
Others

Dietary Counseling

Nutrition and hydration optimal for child
Weight maintained/gain _____ lbs.
Weight stable for patient
Other

Pharmacist

Multiple medication regimens reviewed for food/drug and drug/drug interactions and problems

Medications and blood level laboratory reports reviewed for therapeutic dosage and safe, effective patient response and reported to physician

Stability and safety in complex multiple medication regimens

Other

6. Skills, Interventions/Services, and Management

Home care clinicians must exercise acute and effective critical thinking, observation, technical, teaching and evaluation skills when performing clinical assessments, interventions, and management of their home care patients.

Nursing

Comprehensive assessment of all systems of infant/child admitted to home care for ____ (specify problem necessitating care)

Instruct parents and caregivers regarding safety and universal precautions in the home

Assess pulmonary status, including dyspnea, changed or abnormal breath sounds, retractions, respiratory rate, flaring, and other symptoms of respiratory compromise

Observe and assess all systems and symptoms every visit

Report changes or new symptoms to physician

Teach parents and caregivers all aspects of wound care, including safe disposal of dressing supplies

Instruct on pet care, avoidance of cross contamination, check with physician on certain types of pets

Weigh patient each visit and review food intake diary

Instruct parents or caregivers regarding prescribed diet

Assess and monitor child's use of and response to aerosol therapy medication

Assess child for candidal diaper rash or oral thrush

Teach child and parents safe use of oxygen therapy

Monitor for adverse effects of medication, particularly steroids

Evaluate caregiving ability, particularly if parents or other caregivers are HIV+

Monitor child's blood pressure and other vital signs

Teach parents and caregivers about new medications

Teach parents and caregivers about the importance of optimal hydration and nutrition

Instruct child, parents, and caregivers in all aspects of effective hand washing techniques and proper care of bodily fluids and excretions

Provide emotional support to child and caregivers with chronic/terminal illness and associated implications, especially if a parent is HIV+

Monitor parenteral feeding catheter site for infection and other problems

Instruct parents and caregivers to call physician for symptoms of fever, increased irritability, vomiting, diarrhea, suspected ear or other infection, decreased appetite, new cough, or any new symptom or complaint

Instruct parents regarding the need to isolate HIV+ child from anyone with known infections, such as other children at school who have chickenpox, measles, or other communicable infections that are life threatening for the child with AIDS

Teach parents and caregivers regarding all aspects of child's needed care for safe and effective management at home

Instruct parents or caregivers on all aspects of medications, including schedule, functions, and side effects

Instruct parents or caregivers regarding signs and symptoms that necessitate calling RN or physician

Observe and assess child with an impaired immune response and multiple system infections

Provide support to child with new tumor, necessitating surgery, chemotherapy, or radiation

Address sexuality concerns with young adolescent with AIDS and the importance of safe sexual expression, including the use of condoms, abstinence, or other techniques
Assess the child's unique response to treatments and interventions and to report changes, unfavorable responses, or reactions to the physician
Assess grief, denial, and guilt of parents and caregivers
Other interventions

Home Health Aide
Personal care
Respite care for relief of family and caregivers
Homemaker services to assist caregiver
Activities of daily living (ADL) assistance
Other activities/tasks as assigned

Medical Social Services
Evaluation of psychosocial factors of the child and family with a chronic and terminal illness
Financial assessment and counseling
Emotional support to child, family, and caregivers
Referral to community resources (e.g., entitlement, nutrition assistance, early intervention/school)
Other interventions

Occupational Therapy
Evaluation
Assess for home modifications for safety and maximum functional independence
Instruct in safety and use of adaptive techniques and assistive devices for maximum independence in ADL
Instruct in energy conservation and diaphragmatic breathing for decreased shortness of breath (SOB) and for maximum independent functioning
Teach home exercise program for maximum upper extremity function

Instruct and establish home program for functional positioning and/or use of splints and/or other devices for minimal pain
Adaptive or assistive devices/supplies as indicated to meet child's needs
Other interventions

Physical Therapy

Evaluation
Home exercise program
Other interventions

Speech-Language Pathology

Evaluation for swallowing problem
Other interventions

Dietary Counseling

Assessment of child with difficulty swallowing and low weight and intake
Other interventions

Pharmacist

Evaluation of child's multiple medication regimens for possible food/drug or drug/drug interaction; medication monitoring regarding therapeutic blood levels and dosages
Other interventions

7. Safety Considerations and Discharge Plans

Infection control/universal precautions
Night-light
Medication safety and storage
Infant/child safety (e.g., car seat, electrical outlets)

Symptoms that necessitate immediate reporting/assistance
Safety related to home medical equipment
Smoke detector and fire evacuation plan
Patient maintained in comfort and safety of home with adequate hydration, nutrition, hygiene, and other needs met by family and caregiver
Discharge with caregivers taught and able to manage patient safely in home under physician supervision
Others, based on the patient's unique condition and environment

8. Tips to Support Medical Necessity, Quality, and Reimbursement

Document any variances to expected outcomes. AIDS is usually not what the home care nurse is specifically addressing. The care provided is directed toward symptom and infection control and treatment. These children and adolescents are usually so ill that there are many skills the professional nurse provides.

Document the coordination occurring among team members based on the POC. The interdisciplinary conference notes should be reflected in the clinical record. Refer to these meetings or communications on any form used by third-party payers (e.g., your program's update form).

In addition:
Write the specific care and teaching instructions provided
Document patient's progress toward goals
Document any exacerbation of symptoms that necessitated another visit and be sure there is a physician order for that visit
Document all POC changes
Document all interactions/communications with the physician

Document the skills used in the provision of professional nursing care practice when caring for the child (e.g., teaching, training, observation, assessment, catheters, IV site care, venipuncture)

9. Tips for Communication with Insurance Case Manager

Present objective patient findings and changes since last update

Meet face-to-face for relationship building when possible

Often these children are closely case managed to identify problems early on; communicate information about the child's and family's statuses and course of care necessitating intervention

Discuss other measurable changes and information that communicate the status of the child and the need for skilled home care services

10. Evidence-Based and other Resources for Practice and Education

www.aidsinfo.nih.gov offers government resource organizations and information. There is a hotline for educational/other information, clinical trial information and telephone consultation.

The Center for Disease Control and Prevention's (CDC) National Prevention Information Network (formerly the AIDS Clearinghouse) (www.cdcnpin.org or 1-800-458-5231) offers information and publications. Resources include a 35-page booklet entitled "Caring for Someone with AIDS at Home." The CDC also offers a National AIDS Hotline: 1-800-342-AIDS (1-800-342-2437).

The Health Resources and Services Administration (HRSA) can be reached at 1-800-ASK-HRSA (1-800-275-4772) or http://hab.hrsa.gov and has information available.

One such resource includes "A Clinical Guide on Supportive and Palliative Care for People with HIV/AIDS" (2003).

The Make-A-Wish Foundation (www.wish.org or 1-800-722-WISH [9474]) fulfills special wishes for children suffering from life-threatening illnesses and their families.

Positively Aware, a journal of the Test Positive Aware Network (TPAN) (www.tpan.com or 1-773-989-9400) provides information on AIDS/HIV medical developments, drug interactions, and more.

Book Resource: McGoldrick, M. (2007). Infection Prevention and Control Program. Saint Simons Island, GA: Home Heath Systems. (www.homecareandhospice.com)

Book Resource: Rhinehart, E., McGoldrick, M. (2006). Infection Control in Home Care and Hospice. Sudbury, MA: Jones and Bartlett. (www.homecareandhospice.com)

ANTEPARTAL CARE

1. General Considerations

The antepartal patient referred to home health care usually has an associated medical problem, such as hypertension or hyperemesis gravidarum that necessitates the initial referral for follow-up.

2. Potential Diagnoses and Codes

The diagnoses and codes listed here include some of the most common conditions seen in antepartal home care patients, and have been alphabetized for easy identification. Keep in mind that the ICD-9-CM system requires a focused review of the patient's medical information in addition to the physician-assigned diagnoses. Should additional information be needed, refer to the coding books or a qualified coder.

Diagnosis	Code
Antepartum bleeding	641.93
Asthma	648.93 and 493.90
Dehydration	276.51
Diabetes, gestational	648.83
Fluid and electrolyte imbalance	276.9
Hyperemesis gravidarum, mild	643.03
Hypertension, complicating pregnancy	642.93
Multiple gestation unspecified	651.93
Pelvic inflammatory disease	646.63 and 614.9
Preeclampsia	642.43
Pregnancy state, incidental	V22.2
Pregnancy, high risk, unspecified	V23.9
Preterm labor	644.03
Urinary tract infection	646.63 and 599.0
Venous, superficial, thrombosis	671.23
Venous, deep, thrombosis	671.33
Others	

3. Associated Nursing Diagnoses (see Part Seven)

4. Supportive Factors for the Determination and Documentation of Homebound Status

The homebound factor may or may not be a criterion for admission, based on the managed care program or the third-party payer involved. However, the following are reasons the antepartal patient might be homebound:

Bed rest with bathroom privileges only
Weakness, legs to be elevated
Decreased activity
Home confinement because of medical problems
Receiving IV care for hyperemesis

5. Potential Goals and Outcomes

The following patient-centered goals/outcomes can be individualized according to the identified needs of the patient and family.

Nursing

Patient/caregiver verbalizes satisfaction with care
Behavioral compliance with home care regimen
Patient symptoms will be controlled to obtain adequate rest (8 to 10 hr/24 hr)
Patient compliant with program of bed rest and delivers healthy full-term infant (specify EDC)
Patient/caregiver will demonstrate _____ percent behavioral compliance with instructions related to medications, diet, and bed rest
Optimal circulation and nutrition for essentially bedbound patient
Mother returned to self-care with healthy infant
Adherence to POC by patient and caregiver and able to demonstrate safe and supportive care

Optimal nutrition/hydration needs maintained/addressed as evidenced by patient's weight maintained/decreased/ increased by _____ pounds

Patient will be maintained in home stating/demonstrating adherence to POC

Successful tocolysis, prolongation of pregnancy to term

Blood pressure stable for patient (specify parameters)

Episodes of emesis decreasing and patient verbalizing feeling better by (specify date)

Laboratory values (specify) will be improved/WNL for patient

Patient/caregiver verbalizes signs/symptoms that necessitate calling the physician and need intervention/ follow-up

Other

Home Health Aide

Effective and safe personal care and hygiene

Safe ADL assistance

Safe home environment maintained

Other

Medical Social Services

Resource identification and financial situation assessed/ addressed, allowing for successful implementation of the ordered POC

Financial/access problems addressed, resources identified as demonstrated by food in the refrigerator and medication availability to patient per POC

Linkage to community services, support groups, and other resources for continued support

Other

6. Skills, Interventions/Services, and Management

Home care clinicians must exercise acute and effective critical thinking, observation, technical, teaching, and evaluation skills when performing clinical assessments, interventions, and management of their home care patients.

Nursing

Comprehensive assessment of all systems of patient admitted to home care for _____ (specify problem necessitating care)
Teach patient and family regarding ordered diet therapy
Teach patient and family regarding decreased sodium diet
Assess physical signs and symptoms of fluid status (e.g., vital signs [VS], weight, skin and mucous membrane condition)
Teach patient safe, correct use of home uterine monitor
Teach patient and family regarding vitamin therapy
Teach patient and family regarding exercise and rest period needs
Instruct patient regarding the potential complications of IV therapy and actions to take
Teach patient and family regarding expected physiological changes
Teaching related to uterine activity monitoring
Teach patient and family regarding symptoms that need immediate physician notification
Teach signs of preterm labor and other symptoms or changes that necessitate notifying the physician and being seen immediately (e.g., bleeding, premature rupture of membranes)
Teach need for optimal nutrition and frequent rest periods
Teach rationale and need for bed rest
Monitor amount and site(s) of edema
Weigh daily and record
Dipstick urine for protein
Emotional support for patient and family
Teach patient self-observational skills (weights, results of urine dipsticks, edema, etc.)
Teaching related to the proper use of equipment and administration of infusion therapy
Other interventions

Home Health Aide

Personal care
ADL assistance
Other activities/tasks as assigned

Medical Social Services

Psychosocial assessment
Problem identifications
Financial counseling assistance, referral(s) to community resources as indicated
Other interventions

7. Safety Considerations and Discharge Plans

Infection control/universal precautions
Night-light
Medication safety and storage
If home infusion patient, access to telephone, refrigerator, adequate electricity
Symptoms that necessitate immediate reporting/assistance
Safety related to home medical equipment
Smoke detector and fire evacuation plan
Delivery of healthy infant
Self-care in the community, under physician's supervision
Others, based on the patient's unique condition and environment

8. Tips to Support Medical Necessity, Quality, and Reimbursement

Document any variances to expected outcomes
Document any abnormal blood pressure findings, protein in urine, or blood results
Document communications with physician in clinical record
Document the care given and the actions of that care
Document the specific teaching accomplished and the behavioral outcomes of that teaching

9. Tips for Communication with Insurance Case Manager

Present objective patient findings and changes since last update
Meet face-to-face for relationship building when possible
Communicate information about the interventions and the patient's response to the care
Discuss other measurable changes and information that communicate the status of the patient and the need for skilled home care services

10. Evidence-Based and other Resources for Practice and Education

HRSA's Maternal and Child Health (www.ask.hrsa.gov/MCH.cfm or 1-888-275-4772) programs promote and improve the health of mothers, infants, children, and adolescents, including low-income families, those with diverse racial and ethnic heritages, and those living in rural or isolated areas without access to care. Materials include topics related to health care, prenatal care and newborn screening, preventive care and research, and more.

MotherRisk (www.motherisk.org) or 1-416-813-6780 in Toronto offers information on conditions during pregnancy, substance abuse, and publications such as "Cancer in Pregnancy; Maternal and Fetal Risks" for women, family, and professionals There are also MotherRisk hotlines: 1-877-327-4636 for the alcohol and substance abuse helpline, 1-800-436-8477 for "morning sickness" information and treatments, or 1-888-246-5840 for the HIV and HIV treatment in pregnancy line.

5

CANCER (CARE OF THE CHILD WITH)

1. General Considerations

Cancer is the second leading cause of death in children aged 1 to 19, surpassed only by death from injuries. The incidence of cancer in children aged 0 to 14 in 2003 was 8530 (14.6/100,000), and there were 1543 deaths (2.5/100,000). Leukemias are the most common cancers diagnosed in children.

Cancer care in children utilizes all facets of nursing skills. Death at any age is sad, but the suffering and death of children magnify the emotional turmoil. Parents know their child best and in this role they are the teachers for care providers. Parental control should be maintained as much as possible.

2. Potential Diagnoses and Codes

The diagnoses and codes listed here include some of the most common conditions seen in children with cancer, and have been alphabetized for easy identification. Keep in mind that the ICD-9-CM system requires a focused review of the patient's medical information in addition to the physician-assigned diagnoses. Should additional information be needed, refer to the coding books or a qualified coder.

Diagnosis	Code
Acute lymphocytic leukemia	204.0X
Acute myelogenous leukemia	205.0X
Aplastic anemia	284.9
Astrocytoma, unspecified site	191.9
Chronic leukemia	208.1X
Chronic myelogenous leukemia	205.1X
Leukopenia	288.0
Neuroblastoma, unspecified site	194.0
Wilms' tumor	189.0
Others	

3. Associated Nursing Diagnoses (see Part Seven)

4. Supportive Factors for the Determination and Documentation of Homebound Status

The homebound factor is not usually a criterion for this patient population; however, the following are the most common reasons the child would be homebound:

Infection protection
Pain
Severe fatigue
SOB during any activity
Medical restrictions to home because of low blood count

NOTE: If the child is in an insurance hospice program, this requirement is usually waived

5. Potential Goals and Outcomes

The following patient-centered goals/outcomes can be individualized according to the identified needs of the patient and family.

Nursing

Support developmental tasks of childhood
Patient/caregiver verbalizes satisfaction with care
Educational tools/plans incorporated in daily care and child/ caregiver verbalizes understanding of safe, needed care
Patient/parent decides on care, interventions, and evaluation
Caregiver effective in care management and knows whom to call for questions/concerns
Parent/caregiver will express satisfaction with hospice or other support received and will experience increased comfort
Child will be made comfortable at home through death in accordance with the patient's wishes
Effective pain control and symptom control communicated by child

Parent/caregiver verbalizes understanding of and adheres to care and medication regimens
Child and family supported through patient's death
Comfort maintained through course of care
The patient and family receive support and care, and family members and friends are able to spend quality time with the patient
Child/caregivers supported through and receive the maximum benefit from surgery, chemotherapy, and/or radiation
Patient/caregiver lists adverse reactions, potential complications, signs/symptoms of infection (e.g., sputum change, chest congestion)
Comfort maintained through death with dignity
Patient has stable respiratory status with patent airway (e.g., no dyspnea, infection-free)
Patient protected from injury and compliant with medication, safety, and care regimens
Comfort and individualized intervention of child with cancer
Spiritual and psychosocial needs met (specify) as defined by child/parent/caregiver throughout course of care
Other

Home Health Aide

Effective and safe personal care and hygiene maintained
Safe ADL assistance
Respite and increased comfort
Other

Medical Social Services

Child/caregiver will cope adaptively with illness and death
Identification and addressing/resolution of problems impeding the successful implementation of the POC
Adaptive adjustment of child to changed body/image
Psychosocial support and counseling offered/initiated to patient and caregivers experiencing grief (if appropriate)
Other

6. Skills, Interventions/Services, and Management

Home care clinicians must exercise acute and effective critical thinking, observation, technical, teaching, and evaluation skills when performing clinical assessments, interventions, and management of their home care patients. Pain management and support/respite for the caregiver(s) are a major focus.

Nursing

Parent/caregiver provided with home safety information and instruction related to _____ and documented in the clinical record
Assess pain and other symptoms
Teach care of the patient
Measure vital signs
Assess cardiovascular, pulmonary, and respiratory status
Assess nutrition and hydration status
Teach new pain and symptom control medication
Diet counseling for patient with anorexia
Check for and remove impaction as needed
Indwelling catheter as indicated
Teach feeding tube care to family and caregiver
Teach caregivers symptom and relief measures
Assess weight as ordered
Measure abdominal girth for ascites and edema, document sites and amount
Oxygen at _____ liter per _____
Assess mental status, sleep disturbance changes
Obtain venipuncture as ordered q _____
Teach medication regimen, including schedule, route, functions, and side effects
Teach importance of around-the-clock medications for pain control
Instruct re: the availability of hospice and other support services for the patient, parents, and caregivers
Pressure ulcer care as indicated

Assess for electrolyte imbalance
Teach catheter care to caregiver
Assess amount and frequency of urinary output
Teach family regarding safety
Teach patient and family regarding conservation of energy techniques
Provide emotional support to patient and family
Anticipate and encourage patient and family input into care regimen(s)
Assess patient's and family's coping skills
Teach symptom control for side effects of radiation or chemotherapy
Teach the importance of optimal nutrition and hydration
Teach caregivers observational aspects of care, including fever, bleeding, bruising, and other signs unique to the disease or treatment, and what to report to care provider
Monitor for seizure activity and perform neurological checks each visit
Teach the importance of effective hand washing and other infection control measures, including the avoidance of infection when possible
Provide emotional support to child and family with chronic or terminal illness and associated implications
Instruct caregiver to call physician for symptoms of fever, irritability, vomiting, diarrhea, suspected ear or other infection, decreased appetite, cough, or other complaint
Assess the child's unique response to treatments and interventions and to report changes or unfavorable responses or reactions to physician
Other interventions

Home Health Aide

Effective personal care
ADL activities
Other tasks/activities as assigned

Medical Social Services

Psychosocial assessment of family with child who has cancer
Problem evaluation
Financial assistance counseling
Support to patient and family
Community resource referral(s) (American Cancer Society, Ronald McDonald House, etc.)
Other interventions

7. Safety Considerations and Discharge Plans

Infection control/universal precautions
Night-light
Medication safety and storage
Child safety considerations (e.g., car seat, electrical outlets)
Symptoms that necessitate immediate reporting/assistance
Safety related to home medical equipment
Smoke detector and fire evacuation plan
Status stable
Discharged when goals achieved
Patient death with dignity maintained and family present
Admitted to acute care facility for 24-hour care
Patient discharged, family able to manage care, under physician's supervision
Referred to pediatric hospice program
Others, based on the patient's unique condition and environment

8. Tips to Support Medical Necessity, Quality, and Reimbursement

Document all care rendered and the outcomes of that care
Document any patient changes and communications with the physician
Document home care in lieu of hospitalization, when applicable

9. Tips for Communication with Insurance Case Manager

Present objective patient findings and changes since last update
Meet face-to-face for relationship building when possible
Communicate information about the interventions and the child's response to the care
Discuss other measurable changes and information that communicate the status of the patient and the need for skilled home care services

10. Evidence-Based and other Resources for Practice and Education

The Agency for Healthcare Research and Quality (AHRQ) (www.ahrq.gov or 1-800-358-9295) offers "Acute Pain Management in Infants, Children, and Adolescents: Operative or Medical Procedures and Trauma (Quick Reference Guide for Clinicians)" (AHCPR 92-0020).
The American Cancer Society (www.cancer.org) (1-800-227-2345) offers information and support groups for children and adolescents with cancer.
The Brain Tumor Society (www.tbts.org or 1-800-770-8287) has information on healthy eating habits and programs such as COPE for patient support.
Children's Hospice International (www.chionline.org or 1-800-242-4453) has information on children's hospice, palliative care, and end-of-life care services and how to locate a program near you. Publications are also available for families and professionals.
The City of Hope National Medical Center (www.cityofhope.org or 1-626-256-4673) offers information on adult and pediatric cancers of all sorts for patients and caregivers, families, and professionals. Information pages on each type of cancer include what the cancer is, what parts of the body the cancer affects and how, and what each stage

of the cancer involves. Information is also available on treatment, patient referral options, and current trials.

Compassionate Friends (www.compassionatefriends.org or 1-877-969-0010) is an organization which offers grief support for families after the death of a child. Chapters across the country hope to offer families an opportunity to work towards a positive resolution after the loss of a child of any age.

The Dougy Center for Grieving Children and Families (www.dougy.org or 1-866-775-5683) offers support for children, teenagers, and their families when dealing with the death of a loved one. Sections are specifically tailored for adults who want to help a grieving child, children, teens, and those working with students. This information is offered through the website and centers across the country.

The Make-A-Wish Foundation (www.wish.org or 1-800-722-WISH [9474]) fulfills special wishes for children with a life-threatening illness and their families.

SuperSibs (www.supersibs.org or 1-866-444-SIBS [7427]) offers support for siblings of children with cancer including scholarships, grief support, and resources for siblings and parents of children with cancer.

CESAREAN SECTION (C/S) POSTCARE

1. General Considerations

The nursing care of the new mother following cesarean section (C/S) surgery is usually directed toward wound care, catheter care, or other complications that necessitate the need for skilled services. Goals are directed to facilitate resolution of the problems to support bonding with the infant during this important perinatal period.

2. Potential Diagnoses and Codes

The diagnoses and codes listed here include some of the most common conditions seen in home care for these patients, and have been alphabetized for easy identification. Keep in mind that the ICD-9-CM system requires a focused review of the patient's medical information in addition to the physician-assigned diagnoses. Should additional information be needed, refer to the coding books or a qualified coder.

Diagnosis	Code
Anemia	648.24 and 285.9
Constipation	674.84 and 564.0
Diabetes mellitus, with complications, type 2 or unspecified, not stated as controlled	648.04 and 250.90
Diabetes mellitus, with complications, type 1	648.04 and 250.91
Hemorrhoids, external	671.84 and 455.3
Hemorrhoids, internal	671.84 and 455.0
Hemorrhoids, postpartum (unspecified)	671.84 and 455.6
Long-term (current) use of insulin	V58.67
Surgical dressing changes	V58.31
Suture removal	V58.32
Urinary infection	646.64 and 599.0
Urinary retention	646.64 and 788.20
Wound dehiscence	674.14
Wound infection	674.34
Others	

3. Associated Nursing Diagnoses (see Part Seven)

4. Supportive Factors for the Determination and Documentation of Homebound Status

Although this is not usually an admission criterion, some managed-care programs will need rationale for why the patient cannot get to the physician's office. The following are some of the reasons the patient would be homebound:

Pain
Severe fatigue
SOB on any activity
Infection protection
Open wound site
Others

5. Potential Goals and Outcomes

The following patient-centered goals/outcomes can be individualized according to the identified needs of the patient and family.

Nursing

Patient/caregiver verbalizes satisfaction with care
Hydration and nutrition optimal for mother and infant
Teaching accomplished related to parenting roles, support and coping, home safety, and self-care after C/S
Pain and symptom control after C/S
Infection-free wound site (specify parameters) by _____
Catheter patent without infection
Patient returned to self-care status
Maternal and family bonding evidenced by loving relationship toward newborn
Mother self-care and able to care for infant effectively
Other

5

Home Health Aide

Effective personal hygiene
Safe ADL assistance
Verbalization of patient feeling clean and comfortable
Other

Medical Social Services

Resource identification and financial situation assessed/ addressed
Linkage with community services and other resources
Referral of patient and family to _____ (specify)
Financial access problems addressed, resources identified as demonstrated by _____ (specify)
Plan of care successfully implemented due to resolution of identified problems impeding progress
Other

6. Skills, Interventions/Services, and Management

Home care clinicians must exercise acute and effective critical thinking, observation, technical, teaching, and evaluation skills when performing clinical assessments, interventions, and management of their home care patients.

Nursing

Patient/caregiver provided with home safety information and instruction related to _____ and documented in the clinical record
Provide aseptic care to open wound site (specify supplies, frequency, other physician's orders)
Observation and assessment of wound site and surrounding skin
Assessment of post-op complications
Teach incision care (keep dry, avoid pressure on site)
Assess patient's pain on an ongoing basis to identify need for change, alteration, addition, or other plan for pain management

Provide emotional support to patient and family
Assess amount and character of lochia
Evaluate patient's bowel patterns, need for stool softeners, laxatives, dietary changes, or increase in fluid
Evaluate pain in relation to other symptoms, including fatigue, constipation, depression, or others
Assessment of breasts and nipples, engorgement, soreness, cracking, or blisters
Prevention and management of pain and constipation
Obtain urine for culture and sensitivity
Instruct new mother regarding breast care comfort techniques
Assess patient and family stress/coping skills
Implement nonpharmacological interventions with medication schedule, including massage, imagery, progressive relaxation exercises, humor, and music therapies
Assess fundus
Teach new parents regarding infant safety measures, parenting skills, bathing, cord care, circumcision care, and well-child care, including need for immunizations at specified time intervals in the future
Assess nutrition and hydration statuses
Venipuncture for complete blood count (CBC) (specify per physician's orders)
Teach patient about wound care and infection control measures
Assess the patient's unique response to ordered interventions and treatments and report changes, unfavorable responses, or reactions to the physician
Teach regarding sexuality and family planning concerns
Management and evaluation of the patient's POC
Other interventions

Home Health Aide

Personal care
ADL assistance
Meal preparation

Infant care
Other tasks/activities as assigned

Medical Social Services

Evaluation of financial/social situation related to follow-up care for infant and adaptive adjustment of teenage mother
Other interventions

7. Safety Considerations and Discharge Plans

Infection control/universal precautions
Medication safety and storage
Surgical precautions (e.g., driving, lifting)
Symptoms that necessitate immediate reporting/assistance
Infant safety information (e.g., car seat, infant sleep position)
Safety related to home medical equipment
Smoke detector and fire evacuation plan
Discharge to care of new parents, with physician follow-up for well-child care, including planned immunization schedule
Others, based on the patient's unique condition and environment

8. Tips to Support Medical Necessity, Quality, and Reimbursement

Document variances to expected outcomes. Some third-party payers will want reasons for continued visits to see the patient when the wound is not infected, although still open. The professional nurse skills, however, are more than the actual hands-on packing of the wound and applying Montgomery straps or whatever the specific orders entail. It is teaching, observation, and assessment that usually justify the nurse's continued involvement before wound healing, closure, or the patient is able to go back to the physician for further care.

Document the specific care and teaching instructions provided
Document your progress toward patient-centered, realistic goals
Document all POC changes and obtain orders for any POC changes

9. Tips for Communication with Insurance Case Manager

Present objective patient findings and changes since last update
Document with pictures to send to case manager
Meet face-to-face for relationship building when possible
Identify education that occurred and where patient will go for follow-up and care
Communicate information about the interventions and the patient's response to the care
Discuss other measurable changes and information that communicate the status of the patient and the need for skilled home care services

10. Evidence-Based and other Resources for Practice and Education

HRSA's Maternal and Child Health (www.ask.hrsa.gov/MCH.cfm or 1-888-275-4772) programs promote and improve the health of mothers, infants, children, and adolescents, including low-income families, those with diverse racial and ethnic heritages, and those living in rural or isolated areas without access to care. Materials include topics related to health care, prenatal care and newborn screening, preventive care and research, and more.

5

CYSTIC FIBROSIS (CARE OF THE CHILD WITH)

1. General Considerations

Cystic fibrosis (CF) is the most common life-threatening genetic disease affecting Caucasians in the U.S.; approximately 30,000 children and adults in the United States are diagnosed with CF, and about 1000 new cases occur each year. CF causes unusually thick, sticky mucus that clogs the lungs and leads to deadly lung infections; it also obstructs the pancreas and stops natural enzymes from helping the body break down and absorb food.

In the 1950s, few children with cystic fibrosis lived to attend elementary school. Today, advances in research and medical treatments have further enhanced and extended life for children and adults with CF. In 2006, the predicted median age of survival was 37 years.

2. Potential Diagnoses and Codes

The diagnoses and codes listed here include some of the most common conditions seen in children with cystic fibrosis, and have been alphabetized for easy identification. Keep in mind that the ICD-9-CM system requires a focused review of the patient's medical information in addition to the physician-assigned diagnoses. Should additional information be needed, refer to the coding books or a qualified coder.

Diagnosis	Code
Anemia	285.9
Bronchitis	490
Bronchopneumonia	485
Cholecystitis	575.10
Chronic obstructive pulmonary disease	496
Cirrhosis, biliary	571.6
Congestive heart failure	428.0
Constipation	564.0
Cor pulmonale	416.9
Cystic fibrosis	277.00
Dehydration	276.51
Diabetes mellitus, with complications, type 2 or unspecified	250.90

Diabetes mellitus, with complications, type 1	250.91
Emphysema	492.8
Failure to thrive, child	783.41
Hemoptysis	786.3
Ileus	560.1
Long-term (current) use of insulin	V58.67
Pancreatic insufficiency	577.8
Peptic ulcer	533.90
Pneumonia	486
Rectum, prolapse of	569.1
Sinusitis	473.9
S/P heart-lung transplant care	V42.1 and V42.6
Others	

3. Associated Nursing Diagnoses(see Part Seven)

4. Supportive Factors for the Determination and Documentation of Homebound Status

Although homebound may or may not be an admission criterion, the following are some of the reasons that the child would be cared for at home:

Child with CF and chest process, physician wants cared for at home for infection control and to protect child from other sick children
SOB on any activity
Child with CF on home antibiotic regimen or total parenteral nutrition (TPN)
Others

5. Potential Goals and Outcomes

The following patient-centered goals/outcomes can be individualized according to the identified needs of the patient and family.

Nursing
Support growth and developmental tasks of childhood
Patient/caregiver verbalizes satisfaction with care

Educational tools/plans incorporated in daily care and child/caregiver verbalizes understanding of safe, needed care
Patient/parent decides on care, interventions, and evaluation
Caregiver effective in care management and knows who should be contacted for questions/concerns
Parent/caregiver verbalizes understanding of and adheres to pulmonary care and medication regimens
Patient/caregiver lists adverse reactions, potential complications, signs/symptoms of infection (e.g., sputum change, chest congestion, fever)

Family demonstrates correct provision of care to child by discharge
Child maintains/increases weight to _____ lbs. by _____ (date)
Hydration and nutrition optimal for child
Maintenance of bowel function or normal habits for child
Patient has stable respiratory status with airway clear of mucus (e.g., no dyspnea, infection free)
Patient protected from injury, further infections, and compliant with medication, safety, and care regimens
Comfort and individualized intervention of child with CF
Other

Home Health Aide

Effective and safe personal care and hygiene maintained
Safe ADL assistance
Respite and increased comfort
Other

Medical Social Services

Child/caregiver will cope adaptively with chronic illness
Identification and addressing/resolution of problems impeding the successful implementation of the POC
Psychosocial support and counseling offered to/initiated with patient and caregivers experiencing grief (if appropriate)
Other

Physical Therapy

Patient using home exercise regimen taught and has _____ percent increase in mobility/function/strength

Maintenance of balance, mobility, and endurance as verbalized and demonstrated by patient
Effective CPT regimen demonstrated by patient
Other

Occupational Therapy
Home modifications for safety will be arranged for completion by _____ (date)
Patient/caregiver will achieve maximum independence and safety with ADLs within pain tolerance
Instruction in use of adaptive techniques and assistive devices by _____ (date)
Patient/caregiver will demonstrate effective use of energy conservation and diaphragmatic breathing by _____ (date)
Patient/caregiver will be independent with program for positioning patient effectively to minimize pain and maximize breathing
Patient will be effective in communicating needs with use of adaptive measures as needed
Other

6. Skills, Interventions/Services, and Management

Home care clinicians must exercise acute and effective critical thinking, observation, technical, teaching and evaluation skills when performing clinical assessments, interventions, and management of their home care patients.

Nursing
Parent/caregiver provided with home safety information and instruction related to _____ and documented in the clinical record
Teach patient/caregiver daily chest care physiotherapy regimen to maintain and help ensure aeration and decrease secretions
Teach the need for the pancreatic enzyme replacements administered with each meal and snack
Teach caregiver signs and symptoms of the CF child that necessitate calling the physician

Instruct about the need for a well-balanced, high-calorie diet to help ensure growth
Teach chest percussion and postural drainage on child
Instruct regarding infection control measures, including effective hand washing techniques and avoiding people with upper respiratory or other infections
Teach caregiver observational skills of weight loss or gain and to weigh and record daily weights
Evaluate home setting and caregiver for safe administration of IV antibiotic therapy with central venous access device
Teach child and caregiver effective conservation of energy techniques
Teach child and caregiver effective coughing techniques
Teach and monitor administration of aerosol bronchodilator medication to assist in expectoration
Assess patient's respiratory status and lung sounds, before and after chest physical therapy (CPT), consisting of clapping, drainage, and aerosol treatment and instructing caregiver about these skills
Observe and assess amount and frequency of stools, abdominal distension, and other gastrointestinal symptoms or complaints
Teach caregiver to watch for symptoms of infection, including change in child's behavior, increased irritability, fever, decreased appetite, or other signs
Assess the child's unique response to treatments and interventions and report changes or unfavorable responses or reactions to the physician
Other interventions

Home Health Aide

Personal care
ADL assistance
Participation in home exercise program
Other tasks/activities as assigned

Medical Social Services

Evaluation of psychosocial factors that have an impact on the family and child with a chronic illness and that impact POC implementation

Counseling regarding financial and food assistance programs

Emotional support to child, family, and caregivers

Referral to community programs

Other interventions

Physical Therapy

Evaluation of patient and learning needs of child, family, and caregiver

Instruct regarding performance of postural drainage, percussion, breathing exercises, and administration of treatments

Home exercise regimen appropriate to developmental stage and strength/conditioning deficits

Other interventions

Occupational Therapy

Evaluation

Assess for home modifications for safety and maximum functional independence

Instruct in safety and use of adaptive techniques and assistive devices for maximum independence in ADLs/IADLs

Assist family in providing appropriate play/leisure activities

Instruct in energy conservation and diaphragmatic breathing for decreased and maximum independent functioning

Teach home exercise program for maximum upper extremity function

Instruct and establish home program for functional positioning and/or use of splints and/or other devices for minimal pain

Assessment and instructions to enable patient to effectively communicate needs

Instructions on functional positioning for maximum comfort, including use of splints and/or other devices
Other interventions

7. Safety Considerations and Discharge Plans

Infection control/universal precautions
Night-light
Medication safety and storage, other child safety information
Signs/symptoms that necessitate immediate reporting/assistance
Safety related to home medical equipment
Smoke detector and fire evacuation plan
Discontinued course of antibiotics
Discharged from home care, under physician's supervision
Caregiver demonstrated ability to keep up with new interventions
Caregiver demonstrated knowledge of daily care, including pulmonary care, discharged from home care
Patient readmitted to hospital with acute exacerbation respiratory problems, discharged from home care
Others, based on the patient's unique condition and environment

8. Tips to Support Medical Necessity, Quality, and Reimbursement

Document any variances to expected outcomes. Document the coordination occurring among team members based on the POC. The interdisciplinary conference notes should be reflected in the clinical record.
In addition:
Write the specific care and teaching instructions provided
Document progress toward patient-centered, realistic goals
Document the nursing actions and responses to the care interventions

Document the specific teaching accomplished and the behavioral outcomes of that teaching
Document the amount and character of secretions
Document any changes in the POC
Document any exacerbation of symptoms that necessitated another visit and be sure that there is a physician's order for that visit in the clinical record
Document the skills used in the provision of professional nursing care practice when caring for the child (e.g., teaching, training, observation, assessment)

9. Tips for Communication with Insurance Case Manager

Present objective patient findings and changes since last update
Meet face-to-face for relationship building when possible
Communicate information about the interventions and the child's response to the care
Discuss other measurable changes and information that communicate the status of the patient and the need for skilled home care services

10. Evidence-Based and other Resources for Practice and Education

The American Association for Respiratory Care (AARC) (www.AARC.org/store.cfm or 1-972-243-2272) offers a video entitled "Breath of Life—A Caregiver's Guide to Pediatric Tracheostomy Care" that was created with input from parents of a child with a tracheostomy.
The Cystic Fibrosis Foundation (www.cff.org or 1-800-344-4823) is available to provide information and educational support to health care professionals and patients with CF, their families, and caregivers.

DIABETES (CARE OF THE CHILD WITH)

1. General Considerations

In 2005, 176,500 people aged 20 years or younger had diabetes, or 0.22 percent of all people in this age group. About one in every 400 to 600 children and adolescents has Type 1 diabetes. Maturity onset diabetes in youth (MODY) now accounts for 30 to 50 percent of childhood onset diabetes.

Children with diabetes are often referred to home health care after a hospitalization or to prevent hospitalization or rehospitalizations. These children and their families have multiple teaching and other intervention needs.

2. Potential Diagnoses and Codes

The diagnoses and codes listed here include some of the most common conditions seen in children with diabetes mellitus, and have been alphabetized for easy identification. Keep in mind that the ICD-9-CM system requires a focused review of the patient's medical information in addition to the physician-assigned diagnoses. Should additional information be needed, refer to the coding books or a qualified coder.

Diagnosis	Code
Dehydration	276.51
Diabetes mellitus, insulin dependent	250.01
Diabetic retinopathy	250.51 and 362.01
Hyperglycemia, uncontrolled	250.03
Hypoglycemia	250.81
Ketoacidosis	250.13
Long-term (current) use of insulin	V58.67
Others	

3. Associated Nursing Diagnoses (see Part Seven)

4. Supportive Factors for the Determination and Documentation of Homebound Status

The homebound factor is usually not a criterion for this patient population, although the following are the most common:

Fatigue
Infection protection
Safety concerns while insulin is being regulated (e.g., rapid changes in blood sugar and associated signs/symptoms)
Others

5. Potential Goals and Outcomes

The following patient-centered goals/outcomes can be individualized according to the identified needs of the patient and family.

Nursing

Patient/caregiver articulates satisfaction with care
Support growth and developmental tasks of childhood
Educational tools/plans incorporated in daily care and child/caregiver verbalizes understanding of safe, needed care
Stable blood sugar levels and health status by _____ (specify)
Self-care related to diabetes care including _____ (specify)
Patient/parent decides on care, interventions, and evaluation
Caregiver effective in care management and knows whom to call for questions/concerns
Parent/caregiver states understanding and adheres to care regimen, including insulin, dietary management, weight management, and emergency measures

Parent/caregiver states understanding and adheres to care regimen, including oral medications, dietary management, weight management, and emergency measures
Mother/caretaker lists sick day care considerations
Family demonstrates correct provision of care to child by discharge
Hydration and nutrition optimal for child
Patient protected from injury and infections and compliant with medication, safety, and care regimens
Child demonstrates ____ percent behavioral compliance with instructions related to blood glucose monitoring, food choices, insulin injections (specify)
Other

Medical Social Services

Child/caregiver will cope adaptively with chronic illness
Identification and addressing/resolution of problems impeding the successful implementation of the POC
Psychosocial support and counseling offered/initiated to patient and caregivers experiencing grief (if appropriate)
Other

Dietary Counseling

Patient/caregiver demonstrate appropriate dietary choices and understanding of diet options
Other

6. Skills, Interventions/Services, and Management

Home care clinicians must exercise acute and effective critical thinking, observation, technical, teaching and evaluation skills when performing clinical assessments, interventions, and management of their home care patients.

Nursing

Parent/caregiver provided with disease process related to Type ____ diabetes, home safety information and instruction related to _____ and documented in the clinical record

Teach parents/patient to draw up and administer insulin

Teach diabetes management regimen(s), including sick day rules and care

Emotional support for child and parents with newly diagnosed diabetes

Teach regarding diet and importance of eating at regular, consistent times

Perform blood glucose monitor checks q _____, call physician if over _____ or less than _____

Teach patient and parents to mix insulins

Teach patient and parents blood glucose monitoring process

Teach signs and symptoms of hyperglycemia and hypoglycemia, teach emergency measures to patient and parents

Venipuncture for FBS as indicated

Teach patient and parents urine check procedures

Teach regarding new insulin and medication regimen

The importance of compliance with all the regimens related to care

Teach action of ordered insulin(s)

Assess long-term ability of patient and parents to comply with regimen

Teach patient and parents regarding site rotation and importance of site rotation

Teach patient and parents regarding dietary management and restrictions

Teach patient and parents regarding stressors that can increase the amount of insulin needed (e.g., infection)

Teach patient/parents importance of weight management

Teach patient/parents regarding activity/exercise safety for play and sports
Assess family and patient ability to integrate diabetes in school day
Coordinate diabetic activities with school nurse
Assess school ability to assist with diabetes management (glucose monitoring, insulin injections, emergency measures, etc.)
Referral to school guidance counselor and/or school nurse
Assess family and patient coping, refer as needed to support group
Other interventions

Medical Social Services

Psychosocial assessment of patient and family with new illness of a chronic nature
Assist parents in care and acceptance of child's diagnosis
Problem identification
Referral to community resource(s)
Financial counseling and assistance
Other interventions

Dietary Counseling

Teaching regarding disease and food choices in home, school and social settings
Other interventions

7. Safety Considerations and Discharge Plans

Infection control/universal precautions
Night-light
Needles/sharps disposal
Child safety information
Refrigeration for insulin storage
Medication safety and storage
Emergency actions related to hyperglycemia/hypoglycemia

Signs/symptoms that necessitate immediate reporting/assistance
Safety related to home medical equipment
Smoke detector and fire evacuation plan
Discharged to self-care (age dependent), under physician's supervision
Discharged, parent and family able to care for patient, with no follow-up
Discharged with peer, parent, and support groups available
Goals achieved, return to self-care status
Others, based on the patient's unique condition and environment

8. Tips to Support Medical Necessity, Quality, and Reimbursement

Document any variances to expected outcomes
Document the actions of your care
Document the specific areas of education and care needed
Obtain a telephone order for any POC change
Document specific teaching accomplished and the behavioral outcomes of that teaching

9. Tips for Communication with Insurance Case Manager

Present objective patient findings and changes since last update
Meet face-to-face for relationship building when possible
Communicate information about the interventions and the child's response to the care
Discuss other measurable changes and information that communicate the status of the patient and the need for skilled home care services

5

10. Evidence-Based and other Resources for Practice and Education

The American Diabetes Association (ADA) (www.diabetes.org, or 1-800-DIABETES [1-800-342-2383]) offers many resources for patients, families, and professionals.

The Centers for Disease Control and Prevention (CDC) (www.cdc.gov/diabetes or 1-800-CDC-INFO [1-800-232-4636]) offers a Public Health Resource page on diabetes with information on diabetes, eating right, and publications including fact sheets and statistics in English and Spanish.

The Diabetes Action Research and Education Foundation (www.diabetesaction.org or 1-202-333-4520) offers numerous resources on their website including healthy recipes, frequently asked questions, an "Ask the Diabetes Educator" page, news updates on research and funding projects, and more.

The Juvenile Diabetes Research Foundation International (www.jdrf.org or 1-800-223-1138 or 1-212-889-7575) promotes education in diabetes and has an online support team available.

The National Diabetes Information Clearinghouse (www.diabetes.niddk.nih.gov or 1-301-654-3327) offers many fact sheets, information packets, and professional publications.

Book Resource

American Association of Diabetes Educators. (2006) The art and science of diabetes self-management. Chicago, IL: American Association of Diabetes Educators.

GESTATIONAL DIABETES

1. General Considerations

Gestational diabetes is a form of glucose intolerance diagnosed in some women during pregnancy, and occurs more frequently among African Americans, Hispanic/Latino Americans, and American Indians. It is also more common among obese women and women with a family history of diabetes. During pregnancy, gestational diabetes requires treatment to normalize maternal blood glucose levels to avoid complications in the infant. According to the National Diabetes Clearinghouse, 5 to 10 percent of women with gestational diabetes are diagnosed with type 2 diabetes, and those who have had gestational diabetes have a 20 to 50 percent chance of developing diabetes in the next 5 to 10 years.

2. Potential Diagnoses and Codes

The diagnoses and codes listed here include some of the most common conditions seen in pregnant women with diabetes, and have been alphabetized for easy identification. Keep in mind that the ICD-9-CM system requires a focused review of the patient's medical information in addition to the physician-assigned diagnoses. Should additional information be needed, refer to the coding books or a qualified coder.

Diagnosis	Code
Dehydration	276.51
Diabetes mellitus, type 1	648.00 and 250.01
Gestational diabetes mellitus, type 2	648.00 and 250.00
Hyperglycemia	790.6
Hypoglycemia	648.00 and 250.80
Long-term (current) use of insulin	V58.67
Pregnancy, high-risk	V23.9
Others	

3. Associated Nursing Diagnoses (see Part Seven)

4. Supportive Factors for the Determination and Documentation of Homebound Status

The homebound factor may or may not be a criterion for admission, based on the managed care program or the third-party payer involved. However, the following are reasons the patient would be homebound:

5

Confined to home because of instability of diabetes
Weakness, SOB
Medically restricted because of high-risk pregnancy
Activity restriction per obstetrician (e.g., patient on bed rest, etc.)
Others

5. Potential Goals and Outcomes

The following patient-centered goals/outcomes can be individualized according to the identified needs of the patient and family.

Nursing

Patient/caregiver articulates satisfaction with care
Educational tools/plans incorporated in daily care and verbalizes understanding of needed care
Stable blood sugar levels and health status by _____ (specify)
Self-care related to diabetes care including _____ (specify)
Patient decides on care, interventions, and evaluation
Well-controlled and continuous blood glucose control as measured through blood test results
Patient lists problems with pregnancy necessitating immediate notification, including vaginal bleeding, membrane rupture, uterine contractions, or decreased fetal activity
Caregiver effective in care management and knows who to call for questions/concerns

Patient/caregiver states understanding and adheres to care regimen, including insulin, dietary, and emergency measures
Hydration and nutrition optimal for developing fetus
Patient protected from injury and infections and compliant with medication, safety, and care regimens
Adherence to POC as demonstrated and reported by patient/caregiver and demonstrated by patient findings
Caregiver effective in care management and knows whom to call for questions/concerns
Patient verbalizes understanding of and adheres to medication regimens
Patient self-care in relation to diabetes regimen
Blood sugar level in normal-for-patient range and patient verbalizes understanding of factors that contribute to avoidance of complications
Optimal nutrition for patient on weight loss regimen and integrated into daily care regimen by _____ (date)
Adherence to diet in relation to blood glucose levels
Other goals/outcomes based on the patient's unique needs and problems

6. Skills, Interventions/Services, and Management

Home care clinicians must exercise acute and effective critical thinking, observation, technical, teaching and evaluation skills when performing clinical assessments, interventions, and management of their home care patients.

Nursing

Patient provided with home safety information and instruction related to _____ and documented in the clinical record
Teach patient or family member to correctly draw up and administer insulin
Teach diabetes management regimen(s)

Teach regarding diet and importance of eating at regular, consistent times
Teach regarding changing need of insulin amount as pregnancy advances
Perform blood glucose checks q _____, call physician if over _____ or less than _____
Teach patient and family to mix insulins
Teach patient and family member blood glucose monitoring process

Teach signs and symptoms of hyperglycemia and hypoglycemia
Teach emergency measures to patient and family
Teach regarding importance of reporting the following symptoms immediately to physician: Nausea, vomiting, and infection
Venipuncture for FBS as ordered
Teach importance of compliance to the diabetic care regimens and keeping scheduled OB and endocrinology appointments
Teach signs/symptoms of labor and other symptoms or changes that necessitate notifying the physician and being seen immediately (e.g., bleeding, premature rupture of membranes)
Teach patient and family urine check procedures for ketones
Teach need for optimal nutrition and frequent rest periods
Teach self-observational skills, including home blood glucose monitoring findings, daily weights, etc.
Teach regarding medication regimen, including insulin
Teach dietary management related to insulin therapy
Teach action of different ordered insulins
Teach signs/symptoms hypoglycemia/hyperglycemia and appropriate interventions, including emergency measures
Reassurance and support to pregnant patient regarding disease and appropriate concerns
Other interventions

Medical Social Services

Psychosocial evaluation
Financial counseling assistance
Referral(s) to community resources
Support to high-risk patient
Other interventions

Dietary Counseling

Nutritional assessment of patient with diabetes during pregnancy
Plan for optimal nutrition
Other interventions

7. Safety Considerations and Discharge Plans

Infection control/universal precautions
Night-light
Needles/sharps disposal and safety
Refrigeration for insulin storage
Medication safety and storage
Emergency actions related to hyperglycemia/hypoglycemia
Symptoms that necessitate immediate reporting/assistance
Safety related to home medical equipment
Smoke detector and fire evacuation plan
Others, based on the patient's unique condition and environment
Return to self-care status, under physician's supervision
Continuing need for home health care because patient remains medically confined to home and needs nursing care to prevent hospitalization
Delivery of infant
Others, based on the patient's unique condition and environment

8. Tips to Support Medical Necessity, Quality, and Reimbursement

Document any variances to expected outcomes
Document your care and the actions of your care
Document any abnormal findings in the clinical record and the notification of the physician
Document initial knowledge level and progress achieved through the teaching process
Document specific teaching accomplished and the behavioral outcomes of that teaching

9. Tips for Communication with Insurance Case Manager

Present objective patient findings and changes since last update
Meet face-to-face for relationship building when possible
Communicate information about the interventions and the patient's response to the care
Discuss other measurable changes and information that communicate the status of the patient and the need for skilled home care services

10. Evidence-Based and other Resources for Practice and Education

The American Diabetes Association (ADA) (www.diabetes.org, or 1-800-DIABETES [1-800-342-2383]) offers many resources for patients, families, and professionals.
The Centers for Disease Control and Prevention (CDC) (www.cdc.gov/diabetes or 1-800-CDC-INFO [1-800-232-4636]) offers a Public Health Resource page on diabetes with information on diabetes, eating right, and publications including fact sheets and statistics in English and Spanish.

The Diabetes Action Research and Education Foundation (www.diabetesaction.org or call 1-202-333-4520) offers numerous resources on their website including healthy recipes, frequently asked questions, an "Ask the Diabetes Educator" page, news updates on research and funding projects, and more.

The Juvenile Diabetes Research Foundation International offers resources for teens, children, and parents living with JD. Visit www.jdrf.org or call 1-800-533-CURE (2873).

The National Diabetes Information Clearinghouse (www.diabetes.niddk.nih.gov or 1-800-891-5388) offers *Understanding Gestational Diabetes: A Practical Guide to a Healthy Pregnancy.*

MEDICALLY FRAGILE CHILD CARE

1. General Considerations

According to the CDC, accidents remain the leading cause of death in children. However, many medically fragile children with congenital problems and other diseases and conditions are cared for at home. Children who have suffered trauma, either head or other injuries, and have extended rehabilitation needs; developmentally challenged children; and those with life-limiting cancers are other examples of medically fragile children cared for at home. The medically fragile child is a growing patient population in home care. Many of these children are "preemies" who have been cared for in neonatal intensive care units (NICUs) for extended periods of time. The home care team members provide skilled care to this special patient population, directed toward health maintenance and supporting the child's growth and development.

2. Potential Diagnoses and Codes

The diagnoses and codes listed here include some of the most common conditions seen in medically fragile children, and have been alphabetized for easy identification. Keep in mind that the ICD-9-CM system requires a focused review of the patient's medical information in addition to the physician-assigned diagnoses. Should additional information be needed, refer to the coding books or a qualified coder.

Diagnosis	Code
Aftercare following surgery	V58.7X
Aftercare following surgery for injury and trauma	V58.43
AIDS	042
Apnea	786.03
Apnea, newborn	770.8X
Asthma	493.90
Bacteriuria	791.9
Biliuria	791.4

Bronchiolitis	466.19
Cardiac dysrhythmia	427.9
Cerebral palsy, unspecified	343.9
Child maltreatment syndrome	995.5X
Cholelithiasis	574.2X
Chronic renal failure	585
Cleft lip	749.1X
Cleft palate	749.0X
Cystic fibrosis	277.0X
Dehydration	276.51
Diabetes, with unspecified complications	250.90
Diarrhea	787.91
Down's syndrome	758.0
Failure to thrive, child	783.41
Fetal bronchopulmonary dysplasia	770.7
Fetal/neonatal jaundice	774.6
Immaturity, extreme	765.0X
Jaundice (not of newborns)	782.4
Metabolism disorder	277.9
Muscular dystrophy, not otherwise specified	359.1
Newborn feeding problems	779.3
Normal delivery	650
Normal physiological development, lack of, in child (failure to thrive)	783.41
Pancreatitis, acute	577.0
Pneumonia	486
Preterm infant, unspecified weight	765.10
Pulmonary insufficiency, newborn	770.8X
Reactive airway disease	493.90
Rectal prolapse	569.1
Respiratory problem, newborn	770.8X
Respiratory syncytial virus	079.6
Seizure disorder	780.39
Sickle cell anemia, unspecified	282.60
Sickle cell crisis	282.62
Sickle cell trait	282.5
Spina bifida	741.9X
Tracheal stenosis	519.1X
Tracheal stenosis, congenital	748.3
Tracheal malacia, congenital	748.3
Tracheomalacia	519.1X
Tracheostomy, attention to	V55.0
Others	

3. Associated Nursing Diagnoses (see Part Seven)

4. Supportive Factors for the Determination and Documentation of Homebound Status

Homebound is usually not a factor with payers regarding children. In fact, many of these infants/children are case managed, and home care may be in lieu of higher-cost inpatient hospital care.

5. Potential Goals and Outcomes.

The following patient-centered goals/outcomes can be individualized according to the identified needs of the patient and family.

Nursing

Support growth and developmental tasks of childhood

Parent/child articulates satisfaction with care

Educational tools/plans related to care of infant with _____ incorporated into care routines (e.g., rest, fluids)

Safe and infection-free delivery of TPN at home

Child remains at home without or with minimal complications

Infant/child is pain free and comfortable

Child will demonstrate an adequate breathing pattern as evidenced by lack of respiratory distress (e.g., no retractions, not using accessory muscles, appears comfortable)

Child will maintain a patent airway and mobilization of secretions by use of respiratory treatments, oral medications, and effective cough

Child will maintain sufficient fluid intake to prevent dehydration (e.g., _____ ml in 24 hours)

Mother/caregiver will identify factors/triggers that seem to cause exacerbations

Prevention of multiple hospital admissions for infusion therapy with case management and phone intervention program by _____ (specify date)
Parent/caregiver will meet the developmental and play needs of child
Parent/caregiver demonstrates the ability to perform taught/learned health-related behaviors
Parent can list medications, their schedule, use, and side effects
Parent able to describe what is abnormal for infant and actions to take regarding apnea monitoring
Infant experiences improved feeding, weight gain; parent experiences decreased worry
Parental and family bonding evidenced by loving relationship with infant
Parent effective in child's health maintenance and knows whom to call for questions/concerns
Other

Home Health Aide

Effective personal care
Safe ADL assistance
Other

Physical Therapy/Occupational Therapy/S-LP Therapy

Evaluation
Provide developmental assessment and therapies to promote postural control, fine and gross motor skills, sensory integration, communication and feeding

Medical Social Services

Resource identification and financial situation assessed/addressed
Linkage to community services and resources
Plan of care successfully implemented because of resolution of problems impeding POC's success
Other

Nutritional and Dietary Counseling

Hydration/nutrition optimal for high-risk infant/child

Weight increased/stabilized at _____ lbs. by _____ (specify date)

Other

6. Skills, Interventions/Services, and Management

Home care clinicians must exercise acute and effective critical thinking, observation, technical, teaching and evaluation skills when performing clinical assessments, interventions, and management of their home care patients.

Nursing

Child/parent provided with home safety information and instruction related to _____ and documented in the clinical record

Comprehensive skilled assessment of all systems of infant/child with _____ (specify) admitted to home care for _____

Support play, growth and development, and health maintenance through length of care

Establish an environment of mutual trust and respect to enhance learning

Communicate only brief amounts of complex information related to the infant's care at any given time

Assess respiratory rate and depth and lung sounds for improvement or deterioration

Administer prescribed medications as ordered, including aerosol treatments, and monitor for adverse effects

Encourage family members to avoid any smoking in the home

Schedule frequent rest periods with activities to promote optimal oxygenation

Review of cardiopulmonary resuscitation (CPR) with parents/caregivers

Instruct on need for phone access into 911 system in event of severe breathing difficulties

Assist willing family members to learn basic life support
Monitor length, weight, head circumference, and review of food diary for infant with failure to thrive
Reinforce feeding techniques and intake and output diary
Teach parent/caregiver management of cardiorespiratory monitor
Teach parent/caregiver oxygen administration and safety considerations with infant at risk for hypoxemia and history of bradycardia and apnea
Instruct regarding medication administration and side effects
Instruct regarding health maintenance, including immunizations
Instruct regarding growth and development information
Teach signs/symptoms that necessitate calling the physician
Teach potential complications of technologies used for child's care (e.g., TPN)
Review home medical equipment vendor's name and number
Other interventions, based on the infant's/child's unique needs

Home Health Aide

Personal care
ADL assistance
Other tasks/activities as assigned

Medical Social Services

Evaluation of family situation of child with chronic illness
Community linkage for access to programs and benefits
Planning for long-term care of infant
Other interventions

Dietary Counseling

Nutritional assessment in child on long-term parenteral nutrition
Plan for optimal nutrition and hydration to facilitate growth and development
Other interventions

5

7. Safety Considerations and Discharge Plans

Infection control/universal precautions
Night-light
Infant/child safety considerations (e.g., car seat, electrical outlet protection, sleeping position, immunizations)
Telephone number of whom to call with a problem
Medication access and storage
Oxygen safety
Equipment safety if there is home medical equipment/technology
Symptoms, problems that necessitate emergency call to 911
If ventilator, TPN, or infusion patient—adequate electricity, refrigerator, clean storage area, and access to a telephone
Smoke detector and fire evacuation plan
Child discharged in care of parents back to the community
Child to receive long-term care due to nature of chronic illness
Child discharged with community linkage and support
Child referred to pediatric hospice for care
Others, based on the patient's unique condition and environment

8. Tips to Support Medical Necessity, Quality, and Reimbursement

Document patient changes and the notification of these changes to the physician; in the documentation write specifically what was discussed and the resolution or change to the plan of care that was the outcome of the update/communication.

Document interdisciplinary care planning (e.g., discussions with the aide or dietitian about the child's care and plan); care planning and care coordination are hallmarks of quality care and can occur face-to-face (team meetings) or may occur on the phone; the goal of care coordination is that everyone involved in the care and planning is working toward common goals.

9. Tips for Communication with Insurance Case Manager

Present objective patient findings and changes since last update

Update regarding blood values, pulse oximetry readings, and other measurable tests

Identify how the plan of care is working toward discharge and how the parent and other caregivers are demonstrating taught care; similarly, if the parent is unable or unwilling to learn, communicate this information to the nurse case manager

10. Evidence-Based and other Resources for Practice and Education

The American Academy of Pediatrics (AAP) (www.aap.org) offers materials and information related to appropriate care for children with special health care needs.

The National Easter Seal Society (www.easterseals.com) offer services to children and adults with disabilities and special needs. Teams of therapists, teachers and other health professionals help each person overcome obstacles to independence and reach his or her personal goals. Easter Seals also includes families as active members of any therapy program, and offers the support families need.

The National Information Center for Children and Youth With Disabilities (NICHCY) (www.nichcy.org or 800-695-0285) offers information and materials.

United Cerebral Palsy (www.ucpa.org) is a leading source of information on cerebral palsy and an advocate for the rights of persons with any disability. They offer a myriad of educational resources for patients, families, and professionals.

NEWBORN CARE

1. General Considerations

According to the Health Resources and Services Administration (HRSA) Maternal and Child Health Bureau, 18,593 infants died before reaching 28 days of age in 2004, representing a neonatal mortality rate of 4.5 deaths per 1000 live births. Neonatal mortality is generally related to short gestation and low birth weight, congenital malformations, and conditions occurring in the perinatal period. New mothers and their infants may be referred to home health care or special programs this and a number of other reasons, including the mother's age or the infant's weight. Many commercial insurers encourage mothers and newborns to receive care at home after shortened inpatient stays (12 to 24 hours).

Home care of the newborn infant includes assessment and intervention related to adequate nutrition, infection protection, and infant-parent attachment (see also Postpartum Care in this Part of this text).

2. Potential Diagnoses and Codes

The diagnoses and codes listed here include some of the most common conditions seen in newborn care, and have been alphabetized for easy identification. Keep in mind that the ICD-9-CM system requires a focused review of the patient's medical information in addition to the physician-assigned diagnoses. Should additional information be needed, refer to the coding books or a qualified coder.

Diagnosis	Code
Biliuria	791.4
Cesarean delivery with complication, affecting newborn	763.4
Delayed development, newborn	783.41
Failure to thrive	783.41
Jaundice, fetal/neonatal	774.6
Newborn apnea	770.8X
Newborn bradycardia	763.83
Newborn feeding problems	779.3
Others	

3. Associated Nursing Diagnoses (see Part Seven)

4. Supportive Factors for the Determination and Documentation of Homebound Status

Usually not a requirement for early discharge maternity program, but the mothers and infants are confined to home for infection control, feeding reasons for the infant, and the increased rest needs of the new postpartal mother.

5. Potential Goals and Outcomes

The following patient-centered goals/outcomes can be individualized according to the identified needs of the patient and family.

Nursing

Parent/caregiver verbalizes satisfaction with care
Educational tools/plans related to newborn incorporated in daily care and parent verbalizes understanding of needed care
Optimal nutrition for growth and development of infant
Safe and supportive care provided by parents
Parent/caregiver effective in care management and knows whom to call for questions/concerns
Cord site clean, drying, infection free
Stable, healthy newborn
Mother/baby demonstrate effective feeding techniques
Parent/caregiver demonstrates positioning of baby on back and verbalizes rationale
Positive relationship demonstrated between newborn, parent, family
Infant protected from injury, infections, and caregiver providing safety and care regimens
Other

Medical Social Services

Identification and addressing/resolution of problems impeding the successful implementation of the POC
Referral/linkage with community resources
Other

6. Skills, Interventions/Services, and Management

Home care clinicians must exercise acute and effective critical thinking, observation, technical, teaching and evaluation skills when performing clinical assessments, interventions, and management of their home care patients.

5

Nursing

Parent/caregiver provided with home safety information and instruction related to _____ and documented in the clinical record
Teach regarding importance of effective hand washing to mother and family
Assess for jaundice and instruct regarding care of same
Weigh infant every visit, lining, and balancing scale
Record infant voiding pattern, noting frequency, color, volume
Assess and record infant's bowel movements, noting frequency, color, consistency, and amount
Measure head circumference each visit
Heel stick to obtain blood per state regulations (e.g., PKU)
Assess head, thorax, skin, and genitals
Assess ability to suck or latch on if breast feeding
Teach breast feeding/bottle feeding procedures
Evaluate reflexes
Care of circumcision site per specific physician orders
Care of cord per specific physician orders
Evaluate baby's total nursing and feeding time(s)
Teach mother and family regarding bathing of infant
Teach mother and family regarding circumcision care
Teach mother and family regarding care of infant skin
Assess skin/sclera coloring for jaundice
Teach mother and family regarding cord care
Teach mother and family regarding infant safety instructions (e.g., car seat, playpen, crib rails)
Teach mother/family to position infant on back to reduce SIDS
Teach mother and family regarding community safety and precaution of infant/child abduction

Teach mother and family regarding clothing and other identified areas needing information
Instruct regarding importance of medical follow-up and keeping pediatrician appointments
Teach signs/symptoms of postpartum depression and coping mechanisms
Teach safety aspects of newborn care, including the projected immunization/well-child schedule
Teach care related to feeding and breast-feeding
Coordinate care with lactation specialist prn
Other care regimens as identified based on the patient's and family's unique needs

Home Health Aide

Personal care
ADL assistance, including bathing and dressing the infant, meal preparation for the family, and assisting with other siblings as indicated
Other tasks/activities as assigned

Medical Social Services

Psychosocial assessment
Referral to community resources
Financial assistance counseling
Other interventions

7. Safety Considerations and Discharge Plans

Infection control/universal precautions
Night-light
Infant safety related to infection, germs, need for hand washing
Safety considerations (e.g., car seat placement, sleeping position)
Symptoms that necessitate immediate reporting/assistance
Safety related to home medical equipment
Smoke detector and fire evacuation plan

Discharged to care of parent(s) and other family, under physician's care
Discharged with continued follow-up with lactation specialist
Others, based on the patient's unique condition and environment

8. Tips to Support Medical Necessity, Quality, and Reimbursement

Document any variances to expected outcomes
Document all nursing care and the actions of that care
Usually there is one clinical record for both mother and infant
Document the feeding schedule in progress notes
Two to three nursing visits are usually covered by insurance, depending on specific policies
Home health aides are usually involved and can stay as long as up to 8 hours daily in some insurance benefit programs

9. Tips for Communication with Insurance Case Manager

Present objective patient findings and changes since last update
Meet face-to-face for relationship building when possible
Communicate information about the infant's status, education provided, and the plans for follow-up care

10. Evidence-Based and other Resources for Practice and Education

The American Academy of Pediatrics (AAP) (www.aap.org or 847-434-4000) offers information on a variety of children's health topics including breastfeeding, the common cold, circumcision, and hearing screenings.
The American Sudden Infant Death Syndrome Institute (www.sids.org or 800-232-SIDS [7437]) offers a pamphlet entitled "Coping with Infant Loss Grief and Bereavement."

HRSA's Maternal and Child Health (www.ask.hrsa.gov/MCH.cfm or 888-275-4772) programs promote and improve the health of mothers, infants, children, and adolescents, including low-income families, those with diverse racial and ethnic heritages, and those living in rural or isolated areas without access to care. Materials include topics related to health care, prenatal care and newborn screening, preventive care and research, and more.

La Leche League International (www.llli.org) offers resources on all facets of breastfeeding from health benefits to legislation concerning breastfeeding in the United States and around the world. Resources are also available for mothers and caregivers dealing with childhood illnesses and problems, including colic and allergies, or issues for the mother such as breast pain and possible toxins in milk.

The National Network for Immunization (www.immunizationinfo.org) offers information on immunizations, including a fact sheet entitled "Are Vaccines Safe?" and a glossary guide to understanding vaccine research terminology. There is also a weekly e-news letter filled with news stories about vaccines called *Immunization Newsbriefs*.

Book Resource:

Shu, Jennifer. (2006). American Academy of Pediatrics Baby and Child Health. Elk Grove, IL: American Academy of Pediatrics.

POSTPARTUM CARE

1. General Considerations

With early maternity discharge programs, postpartum and newborn care is increasingly being provided by HHAs. Usually the mothers and infants go home within 24 hours after birth and the home health nurse evaluates the mother and baby the next day (see also Newborn Care in this Part of this text).

2. Potential Diagnoses and Codes

The diagnoses and codes listed here include some of the most common conditions seen in postpartum care, and have been alphabetized for easy identification. Keep in mind that the ICD-9-CM system requires a focused review of the patient's medical information in addition to the physician-assigned diagnoses. Should additional information be needed, refer to the coding books or a qualified coder.

Diagnosis	Code
Cesarean delivery for fetal distress	656.30
Cesarean delivery without mention of indication	669.70
Cesarean delivery for excessive fetal growth	656.60
Cesarean delivery, previous	654.20
Mastitis	611.0
Mastitis, postpartum	675.24
Normal delivery	650
Pelvic inflammatory disease	646.64 and 614.9
Postpartum endometritis	670.04
Others	

3. Associated Nursing Diagnoses (see Part Seven)

4. Supportive Factors for the Determination and Documentation of Homebound Status

Usually not a requirement for early discharge maternity program, but the mothers and infants are confined to home for infection control, feeding reasons for the infant, and the increased rest needs of the new postpartum mother.

5. Potential Goals and Outcomes

The following patient-centered goals/outcomes can be individualized according to the identified needs of the patient and family.

Nursing

Patient articulates satisfaction with care
Educational tools/plans related to postpartum care incorporated in daily care routines (e.g., rest, fluids, increased nutritional needs if breast-feeding)
Nutrition and hydration optimal for health maintenance and milk supply
Patient effective in own and infant's care and knows whom to call for questions/concerns
Pain-free and infection-free postpartum patient
Positive relationship with infant seen by team members during visits
Healing, infection-free episiotomy or laceration site
Patient verbalizes signs (e.g., bleeding, infection) that necessitate calling the physician
Other

Home Health Aide

Effective personal care
ADL assistance and respite
Other

Medical Social Services

Identification and addressing/resolution of problems impeding the successful implementation of the POC
Referral/linkage with community resources
Other

6. Skills, Interventions/Services, and Management

Home care clinicians must exercise acute and effective critical thinking, observation, technical, teaching and evaluation skills when performing clinical assessments, interventions, and management of their home care patients.

Nursing

Patient provided with home safety information and instruction related to _____ and documented in the clinical record

Assessment of breasts and nipples, engorgement, soreness, cracking, blisters

Assessment of Homans' sign

Assess patient's pain on an ongoing basis to identify need for change, alteration addition, or other plan for pain management

Vital signs, including pain assessment each visit

Instruct regarding management of pain, including hemorrhoid discomfort and episiotomy pain

Teach new parents regarding infant care and safety measures, back positioning, parenting skills, bathing, cord care, circumcision care, and well-child care, including immunizations

Obtain urine for culture and sensitivity

Assessment of amount, character of lochia

Assessment of episiotomy site

Check fundus

Teach regarding parenting

Teach regarding breast-care regimen(s) and uterine involution process

Teach breast feeding techniques, and care of breasts for breast feeding

Teach regarding activity level

Teach regarding exercise level

Teach regarding family planning

Teach regarding sexuality questions

Maternal support related to caring for infant
Teach importance of optimal hydration, nutrition, and rest for healing and breast-feeding
Teach infection control, including effective hand washing
Teach indications for sitz bath, and procedure as indicated
Teach nutrition, especially if breast feeding
Teach importance of medical follow-up
Teach sign/symptoms of postpartum depression and coping mechanisms
Consult lactation specialist prn
Other aspects of care related to the patient's unique needs

Home Health Aide

Personal care
ADL assistance, may assist mother with meal preparation, light housekeeping, assisting with other siblings as indicated
Other tasks/activities as assigned

Medical Social Services

Psychosocial evaluation
Referral to community resources
Financial assistance counseling
Home safety assessment and counseling
Other interventions

7. Safety Considerations and Discharge Plans

Infection control/universal precautions
Night-light
Infant safety related to infection, germs, need for hand washing
Safety considerations (e.g., car seat placement, sleeping position)
Signs/symptoms that necessitate immediate reporting/ assistance

Safety related to home medical equipment
Smoke detector and fire evacuation plan
Return mother to self-care status in community, effectively caring for infant, under MD or public health supervision with lactation consultation as needed
Others, based on the patient's unique condition and environment

8. Tips to Support Medical Necessity, Quality, and Reimbursement

Document any variances to expected outcomes
Document all nursing care and the actions of that care
Two to three nursing visits are usually covered by insurance, depending on specific policies
Home health aides are sometimes involved and can stay up to 8 hours daily in some insurance benefit programs

9. Tips for Communication with Insurance Case Manager

Present objective patient findings and changes since last update
Meet face-to-face for relationship building when possible
Communicate information about the infant's status, education provided to parent, and the plans for follow-up care

10. Evidence-Based and other Resources for Practice and Education.

The American Academy of Pediatrics (AAP) (www.aap.org or 847-434-4000) offers information on a variety of children's health topics including breastfeeding, the common cold, circumcision, and hearing screenings.
HRSA's Maternal and Child Health (www.ask.hrsa.gov/MCH.cfm or 888-275-4772) programs promote and improve the health of mothers, infants, children, and adolescents,

including low-income families, those with diverse racial and ethnic heritages, and those living in rural or isolated areas without access to care. Materials include topics related to health care, prenatal care and newborn screening, preventive care and research, and more.

La Leche League International (www.llli.org) offers resources on all facets of breastfeeding from health benefits to legislation concerning breastfeeding in the United States and around the world. Resources are also available for mothers and caregivers dealing with childhood illnesses and problems, including colic and allergies, or issues for the mother such as breast pain and possible toxins in milk.

SICKLE CELL ANEMIA (CARE OF THE CHILD WITH)

1. General Considerations

Children and adolescents with sickle cell anemia are occasionally referred to home health organizations for follow-up after hospitalization. The emphasis at home utilizes nursing teaching skills.

2. Potential Diagnoses and Codes

The diagnoses and codes listed here include some of the most common conditions seen in children with sickle cell anemia, and have been alphabetized for easy identification. Keep in mind that the ICD-9-CM system requires a focused review of the patient's medical information in addition to the physician-assigned diagnoses. Should additional information be needed, refer to the coding books or a qualified coder.

Acute chest pain	786.50
Dehydration	276.51
Sickle cell anemia	282.60
Sickle cell crisis	282.62
Sickle cell trait	282.5
Others	

3. Associated Nursing Diagnoses (see Part Seven)

4. Supportive Factors for Determination and Documentation of Homebound Status

The homebound factor may or may not be a criterion for admission, based on the managed care program or the third-party payer involved. However, the following are reasons the patient would be homebound:

Pain, weakness
Decreased activity, bed rest to decrease oxygen need
Others

5. Potential Goals and Outcomes

The following patient-centered goals/outcomes can be individualized according to the identified needs of the patient and family.

Nursing

Patient verbalizes satisfaction with care
Support growth and developmental tasks of childhood
Educational tools/plans related to sickle cell disease incorporated into care routines (e.g., rest, increased fluids)
Nutrition and hydration optimal for health maintenance
Patient effective in self-care by discharge _____ and knows whom to call for questions/concerns
Pain free and infection free after sickle cell exacerbation
Patient verbalizes signs (e.g., increased pain, swelling) that necessitate calling the physician
Effective pain management as verbalized by patient
Prevention of multiple hospital admissions for IV fluids and pain medication with case management/phone intervention program by _____ (specify date)
Patient comfortable, pain free, and hydrated at home
Other

Home Health Aide

Effective personal care.
ADL assistance
Other

Medical Social Services

Identification and addressing/resolution of problems impeding the successful implementation of the POC
Referral/linkage with community resources
Other

Occupational Therapy

ADL level maintained at patient's optimal level
Optimal functional, safe mobility maintained
Quality of life improved through assistive/adaptive devices and energy-conservation techniques
Other

6. Skills, Interventions/Services, and Management

Home care clinicians must exercise acute and effective critical thinking, observation, technical, teaching and evaluation skills when performing clinical assessments, interventions, and management of their home care patients.

Nursing

Comprehensive assessment of all systems of child admitted to home care for _____ (specify problem necessitating care)
Assess pain medication regimen and response to therapy
Assess respiratory status
Assist with management of sickle cell crisis
Encourage nutritional supplements as ordered
Assess amount and site of any swelling
Teach regarding importance of contacting RN and physician regarding fever, SOB, or crisis onset
Teach patient to avoid factors that may predispose to crisis episode
Assess patient for signs and symptoms of infection, S/P multiple blood transfusions
Monitor amount and site of pain
Observe for chronic leg ulcers and other sites of thrombosis
Counsel patient on importance of adequate hydration, nutrition, rest, and infection resolution and control
Teach patient about safe, effective use of oxygen therapy
Observe and assess patient for signs of impending crisis
Monitor patient's respiratory, mental status, and other functions for evidence of change or impending crisis

Monitor vital signs
Venipuncture for CBC, sedimentation rate (specify frequency ordered)
Monitor patient's weight
Start and monitor IV of _____ for hydration (per specific physician's orders)
Assess IV's patency and site for redness, tenderness, swelling, or other signs of infection/infiltration
Monitor intake and output and pain management of patient recently discharged from the hospital S/P crisis
Dress leg wound sites with (specify per physician's orders) each (specify frequency)
Monitor patient's pain control regimen, including teaching caregivers the importance of adherence to the ordered and fixed medication schedule
Teach patient relaxation techniques, imagery, and other nonpharmacologic interventions that may assist relief
Instruct in how to avoid infections
Instruct importance of medical follow-up
Refer to support groups in the community that are available to patients and their caregivers
Other interventions

Home Health Aide
Personal care
ADL assistance
Other tasks/activities as assigned

Medical Social Services
Psychosocial assessment
Problem identification
Referral for genetic counseling
Financial assistance counseling
Referral(s) to community resources
Home safety assessment
Other interventions

5

Occupational Therapy

Evaluation
Assess home safety
Conservation of energy techniques
Selection of appropriate play activities
Adaptive/assistive devices as indicated
Other interventions

Physical Therapy

Evaluation
Therapeutic exercise program
Safe transfer training/locomotion
Instruct, supervise, and teach caregiver home exercise program
Assess for DME needs
Modalities/manual therapies for pain management
Other interventions

7. Safety Considerations and Discharge Plans

Infection control/universal precautions
Night-light, other child safety information
Avoidance, where possible, of precipitating factors
Symptoms that necessitate immediate reporting/assistance
Safety related to home medical equipment
Smoke detector and fire evacuation plan
Discharged, family able to provide care, under physician's supervision
Discharged to 24-hour acute facility for pain-control management
Others, based on the patient's unique condition and environment

8. Tips to Support Medical Necessity, Quality, and Reimbursement

Document hematocrit and hemoglobin values
Ultimately, any organs can be affected and have clinical involvement, document these changes

Document the nursing care provided and the outcomes of that care

Document the specific teaching accomplished and the behavioral outcomes of that teaching

Patients with sickle cell disease have a long history of interactions with health care settings and professionals. The patients know their histories, what pain medications bring relief most effectively, and other important information that assists the home care nurse in meeting patient and home care goals.

9. Tips for Communication with Insurance Case Manager

Present objective patient findings and changes since last update

Meet face-to-face for relationship building when possible

Communicate information about the patient's status, including pain management, resolution of crisis, education provided to parent, and the plans for follow-up care

10. Evidence-Based and other Resources for Practice and Education

The Agency for Healthcare Research and Quality (AHRQ) (www.ahrq.gov or 800-358-9295) offers "Acute Pain Management in Infants, Children, and Adolescents: Operative or Medical Procedures and Trauma (Quick Reference Guide for Clinicians)" (AHCPR 92-0020).

Sickle Cell Disease Association of America (www.sicklecelldisease.org or 800-421-8453) has regional chapters and provides support, information, and other resources for clinicians, patients, and families.

5

SURGICAL (POSTOPERATIVE) CARE OF THE CHILD

1. General Considerations

The Centers for Disease Control and Prevention report that accidents continue to be the leading cause of death in children younger than 18 years. The care of the child at home after hospitalization and surgery is often the result of trauma, particularly car accidents. Depending on the circumstances, care will usually be directed toward wound healing, restorative nursing, and rehabilitation goals (see also Medically Fragile Child Care guideline in this Part of this text).

2. Potential Diagnoses and Codes

The diagnoses and codes listed here include some of the most common conditions seen in children post-surgery, and have been alphabetized for easy identification. Keep in mind that the ICD-9-CM system requires a focused review of the patient's medical information in addition to the physician-assigned diagnoses. Should additional information be needed, refer to the coding books or a qualified coder.

Diagnosis	Code
Aftercare following surgery to ______ system	V58.7X
Amputation, status, infected right or left BKA	997.62 and V49.75
Appendicitis, perforation with abscess	540.1
Attention to other artificial opening of urinary tract	V55.6
Bone marrow transplant (surgical)	41.00
Bowel impaction	560.30
Cellulitis, right lower extremity, left lower extremity	682.9
Colitis	558.9
Colostomy, attention to	V55.3
Constipation	564.0
Crohn's disease	555.9

Cystocele, female	618.0
Cystocele, male	596.8
Dehydration	276.5
Depression, reactive	300.4
Diabetes mellitus, with unspecified complications, type 1	250.91
Fitting and adjustment of urinary devices	V53.6
Hemiplegia	342.90
Hypertension	401.9
Ileus	560.1
Ileus, postoperative	997.4
Incontinence of urine	788.30
Long-term (current) use of antibiotics	V58.62
Osteomyelitis, lower leg	730.26
Other aftercare following surgery	V58.49
Paraplegia	344.1
Peritonitis	567.9
Peritonitis, postoperative infection	998.59 and 567.9
Pneumonia	486
Quadriplegia	344.00
Surgical dressing change	V58.31
Suture removal	V58.32
Urinary tract infection	599.0
Wound dehiscence	998.3
Wound infection, postoperative	998.59
Others	

3. Associated Nursing Diagnoses (see Part Seven)

4. Supportive Factors for Determination and Documentation of Homebound Status

The homebound factor may or may not be a criterion for admission, based on the managed care program or the third-party payer involved. However, the following are reasons the child would be homebound:

Patient is status post _____ surgery (specify) and has weakness and pain

Patient is medically restricted for 4 weeks; not to leave home except for scheduled visits with vascular surgeon for flap assessment
Patient has open wound site and is unable to leave home without assistance
Patient is only partial or non-weight bearing
Patient is receiving IV antibiotics to treat infection
Others

5. Potential Goals and Outcomes.

The following patient-centered goals/outcomes can be individualized according to the identified needs of the patient and family.

Nursing
Patient/caregiver verbalizes satisfaction with care
Support growth and developmental tasks of childhood
Behavioral compliance with home care regimen
Educational tools/plans related to postoperative wound care incorporated into care routines (e.g., rest, increased fluids)
Parent/caregiver will meet developmental needs of the child
Parent/caregiver will demonstrate the ability to perform recently learned health-related behaviors
Nutrition and hydration optimal for health maintenance
Child/parent effective in self-care by discharge _____ and knows whom to call for questions/concerns
Parent verbalizes signs (e.g., increased pain, swelling) that necessitate calling the physician
Effective pain management as verbalized by patient
Child/caregiver will demonstrate _____ percent behavioral compliance with instructions related to medications, diet, and activity
Adherence to POC by patient and caregivers, and able to demonstrate safe and supportive care
Optimal nutrition/hydration needs maintained/addressed as evidenced by patient's weight maintained/increased by _____ lbs.

Infection-free wound site (specify parameters) by _____
Patient will be maintained in home stating/demonstrating adherence to POC
Blood pressure stable for patient (specify parameters)
Laboratory values (specify) will be improved/WNL for patient
Caregiver/patient verbalizes symptoms that necessitate calling the physician and need intervention/follow-up
Other

Home Health Agency
Effective and safe personal care and hygiene
Safe ADL assistance
Safe home environment maintained
Other

Medical Social Services
Resource identification and financial situation assessed/addressed allowing for successful implementation of the ordered POC
Financial/access problems addressed, resources identified as demonstrated by food in the refrigerator and medication availability to patient per POC
Linkage to community services and other resources for continued support and health maintenance
Other

Occupational Therapy
ADL level maintained at patient's optimal level
Optimal functional, safe mobility maintained
Quality of life improved through assistive/adaptive devices, energy-conservation techniques, and leisure/play activities
Restoration of age age-appropriate fine motor and ADL skills
Other

Physical Therapy

Increased endurance and comfort as expressed by patient

Caregiver/child compliance with exercise regimen including ROM, strength, coordination, and safety

Restoration of age appropriate gross motor skills

Other

6. Skills, Interventions/Services, and Management

Home care clinicians must exercise acute and effective critical thinking, observation, technical, teaching and evaluation skills when performing clinical assessments, interventions, and management of their home care patients.

Nursing

Parent/caregiver provided with home safety information and instruction related to _____ and documented in the clinical record

Teach child and caregiver about all medications, including schedule, functions, and side effects

Assess lower extremities for signs and symptoms of compromised circulation or decreased sensation

Skilled observation and assessment of wound and other (specify)

Perform wound care as ordered

Teach wound care, dressing change as ordered and disposal of dressings

Evaluate patient pain and implement pain control/relief regimen per physician's orders

Teach parent and caregiver safe use and care of PCA pump

Observation and assessment of postoperative patient's bowel patterns, including frequency and evaluation of need for stool softener, laxatives, or dietary changes

Assessment of blood pressure and other vital signs

Pain management and evaluation each visit

Teach patient/caregiver pain management techniques

Teach infection control
Instruct importance of medical follow-up
Instruct in self-care observational aspects of care, particularly for the wound or other (specify) site
Refer to support groups in the community that are available to patients and their caregivers
Instruct parents regarding the child's need to continue in growth and development phases, including seeing peers, stimulation, and maintaining or completing schoolwork
Teach caregiver importance of nutrition and dietary regimen and requirements postsurgery
Teach child and caregiver about safe postoperative care; no pushing, pulling, lifting, roughhousing, or horseplay with siblings
Observe for signs/symptoms of infection
Instruct caregiver on signs and symptoms to watch for that would necessitate calling nurse or physician
Consult with wound specialist about wounds with surrounding skin involvement
Teach family how to safely care for patient in traction or with pins
Assess and monitor pain, patient's response to interventions, and effective pain relief measures
Medicate patient with (specify physician's order) for pain relief before extensive dressing change
Teach caregivers care of the adolescent in *halo* brace traction
Assess hydration and nutrition through review of food diary, intake and output records, and ordered weights
Assess child's unique response to treatments and interventions and report changes, unfavorable responses, or reactions to the physician
Instruct on signs and symptoms, infection control, and the avoidance of those with upper respiratory or other infections
Teach child and caregivers effective hand washing techniques and other infection control measures
Other interventions

Home Health Aide

Personal care
ADL assistance
Meal preparation
Home exercise program
Other tasks/activities as assigned

Medical Social Services

Evaluation
Assessment of the social and emotional factors impacting effective POC implementation
Determination of factors impeding POC from being successful
Psychosocial assessment of the child and family with multiple social problems
Financial counseling
Community resources referral
Facilitation of school reconnection or identification for tutoring needed for missed schoolwork
Other interventions

Occupational Therapy

Evaluation
Conservation of energy techniques
ADL assistance and retraining
Assessment of patient and home for assistive/adaptive devices or equipment
Other interventions

Physical Therapy

Evaluation
Home exercise strengthening program
Safe transfer training
Instruct, supervise, and teach caregiver home exercise regimen
Evaluate patient for overbed trapeze to facilitate bed mobility
Gait training
Other interventions

7. Safety Considerations and Discharge Plans

Infection control/universal precautions
Night-light, other child safety information
Symptoms that necessitate immediate reporting/assistance
Safety related to home medical equipment
Smoke detector and fire evacuation plan
Patient-centered, realistic goals achieved, discharge from home care, self-care under physician's supervision
Can get to outpatient clinic for care and will have peer-support groups available, discharge per physician's order
Others, based on the patient's unique condition and environment

8. Tips to Support Medical Necessity, Quality, and Reimbursement

Document progress toward wound healing or other specified, patient-centered goals
Document patient or wound deterioration or problems
Document the specific nursing care and teaching instructions provided
Document the patient's and caregiver's response to care interventions
Document any exacerbation of symptoms or problems that necessitated additional visits and be sure that there are orders for all visits
Document all POC changes
Document all the skills used in the provision of professional nursing care practice when caring for the child (e.g., teaching, training, observation and assessment, catheters, IV site care, venipuncture, etc.)
Document the coordination occurring, based on the POC, among team members; the interdisciplinary conference notes should be reflected in the clinical record; refer to these meetings or communications on the forms used by the insurer as an update on the patient's status

9. Tips for Communication with Insurance Case Manager

Present objective patient findings and changes since last update

Meet face-to-face for relationship building, when possible

Communicate information about the child's status, including pain management, surgical site intervention, education provided parent, and plans for follow-up care

10. Evidence-Based and other Resources for Practice and Education

The Agency for Healthcare Research and Quality (AHRQ) (www.ahrq.gov or 1-800-358-9295) offers "Acute Pain Management in Infants, Children, and Adolescents: Operative or Medical Procedures and Trauma (Quick Reference Guide for Clinicians)" (AHCPR 92-0020).

The American Association for Respiratory Care (AARC) www. AARC.org/store.cfm or 972-243-2272 offers a video entitled "Breath of Life—A Caregiver's Guide to Pediatric Tracheostomy Care" that was created with input from parents of a child with a tracheostomy.

PART SIX

MEDICARE HOME CARE GUIDELINES FOR COVERAGE OF SERVICES

Medicare Benefit Policy Manual: Chapter 7—Home Health Services

6

The following is from Chapter 7—Home Health Services in the Medicare Benefit Policy Manual found in the Internet-Only Manuals (IOMs) (http://www.cms.hhs.gov/manuals/Downloads/bp102c07.pdf).

20 - Conditions to Be Met for Coverage of Home Health Services
(Rev. 1, 10-01-03)
A3-3116, HHA-203

Medicare covers HHA services when the following criteria are met:

1. The person to whom the services are provided is an eligible Medicare beneficiary;
2. The HHA that is providing the services to the beneficiary has in effect a valid agreement to participate in the Medicare program;
3. The beneficiary qualifies for coverage of home health services as described in §30;
4. The services for which payment is claimed are covered as described in §§40 and 50;
5. Medicare is the appropriate payer; and
6. The services for which payment is claimed are not otherwise excluded from payment.

20.1 - Reasonable and Necessary Services
(Rev. 1, 10-01-03)
A3-3116.1. HHA-203.1

20.1.1 - Background
(Rev. 1, 10-01-03)
A3-3116.1A, HHA-203.1A

In enacting the Medicare program, Congress recognized that the physician would play an important role in determining utilization of services. The law requires that payment can be made only if a physician certifies the need for services and establishes a plan of care. The Secretary is responsible for ensuring that Medicare covers the claimed services, including determining whether they are "reasonable and necessary."

20.1.2 - Determination of Coverage
(Rev. 1, 10-01-03)
A3-3113.1.B, HHA-203.1.B

The intermediary's decision on whether care is reasonable and necessary is based on information reflected in the home health plan of care, the OASIS as required by 42 CFR 484.55 or a medical record of the individual patient. Medicare does not deny coverage solely on the basis of the reviewer's general inferences about patients with similar diagnoses or on data related to utilization generally, but bases it upon objective clinical evidence regarding the patient's individual need for care.

20.2 - Impact of Other Available Caregivers and Other Available Coverage on Medicare Coverage of Home Health Services
(Rev. 1, 10-01-03)
A3-3116.2, HHA-203.2

Where the Medicare criteria for coverage of home health services are met, patients are entitled by law to coverage of reasonable and necessary home health services. Therefore, a patient is entitled to have the costs of reasonable and necessary services reimbursed by Medicare without regard to whether there is someone available to furnish the services. However, where a family member or other person is or will be providing services that adequately meet the patient's needs, it would not be reasonable and necessary for HHA personnel to furnish such services. Ordinarily it can be presumed that there is no able and willing person in the home to provide the services being rendered by the HHA unless the patient or family indicates otherwise and objects to the provision of the services by the HHA, or unless the HHA has first hand knowledge to the contrary.

EXAMPLE 1: A patient who lives with an adult daughter and otherwise qualifies for Medicare coverage of home health services, requires the assistance of a home health aide for bathing and assistance with an exercise program to improve endurance. The daughter is unwilling to bathe her elderly father and assist him with the exercise program. Home health aide services would be reasonable and necessary.

Similarly, a patient is entitled to have the costs of reasonable and necessary home health services reimbursed by Medicare even if the patient would qualify for institutional care (e.g., hospital care or skilled nursing facility care).

EXAMPLE 2: A patient who is being discharged from a hospital with a diagnosis of osteomyelitis and requires continuation of the I.V. antibiotic therapy that was begun in the hospital was found to meet the criteria for Medicare coverage of skilled nursing facility services. If the patient also meets the qualifying criteria for coverage of home health services, payment may be made for the reasonable and necessary home health services the patient needs, notwithstanding the availability of coverage in a skilled nursing facility.

Medicare payment should be made for reasonable and necessary home health services where the patient is also receiving supplemental services that do not meet Medicare's definition of skilled nursing care or home health aide services.

EXAMPLE 3: A patient who needs skilled nursing care on an intermittent basis also hires a licensed practical (vocational) nurse to provide nighttime assistance while family members sleep. The care provided by the nurse, as respite to the family members, does not require the skills of a licensed nurse (as defined in §40.1) and therefore has no impact on the beneficiary's eligibility for Medicare payment of home health services even though another third party insurer may pay for that nursing care.

20.3 - Use of Utilization Screens and "Rules of Thumb"
(Rev. 1, 10-01-03)
A3-3116.3, HHA-203.3

Medicare recognizes that determinations of whether home health services are reasonable and necessary must be based on an assessment of each beneficiary's individual care needs. Therefore, denial of services based on numerical utilization screens, diagnostic screens, diagnosis, or specific treatment norms is not appropriate.

30 - Conditions Patient Must Meet to Qualify for Coverage of Home Health Services
(Rev. 1, 10-01-03)
A3-3117, HHA-204, A-98-49

To qualify for the Medicare home health benefit, under §§1814(a)(2)(C) and 1835(a)(2)(A) of the Act, a Medicare beneficiary must meet the following requirements:

- Be confined to the home;
- Under the care of a physician;
- Receiving services under a plan of care established and periodically reviewed by a physician;
- Be in need of skilled nursing care on an intermittent basis or physical therapy or speech-language pathology; or
- Have a continuing need for occupational therapy.

For purposes of benefit eligibility, under §§1814(a)(2)(C) and 1835(a)(2)(A) of the Act "intermittent" means skilled nursing care that is either provided or needed on fewer than 7 days each week or less than 8 hours of each day for periods of 21 days or less (with extensions in exceptional circumstances when the need for additional care is finite and predictable).

A patient must meet each of the criteria specified in this section. Patients who meet each of these criteria are eligible to have payment made on their behalf for services discussed in §§40 and 50.

30.1 - Confined to the Home
(Rev. 1, 10-01-03)
A3-3117.1, HHA-204.1

30.1.1 - Patient Confined to the Home
(Rev. 1, 10-01-03)
A3-3117.1.A, HHA-204.1.A, A-01-21

In order for a patient to be eligible to receive covered home health services under both Part A and Part B, the law requires that a physician certify in all cases that the patient is confined to his/her home. An individual does not have to be bedridden to be considered confined to the home. However, the condition of these patients should be such that there exists a normal inability to leave home and, consequently, leaving home would require a considerable and taxing effort.

If the patient does in fact leave the home, the patient may nevertheless be considered homebound if the absences from the home are infrequent or for periods of relatively short duration, or are attributable to the need to receive health care treatment. Absences attributable to the need to receive health care treatment include, but are not limited to:

- Attendance at adult day centers to receive medical care;
- Ongoing receipt of outpatient kidney dialysis; or
- The receipt of outpatient chemotherapy or radiation therapy.

Any absence of an individual from the home attributable to the need to receive health care treatment, including regular absences for the purpose of participating in therapeutic, psychosocial, or medical treatment in an adult day-care program that is licensed or certified by a State, or accredited to furnish adult day-care services in a State, shall not disqualify an individual from being considered to be confined to his home. Any other absence of an individual from the home shall not so disqualify an individual if the absence is of an infrequent or of relatively short duration. For purposes of the preceding sentence, any absence for the purpose of attending a religious service shall be deemed to be an absence of infrequent or short duration. It is expected that in most instances, absences from the home that occur will be for the purpose of receiving health care treatment. However, occasional absences from the home for nonmedical purposes, e.g., an occasional trip to the barber, a walk around the block or a drive, attendance at a family reunion, funeral, graduation, or other infrequent or unique event would not necessitate a finding that the patient is not homebound if the absences are undertaken on an infrequent basis or are of relatively short duration and do not indicate that the patient has the capacity to obtain the health care provided outside rather than in the home.

Generally speaking, a patient will be considered to be homebound if they have a condition due to an illness or injury that restricts their ability to leave their place of residence except with the aid of supportive devices, such as crutches, canes, wheelchairs, and walkers; the use of special transportation; or the assistance of another person; or if leaving home is medically contraindicated.

Some examples of homebound patients that illustrate the factors used to determine whether a homebound condition exists would be:

- A patient paralyzed from a stroke who is confined to a wheelchair or requires the aid of crutches in order to walk;
- A patient who is blind or senile and requires the assistance of another person in leaving their place of residence;
- A patient who has lost the use of their upper extremities and, therefore, is unable to open doors, use handrails on stairways, etc., and requires the assistance of another individual to leave their place of residence;
- A patient in the late stages of ALS or a neurodegenerative disability. In determining whether the patient has the general inability to leave the home and leaves the home only infrequently or for periods of

short duration, it is necessary (as is the case in determining whether skilled nursing services are intermittent) to look at the patient's condition over a period of time rather than for short periods within the home health stay. For example, a patient may leave the home (under the conditions described above, e.g., with severe and taxing effort, with the assistance of others) more frequently during a short period when, for example, the presence of visiting relatives provides a unique opportunity for such absences, than is normally the case. So long as the patient's overall condition and experience is such that he or she meets these qualifications, he or she should be considered confined to the home.

- A patient who has just returned from a hospital stay involving surgery who may be suffering from resultant weakness and pain and, therefore, their actions may be restricted by their physician to certain specified and limited activities such as getting out of bed only for a specified period of time, walking stairs only once a day, etc.;
- A patient with arteriosclerotic heart disease of such severity that they must avoid all stress and physical activity; and
- A patient with a psychiatric illness that is manifested in part by a refusal to leave home or is of such a nature that it would not be considered safe for the patient to leave home unattended, even if they have no physical limitations.

The aged person who does not often travel from home because of feebleness and insecurity brought on by advanced age would not be considered confined to the home for purposes of receiving home health services unless they meet one of the above conditions.

Although a patient must be confined to the home to be eligible for covered home health services, some services cannot be provided at the patient's residence because equipment is required that cannot be made available there. If the services required by an individual involve the use of such equipment, the HHA may make arrangements with a hospital, skilled nursing facility (SNF), or a rehabilitation center to provide these services on an outpatient basis. (See §50.6.) However, even in these situations, for the services to be covered as home health services the patient must be considered as confined to home; and to receive such outpatient services a homebound patient will generally require the use of supportive devices, special transportation, or the assistance of another person to travel to the appropriate facility.

If a question is raised as to whether a patient is confined to the home, the HHA will be requested to furnish the intermediary with the information necessary to establish that the patient is homebound as defined above.

30.1.2 - Patient's Place of Residence
(Rev. 1, 10-01-03)
A3-3117.1.B, HHA-204.1.B

A patient's residence is wherever he or she makes his or her home. This may be his or her own dwelling, an apartment, a relative's home, a home for the aged, or some other type of institution. However, an institution may not be considered a patient's residence if the institution meets the requirements of §§1861(e)(1) or 1819(a)(1) of the Act. Included in this group are hospitals and skilled nursing facilities, as well as most nursing facilities under Medicaid. (See the Medicare State Operations Manual, §2166.)

Thus, if a patient is in an institution or distinct part of an institution identified above, the patient is not entitled to have payment made for home health services under either Part A or Part B since such an institution may not be considered their residence. When a patient remains in a participating SNF following their discharge from active care, the facility may not be considered their residence for purposes of home health coverage.

A patient may have more than one home and the Medicare rules do not prohibit a patient from having one or more places of residence. A patient, under a Medicare home health plan of care, who resides in more than one place of residence during an episode of Medicare covered home health services will not disqualify the patient's homebound status for purposes of eligibility. For example, a person may reside in a principal home and also a second vacation home, mobile home, or the home of a caretaker relative. The fact that the patient resides in more than one home and, as a result, must transit from one to the other, is not in itself, an indication that the patient is not homebound. The requirements of homebound must be met at each location (e.g., considerable taxing effort etc).

A. Assisted Living Facilities, Group Homes, and Personal Care Homes

An individual may be "confined to the home" for purposes of Medicare coverage of home health services if he or she resides in an institution that is not primarily engaged in providing to inpatients:

- Diagnostic and therapeutic services for medical diagnosis;
- Treatment;
- Care of disabled or sick persons;
- Rehabilitation services for the rehabilitation of injured, disabled, or sick persons;
- Skilled nursing care or related services for patients who require medical or nursing care; or
- Rehabilitation services for the rehabilitation of injured, sick, or disabled persons.

If it is determined that the assisted living facility (also called personal care homes, group homes, etc.) in which the individuals reside are not primarily engaged in providing the above services, then Medicare will cover reasonable and necessary home health care furnished to these individuals.

If it is determined that the services furnished by the home health agency are duplicative of services furnished by an assisted living facility (also called personal care homes, group homes, etc.) when provision of such care is required of the facility under State licensure requirements, claims for such services should be denied under §1862(a)(1)(A) of the Act. Section 1862(a)(1)(A) excludes services that are not necessary for the diagnosis or treatment of illness or injury or to improve the functioning of a malformed body member from Medicare coverage. Services to people who already have access to appropriate care from a willing caregiver would not be considered reasonable and necessary to the treatment of the individual's illness or injury.

Medicare coverage would not be an optional substitute for the services that a facility that is required to provide by law to its patients or where the services are included in the base contract of the facility. An individual's choice to reside in such a facility is also a choice to accept the services it holds itself out as offering to its patients.

B. Day Care Centers and Patient's Place of Residence

The current statutory definition of homebound or confined does not imply that Medicare coverage has been expanded to include adult day care services.

The law does not permit an HHA to furnish a Medicare covered billable visit to a patient under a home health plan of care outside his or her home, except in those limited circumstances where the patient needs to use medical equipment that is too cumbersome to bring to the home. Section 1861(m) of the Act stipulates that home health services provided to a patient be provided to the patient on a visiting basis in a place of residence used as the individual's home. A licensed/certified day care center does not meet the definition of a place of residence.

C. State Licensure/Certification of Day Care Facilities

Section 1861(m) of the Act, an adult day care center must be either licensed or certified by the State or accredited by a private accrediting body. State licensure or certification as an adult day care facility must be based on State interpretations of its process. For example, several States do not license adult day care facilities as a whole, but do certify some entities as Medicaid certified centers for purposes of providing adult day care under the Medicaid home and community based waiver program. It is the responsibility of the State to determine the necessary criteria for "State certification" in such a situation. A State could determine that Medicaid certification is an acceptable standard and consider its Medicaid certified adult day care facilities to be "State certified." On the other hand, a State could determine

Medicaid certification to be insufficient and require other conditions to be met before the adult day care facility is considered "State certified."

D. Determination of the Therapeutic, Medical or Psychosocial Treatment of the Patient at the Day Care Facility

It is not the obligation of the HHA to determine whether the adult day care facility is providing psychosocial treatment, but only to assure that the adult day care center is licensed/certified by the State or accrediting body. The intent of the law, in extending the homebound exception status to attendance at such adult day care facilities, recognizes that they ordinarily furnish psychosocial services.

30.2 - Services Are Provided Under a Plan of Care Established and Approved by a Physician
(Rev. 1, 10-01-03)
A3-3117.2, HHA-204.2

30.2.1 - Content of the Plan of Care
(Rev. 1, 10-01-03)
A3-3117.2.A, HHA-204.2.A

The plan of care must contain all pertinent diagnoses, including:

- The patient's mental status;
- The types of services, supplies, and equipment required;
- The frequency of the visits to be made;
- Prognosis;
- Rehabilitation potential;
- Functional limitations;
- Activities permitted;
- Nutritional requirements;
- All medications and treatments;
- Safety measures to protect against injury;
- Instructions for timely discharge or referral; and
- Any additional items the HHA or physician choose to include.

30.2.2 - Specificity of Orders
(Rev. 1, 10-01-03)
A3-3117.2.B, HHA-204.2.B

The orders on the plan of care must indicate the type of services to be provided to the patient, both with respect to the professional who will provide them and the nature of the individual services, as well as the frequency of the services.

EXAMPLE 1: SN x 7/wk x 1 wk; 3/wk x 4 wk; 2/wk x 3 wk, (skilled nursing visits 7 times per week for 1 week; 3 times per week for 4 weeks; and 2 times per week for 3 weeks) for skilled observation and evaluation of the surgical site, for teaching sterile dressing changes and to perform sterile dressing changes. The sterile change consists of (detail of procedure).

Orders for care may indicate a specific range in the frequency of visits to ensure that the most appropriate level of services is provided during the 60-day episode to home health patients. When a range of visits is ordered, the upper limit of the range is considered the specific frequency.

EXAMPLE 2: SN x 2-4/wk x 4 wk; 1-2/wk x 4 wk for skilled observation and evaluation of the surgical site.

Orders for services to be furnished "as needed" or "PRN" must be accompanied by a description of the patient's medical signs and symptoms that would occasion a visit and a specific limit on the number of those visits to be made under the order before an additional physician order would have to be obtained.

30.2.3 - Who Signs the Plan of Care
(Rev. 1, 10-01-03)
A3-3117.2.C, HHA-204-2.C

The physician who signs the plan of care must be qualified to sign the physician certification as described in 42 CFR 424.22.

30.2.4 - Timeliness of Signature
(Rev. 1, 10-01-03)
A3-3117.2.D, HHA-204-2.D

A. Initial Percentage Payment

If a physician signed plan of care is not available at the beginning of the episode, the HHA may submit a RAP for the initial percentage payment based on physician verbal orders OR a referral prescribing detailed orders for the services to be rendered that is signed and dated by the physician. If the RAP submission is based on physician verbal orders, the verbal order must be recorded in the plan of care, include a description of the patient's condition and the services to be provided by the home health agency, include an attestation (relating to the physician's orders and the date received per 42 CFR 409.43), and the plan of care is copied and immediately submitted to the physician. A billable visit must be rendered prior to the submission of a RAP.

B. Final Percentage Payment

The plan of care must be signed and dated by a physician as described who meets the certification and recertification requirements of 42 CFR 424.22 and before the claim for each episode for services is submitted for the final percentage payment. Any changes in the plan of care must be signed and dated by a physician.

30.2.5 - Use of Oral (Verbal) Orders
(Rev. 1, 10-01-03)
A3-3117.2.E, HHA-204-2.E

When services are furnished based on a physician's oral order, the orders may be accepted and put in writing by personnel authorized to do so by applicable State and Federal laws and regulations as well as by the HHA's internal policies. The orders must be signed and dated with the date of receipt by the registered nurse or qualified therapist (i.e., physical therapist, speech-language pathologist, occupational therapist, or medical social worker) responsible for furnishing or supervising the ordered services. The orders may be signed by the supervising registered nurse or qualified therapist after the services have been rendered, as long as HHA personnel who receive the oral orders notify that nurse or therapist before the service is rendered. Thus, the rendering of a service that is based on an oral order would not be delayed pending signature of the supervising nurse or therapist. Oral orders must be countersigned and dated by the physician before the HHA bills for the care in the same way as the plan of care.

Services which are provided from the beginning of the 60-day episode certification period based on a request for anticipated payment and before the physician signs the plan of care are considered to be provided under a plan of care established and approved by the physician where there is an oral order for the care prior to rendering the services which is documented in the medical record and where the services are included in a signed plan of care.

EXAMPLE 1: The HHA acquires an oral order for I.V. medication administration for a patient to be performed on August 1. The HHA provides the I.V. medication administration August 1 and evaluates the patient's need for continued care. The physician signs the plan of care for the I.V. medication administration on August 15. The visit is covered since it is considered provided under a plan of care established and approved by the physician, and the HHA had acquired an oral order prior to the delivery of services.

Services that are provided in the subsequent 60-day episode certification period are considered provided under the plan of care of the subsequent 60-day episode where there is an oral order before the services provided in the subsequent period are furnished and the order is reflected in the medical record. However, services that are provided after the expiration of a plan of care, but before the acquisition of an oral order or a signed plan of care are not considered provided under a plan of care.

EXAMPLE 2: The patient is under a plan of care in which the physician orders I.V. medication administration every two weeks. The last day covered by the initial plan of care is July 31. The patient's next I.V. medication administration is scheduled for August 5 and the physician signs the plan of care for the new period on August 1. The I.V. medication administration on August 5 was provided under a plan of care established and approved by the physician. The episode begins on the 61 day regardless of the date of the first covered visit.

EXAMPLE 3: The patient is under a plan of care in which the physician orders I.V. medication administration every two weeks. The last day covered by the plan of care is July 31. The patient's next I.V. medication administration is scheduled for August 5 and the physician does not sign the plan of care until August 6. The HHA acquires an oral order for the I.V. medication administration before the August 5 visit, and therefore the visit is considered to be provided under a plan of care established and approved by the physician. The episode begins on the 61 day regardless of the date of the first covered visit.

Any increase in the frequency of services or addition of new services during a certification period must be authorized by a physician by way of a written or oral order prior to the provision of the increased or additional services.

30.2.6 - Frequency of Review of the Plan of Care
(Rev. 1, 10-01-03)
A3-3117.2.F, HHA-204.2.F

The plan of care must be reviewed and signed by the physician who established the plan of care, in consultation with HHA professional personnel, at least every 60 days. Each review of a patient's plan of care must contain the signature of the physician and the date of review.

30.2.7 - Facsimile Signatures
(Rev. 1, 10-01-03)
A3-3117.2.G, HHA-204.2.G

The plan of care or oral order may be transmitted by facsimile machine. The HHA is not required to have the original signature on file. However, the HHA is responsible for obtaining original signatures if an issue surfaces that would require verification of an original signature.

30.2.8 - Alternative Signatures
(Rev. 1, 10-01-03)
A3-3117.2.H, HHA-204.2.H

HHAs that maintain patient records by computer rather than hard copy may use electronic signatures. However, all such entries must be appropriately authenticated and dated. Authentication must include signatures, written initials, or computer secure entry by a unique identifier of a primary author who has reviewed and approved the entry. The HHA must have safeguards to prevent unauthorized access to the records and a process for reconstruction of the records in the event of a system breakdown.

30.2.9 - Termination of the Plan of Care - Qualifying Services
(Rev. 1, 10-01-03)
A3-3117.2.I, HHA-204.2.I

The plan of care is considered to be terminated if the patient does not receive at least one covered skilled nursing, physical therapy, speech-language pathology service, or occupational therapy visit in a 60-day period since these are qualifying services for the home health benefit. An exception is if the physician documents that the interval without such care is appropriate to the treatment of the patient's illness or injury.

30.2.10 - Sequence of Qualifying Services and Other Medicare Covered Home Health Services
(Rev. 1, 10-01-03)
A3-3117.2.J, HHA-204.2.J

Once patient eligibility has been confirmed and the plan of care contains physician orders for the qualifying service as well as other Medicare covered home health services, the qualifying service does not have to be rendered prior to the other Medicare covered home health services ordered in the plan of care. The sequence of visits performed by the disciplines must be dictated by the individual patient's plan of care. For example, for an eligible patient in an initial 60-day episode that has both physical therapy and occupational therapy orders in the plan of care, the sequence of the delivery of the type of therapy is irrelevant as long as the need for the qualifying service is established prior to the delivery of other Medicare covered services and the qualifying discipline provides a billable visit prior to transfer or discharge in accordance with 42 CFR 409.43(f).

NOTE: Dependent services provided after the final qualifying skilled service are not covered under the home health benefit, except when the dependent service was followed by a qualifying skilled service as a result of the unexpected inpatient admission or death of the patient or due to some other unanticipated event.

30.3 - Under the Care of a Physician
(Rev. 1, 10-01-03)
A3-3117.3, HHA-204.3

The patient must be under the care of a physician who is qualified to sign the physician certification and plan of care in accordance with 42 CFR 424.22.

A patient is expected to be under the care of the physician who signs the plan of care and the physician certification. It is expected, but not required for coverage, that the physician who signs the plan of care will see the patient, but there is no specified interval of time within which the patient must be seen.

30.4 - Needs Skilled Nursing Care on an Intermittent Basis (Other than Solely Venipuncture for the Purposes of Obtaining a Blood Sample), Physical Therapy, Speech-Language Pathology Services, or Has Continued Need for Occupational Therapy
(Rev. 1, 10-01-03)
A3-3117.4, HHA-204.4

The patient must need one of the following types of services:

1. Skilled nursing care that is

- Reasonable and necessary as defined in §40.1;
- Needed on an "intermittent" based as defined in §40.1; and
- Not solely needed for venipuncture for the purposes of obtaining blood sample as defined in §40.1.2.13;or

2. Physical therapy as defined in §40.2.2; or
3. Speech-language pathology services as defined in §40.2.3; or
4. Have a continuing need for occupational therapy as defined in §§40.2.4. The patient has a continued need for occupational therapy when:

1. The services which the patient requires meet the definition of "occupational therapy" services of §40.2, and

2. The patient's eligibility for home health services has been established by virtue of a prior need for skilled nursing care (other than solely venipuncture for the purposes of obtaining a blood sample), speech-language pathology services, or physical therapy in the current or prior certification period.

EXAMPLE: A patient who is recovering from a cerebrovascular accident (CVA) has an initial plan of care that called for physical therapy, speech-language pathology services, and home health aide services. In the next certification period, the physician orders only occupational therapy and home health aide services because the patient no longer needs the skills of a physical therapist or a speech-language pathologist, but needs the services provided by the occupational therapist. The patient's need for occupational therapy qualifies him for home health services, including home health aide services (presuming that all other qualifying criteria are met).

30.5 - Physician Certification
(Rev. 1, 10-01-03)
A3-3117.5, HHA-204.5

The HHA must be acting upon a physician certification that is part of the plan of care (Form CMS-485) and meets the requirements of this section for HHA services to be covered.

30.5.1 - Content of the Physician Certification
(Rev. 1, 10-01-03)
A3-3117.5.A, HHA-204.5.A

The physician must certify that:

1. The home health services are or were needed because the patient is or was confined to the home as defined in §20.1;
2. The patient needs or needed skilled nursing services on an intermittent basis (other than solely venipuncture for the purposes of obtaining a blood sample), or physical therapy, or speech-language pathology services; or continues to need occupational therapy after the need for skilled nursing care, physical therapy, or speech-language pathology services ceased;
3. A plan of care has been established and is periodically reviewed by a physician; and
4. The services are or were furnished while the patient is or was under the care of a physician.

30.5.2 - Periodic Recertification
(Rev. 1, 10-01-03)
A3-3117.5.B, HHA-204.5.B

At the end of the 60-day episode, a decision must be made whether or not to recertify the patient for a subsequent 60-day episode. An eligible beneficiary who qualifies for a subsequent 60-day episode would start the subsequent 60-day episode on day 61. Under HH PPS, the plan of care must be reviewed and signed by the physician every 60 days unless one of the following occurs:

- A beneficiary transfers to another HHA;
- A SCIC (significant change in condition) resulting in a change in the assigned case-mix; or
- A discharge and return to the same HHA during the 60-day episode.

Medicare does not limit the number of continuous episode recertifications for beneficiaries who continue to be eligible for the home health benefit. The physician certification may cover a period less than but not greater than 60 days.

See §10.4 for counting initial and subsequent 60-day episodes and recertifications. See §10.5 for recertifications for split percentage payments.

30.5.3 - Who May Sign the Certification
(Rev. 1, 10-01-03)
A3-3117.5.C, HHA-204.5.C

The physician who signs the certification must be permitted to do so by 42 CFR 424.22.

40 - Covered Services Under a Qualifying Home Health Plan of Care
(Rev. 1, 10-01-03)
A3-3118, HHA-205

Section 1861(m) of the Act governs the Medicare home health services that may be provided to eligible beneficiaries by or under arrangements made by a participating home health agency (HHA). Section 1861(m) describes home health services as

- Part-time or intermittent skilled nursing care (other than solely venipuncture for the purposes of obtaining a blood sample);
- Part-time or intermittent home health aide services;
- Physical therapy;
- Speech-language pathology;
- Occupational therapy;
- Medical social services;
- Medical supplies including catheters, catheter supplies, ostomy bags, supplies related to ostomy care, and a covered osteoporosis drug (as defined in §1861(kk) of the Act), but excluding other drugs and biologicals;
- Durable medical equipment while under the plan of care established by physician;
- Medical services provided by an intern or resident-in-training under an approved teaching program of the hospital in the case of an HHA which is affiliated or under common control with a hospital; and
- Services at hospitals, skilled nursing facilities, or rehabilitation centers when they involve equipment too cumbersome to bring to the home.

The term "part-time or intermittent" for purposes of coverage under §1861(m) of the Act means skilled nursing and home health aide services furnished any number of days per week as long as they are furnished (combined) less than 8 hours each day and 28 or fewer hours each week (or, subject to review on a case-by-case basis as to the need for care, less than 8 hours each day and 35 or fewer hours per week). See §50.7.

For any home health services to be covered by Medicare, the patient must meet the qualifying criteria as specified in §30, including having a need for skilled nursing care on an intermittent basis, physical therapy, speech-language pathology services, or a continuing need for occupational therapy as defined in this section.

40.1 - Skilled Nursing Care
(Rev. 1, 10-01-03)
A3-3118.1, HHA-205.1

To be covered as skilled nursing services, the services must require the skills of a registered nurse, or a licensed practical (vocational) nurse under the supervision of a registered nurse, must be reasonable and necessary to the treatment of the patient's illness or injury as discussed in §40.1.1, below, and must be intermittent as discussed in §40.1.3.

40.1.1 - General Principles Governing Reasonable and Necessary Skilled Nursing Care
(Rev. 1, 10-01-03)
A3-3118.1, HHA-205.1

A skilled nursing service is a service that must be provided by a registered nurse or a licensed practical (vocational) nurse under the supervision of a registered nurse to be safe and effective. In determining whether a service requires the skills of a nurse, the reviewer considers both the inherent complexity of the service, the condition of the patient and accepted standards of medical and nursing practice.

Some services may be classified as a skilled nursing service on the basis of complexity alone, e.g., intravenous and intramuscular injections or insertion of catheters, and if reasonable and necessary to the treatment of the patient's illness or injury, would be covered on that basis. However, in some cases, the condition of the patient may cause a service that would ordinarily be considered unskilled to be considered a skilled nursing service. This would occur when the patient's condition is such that the service can be safely and effectively provided only by a nurse.

EXAMPLE 1: The presence of a plaster cast on an extremity generally does not indicate a need for skilled nursing care. However, the patient with a preexisting peripheral vascular or circulatory condition might need skilled nursing care to observe for complications, monitor medication administration for pain control, and teach proper skin care to preserve skin integrity and prevent breakdown.

EXAMPLE 2: The condition of a patient, who has irritable bowel syndrome or is recovering from rectal surgery, may be such that he or she can be given an enema safely and effectively only by a nurse. If the enema were necessary to treat the illness or injury, then the visit would be covered as a skilled nursing visit.

A service is not considered a skilled nursing service merely because it is performed by or under the direct supervision of a nurse. If a service can be safely and effectively performed (or self-administered) by a nonmedical person, without the direct supervision of a nurse, the service cannot be regarded as a skilled nursing service although a nurse actually provides the service. Similarly, the unavailability of a competent person to provide a nonskilled service, notwithstanding the importance of the service to the patient, does not make it a skilled service when a nurse provides the service.

EXAMPLE 1: Giving a bath does not ordinarily require the skills of a nurse and, therefore, would not be covered as a skilled nursing service unless the patient's condition is such that the bath could be given safely and effectively only by a nurse (as discussed in §30.1 above).

EXAMPLE 2: A patient with a well-established colostomy absent complications may require assistance changing the colostomy bag because they cannot do it themselves and there is no one else to change the bag. Notwithstanding the need for the routine colostomy care, the care does not become a skilled nursing service when the nurse provides it.

A service which, by its nature, requires the skills of a nurse to be provided safely and effectively continues to be a skilled service even if it is taught to the patient, the patient's family, or other caregivers. Where the patient needs the skilled nursing care and there is no one trained, able and willing to provide it, the services of a nurse would be reasonable and necessary to the treatment of the illness or injury.

EXAMPLE 3: A patient was discharged from the hospital with an open draining wound that requires irrigation, packing, and dressing twice each day. The HHA has taught the family to perform the dressing changes. The HHA continues to see the patient for the wound care that is needed during the time that the family is not available and willing to provide the dressing changes. The wound care continues to be skilled nursing care, notwithstanding that the family provides it part of the time, and may be covered as long as the patient requires it.

4. The skilled nursing service must be reasonable and necessary to the diagnosis and treatment of the patient's illness or injury within the context of the patient's unique medical condition. To be considered reasonable and necessary for the

6

diagnosis or treatment of the patient's illness or injury, the services must be consistent with the nature and severity of the illness or injury, the patient's particular medical needs, and accepted standards of medical and nursing practice. A patient's overall medical condition is a valid factor in deciding whether skilled services are needed. A patient's diagnosis should never be the sole factor in deciding that a service the patient needs is either skilled or not skilled.

The determination of whether the services are reasonable and necessary should be made in consideration that a physician has determined that the services ordered are reasonable and necessary. The services must, therefore, be viewed from the perspective of the condition of the patient when the services were ordered and what was, at that time, reasonably expected to be appropriate treatment for the illness or injury throughout the certification period.

EXAMPLE 1: A physician has ordered skilled nursing visits for a patient with a hairline fracture of the hip. In the absence of any underlying medical condition or illness, nursing visits would not be reasonable and necessary for treatment of the patient's hip injury.

EXAMPLE 2: A physician has ordered skilled nursing visits for injections of insulin and teaching of self-administration and self-management of the medication regimen for a patient with diabetes mellitus. Insulin has been shown to be a safe and effective treatment for diabetes mellitus, and therefore, the skilled nursing visits for the injections and the teaching of self-administration and management of the treatment regimen would be reasonable and necessary.

The determination of whether a patient needs skilled nursing care should be based solely upon the patient's unique condition and individual needs, without regard to whether the illness or injury is acute, chronic, terminal, or expected to extend over a long period of time. In addition, skilled care may, depending on the unique condition of the patient, continue to be necessary for patients whose condition is stable.

EXAMPLE 3: Following a cerebrovascular accident (CVA), a patient has an in-dwelling Foley catheter because of urinary incontinence, and is expected to require the catheter for a long and indefinite period. Periodic visits to change the catheter as needed, treat the symptoms of catheter malfunction, and teach proper patient care would be covered as long as they are reasonable and necessary, although the patient is stable and there is an expectation that the care will be needed for a long and indefinite period.

EXAMPLE 4: A patient with advanced multiple sclerosis undergoing an exacerbation of the illness needs skilled teaching of medications, measures to overcome urinary retention, and the establishment of a program designed to minimize the adverse impact of the exacerbation. The skilled nursing care the patient needs for a short period would be covered despite the chronic nature of the illness.

EXAMPLE 5: A patient with malignant melanoma is terminally ill, and requires skilled observation, assessment, teaching, and treatment. The patient has not elected coverage under Medicare's hospice benefit. The skilled nursing care that the patient requires would be covered, notwithstanding that the condition is terminal, because the services require the skills of a nurse.

40.1.2 - Application of the Principles to Skilled Nursing Services
(Rev. 1, 10-01-03)
A3-3118.1.B, HHA-205.1.B

The following discussion of skilled nursing services applies the foregoing principles to specific skilled nursing services about which questions are most frequently raised.

40.1.2.1 - Observation and Assessment of the Patient's Condition When Only the Specialized Skills of a Medical Professional Can Determine Patient's Status
(Rev. 1, 10-01-03)
A3-3118.1.B.1, HHA-205.1.B.1

Observation and assessment of the patient's condition by a nurse are reasonable and necessary skilled services when the likelihood of change in a patient's condition requires skilled nursing personnel to identify and evaluate the patient's need for possible modification of treatment or initiation of additional medical procedures until the patient's treatment regimen is essentially stabilized. Where a patient was admitted to home health care for skilled observation because there was a reasonable potential of a complication or further acute episode, but did not develop a further acute episode or complication, the skilled observation services are still covered for three weeks or so long as there remains a reasonable potential for such a complication or further acute episode.

Information from the patient's medical history may support the likelihood of a future complication or acute episode and, therefore, may justify the need for continued skilled observation and assessment beyond the 3-week period. Moreover, such indications as abnormal/fluctuating vital signs, weight changes, edema, symptoms of drug toxicity, abnormal/fluctuating lab values, and respiratory changes on auscultation may justify skilled observation and assessment. Where these indications are such that it is likely that skilled observation and assessment by a licensed nurse will result in changes to the treatment of the patient, then the services would be covered. There are cases where patients who are stable continue to require skilled observation and assessment. (See examples below.) However, observation and assessment by a nurse is not reasonable and necessary to the treatment of the illness or injury where these indications are part of a longstanding pattern of the patient's condition, and there is no attempt to change the treatment to resolve them.

EXAMPLE 1: A patient with atherosclerotic heart disease with congestive heart failure requires observation by skilled nursing personnel for signs of decompensation or adverse effects resulting from prescribed medication. Skilled observation is needed to determine whether the drug regimen should be modified or whether other therapeutic measures should be considered until the patient's treatment regimen is essentially stabilized.

EXAMPLE 2: A patient has undergone peripheral vascular disease treatment including a revascularization procedure (bypass). The incision area is showing signs of potential infection (e.g., heat, redness, swelling, drainage) and the patient has elevated body temperature. Skilled observation and monitoring of the vascular supply of the legs and the incision site is required until the signs of potential infection have abated and there is no longer a reasonable potential of infection.

EXAMPLE 3: A patient was hospitalized following a heart attack, and following treatment but before mobilization, is discharged home. Because it is not known whether exertion will exacerbate the heart disease, skilled observation is reasonable and necessary as mobilization is initiated until the patient's treatment regimen is essentially stabilized.

EXAMPLE 4: A frail 85-year old man was hospitalized for pneumonia. The infection was resolved, but the patient, who had previously maintained adequate nutrition, will not eat or eats poorly. The patient is discharged to the HHA for monitoring of fluid and nutrient intake and assessment of the need for tube feeding. Observation and monitoring by skilled nurses of the patient's oral intake, output and hydration status is required to determine what further treatment or other intervention is needed.

EXAMPLE 5: A patient with glaucoma and a cardiac condition has a cataract extraction. Because of the interaction between the eye drops for the glaucoma and cataracts and the beta-blocker for the cardiac condition, the patient is at risk for serious cardiac arrhythmia. Skilled observation and monitoring of the drug actions is reasonable and necessary until the patient's condition is stabilized.

EXAMPLE 6: A patient with hypertension suffered dizziness and weakness. The physician found that the blood pressure was too low and discontinued the hypertension medication. Skilled observation and monitoring of the patient's blood pressure and medication regimen is required until the blood pressure remains stable and in a safe range.

40.1.2.2 - Management and Evaluation of a Patient Care Plan
(Rev. 1, 10-01-03)
A3-3118.1.B.2, HHA-205.1.B.2

Skilled nursing visits for management and evaluation of the patient's care plan are also reasonable and necessary where underlying conditions or complications require that only a registered nurse can ensure that essential nonskilled care is achieving its purpose. For skilled nursing care to be reasonable and necessary for management and evaluation of the patient's plan of care, the complexity of the necessary unskilled services that are a necessary part of the medical treatment must require the involvement of skilled nursing personnel to promote the patient's recovery and medical safety in view of the patient's overall condition.

EXAMPLE 1: An aged patient with a history of diabetes mellitus and angina pectoris is recovering from an open reduction of the neck of the femur. He requires, among other services, careful skin care, appropriate oral medications, a diabetic diet, a therapeutic exercise program to preserve muscle tone and body condition, and observation to notice signs of deterioration in his condition or complications resulting from his restricted, but increasing mobility. Although a properly instructed person could perform any of the required services, that person would not have the capability to understand the relationship among the services and their effect on each other. Since the combination of the patient's condition, age, and immobility create a high potential for serious complications, such an understanding is essential to ensure the patient's recovery and safety. The management of this plan of care requires skilled nursing personnel until the patient's treatment regimen is essentially stabilized.

EXAMPLE 2: An aged patient with a history of mild dementia is recovering from pneumonia which has been treated at home. The patient has had an increase in disorientation, has residual chest congestion, decreased appetite, and has remained in bed, immobile, throughout the episode with pneumonia. While the residual chest congestion and recovery from pneumonia alone would not represent a high risk factor, the patient's immobility and increase in confusion could create a high probability of a relapse. In this situation, skilled oversight of the nonskilled services would be reasonable and necessary pending the elimination of the chest congestion and resolution of the persistent disorientation to ensure the patient's medical safety.

Where visits by a licensed nurse are not needed to observe and assess the effects of the nonskilled services being provided to treat the illness or injury, skilled nursing care would not be considered reasonable and necessary to treat the illness or injury.

EXAMPLE 3: A physician orders one skilled nursing visit every two weeks and three home health aide visits each week for bathing and washing hair for a patient whose recovery from a CVA has left him with residual weakness on the left side. The cardiovascular condition is stable and the patient has reached the maximum restoration potential. There are no underlying conditions that would necessitate the skilled supervision of a licensed nurse in assisting with bathing or hair washing. The skilled nursing visits are not necessary to manage and supervise the home health aide services and would not be covered.

40.1.2.3 - Teaching and Training Activities
(Rev. 1, 10-01-03)
A3-3118.1.B.3, HHA-205.1.B.3

Teaching and training activities that require skilled nursing personnel to teach a patient, the patient's family, or caregivers how to manage the treatment regimen would constitute skilled nursing services. Where the teaching or training is reasonable and necessary to the treatment of the illness or injury, skilled nursing visits for

6

teaching would be covered. The test of whether a nursing service is skilled relates to the skill required to teach and not to the nature of what is being taught. Therefore, where skilled nursing services are necessary to teach an unskilled service, the teaching may be covered. Skilled nursing visits for teaching and training activities are reasonable and necessary where the teaching or training is appropriate to the patient's functional loss, illness, or injury.

Where it becomes apparent after a reasonable period of time that the patient, family, or caregiver will not or is not able to be trained, then further teaching and training would cease to be reasonable and necessary. The reason why the training was unsuccessful should be documented in the record. Notwithstanding that the teaching or training was unsuccessful, the services for teaching and training would be considered to be reasonable and necessary prior to the point that it became apparent that the teaching or training was unsuccessful, as long as such services were appropriate to the patient's illness, functional loss, or injury.

EXAMPLE 1: A physician has ordered skilled nursing care for teaching a diabetic who has recently become insulin dependent. The physician has ordered teaching of self-injection and management of insulin, signs, and symptoms of insulin shock, and actions to take in emergencies. The teaching services are reasonable and necessary to the treatment of the illness or injury.

EXAMPLE 2: A physician has ordered skilled nursing care to teach a patient to follow a new medication regimen (in which there is a significant probability of adverse drug reactions due to the nature of the drug and the patient's condition), signs and symptoms of adverse reactions to new medications, and necessary dietary restrictions. After it becomes apparent that the patient remains unable to take the medications properly, cannot demonstrate awareness of potential adverse reactions, and is not following the necessary dietary restrictions, skilled nursing care for further teaching would not be reasonable and necessary, since the patient has demonstrated an inability to be taught.

EXAMPLE 3: A physician has ordered skilled nursing visits to teach self-administration of insulin to a patient who has been self-injecting insulin for 10 years and there is no change in the patient's physical or mental status that would require re-teaching. The skilled nursing visits would not be considered reasonable and necessary since the patient has a longstanding history of being able to perform the service.

EXAMPLE 4: A physician has ordered skilled nursing visits to teach self-administration of insulin to a patient who has been self-injecting insulin for 10 years because the patient has recently lost the use of the dominant hand and must be retrained to use the other hand. Skilled nursing visits to re-teach self-administration of the insulin would be reasonable and necessary.

In determining the reasonable and necessary number of teaching and training visits, consideration must be given to whether the teaching and training provided constitutes reinforcement of teaching provided previously in an institutional setting or in the home or whether it represents initial instruction. Where the teaching represents initial instruction, the complexity of the activity to be taught and the unique abilities of the patient are to be considered. Where the teaching constitutes reinforcement, an analysis of the patient's retained knowledge and anticipated learning progress is necessary to determine the appropriate number of visits. Skills taught in a controlled institutional setting often need to be reinforced when the patient returns home. Where the patient needs reinforcement of the institutional teaching, additional teaching visits in the home are covered.

EXAMPLE 5: A patient recovering from pneumonia is being sent home requiring I.V. infusion of antibiotics four times per day. The patient's spouse has been shown how to administer the drug during the hospitalization and has been told the signs and symptoms of infection. The physician has ordered home health services for a nurse to teach the administration of the drug and the signs and symptoms requiring immediate medical attention.

Re-teaching or retraining for an appropriate period may be considered reasonable and necessary where there is a change in the procedure or the patient's condition that requires re-teaching, or where the patient, family, or caregiver is not properly carrying out the task. The medical record should document the reason that the re-teaching or retraining is required.

EXAMPLE 6: A spouse who has been taught to perform a dressing change for a post-surgical patient may need to be re-taught wound care if the spouse demonstrates improper performance of wound care.

NOTE: There is no requirement that the patient, family or other caregiver be taught to provide a service if they cannot or choose not to provide the care.

Teaching and training activities that require the skills of a licensed nurse include, but **are not limited to,** the following:

1. Teaching the self-administration of injectable medications, or a complex range of medications;
2. Teaching a newly diagnosed diabetic or caregiver all aspects of diabetes management, including how to prepare and to administer insulin injections, to prepare and follow a diabetic diet, to observe foot-care precautions, and to observe for and understand signs of hyperglycemia and hypoglycemia;
3. Teaching self-administration of medical gases;
4. Teaching wound care where the complexity of the wound, the overall condition of the patient or the ability of the caregiver makes teaching necessary;
5. Teaching care for a recent ostomy or where reinforcement of ostomy care is needed;
6. Teaching self-catheterization;
7. Teaching self-administration of gastrostomy or enteral feedings;
8. Teaching care for and maintenance of peripheral and central venous lines and administration of intravenous medications through such lines;
9. Teaching bowel or bladder training when bowel or bladder dysfunction exists;
10. Teaching how to perform the activities of daily living when the patient or caregiver must use special techniques and adaptive devices due to a loss of function;
11. Teaching transfer techniques, e.g., from bed to chair, that are needed for safe transfer;
12. Teaching proper body alignment and positioning, and timing techniques of a bed-bound patient;
13. Teaching ambulation with prescribed assistive devices (such as crutches, walker, cane, etc.) that are needed due to a recent functional loss;
14. Teaching prosthesis care and gait training;
15. Teaching the use and care of braces, splints and orthotics and associated skin care;
16. Teaching the preparation and maintenance of a therapeutic diet; and
17. Teaching proper administration of oral medication, including signs of side-effects and avoidance of interaction with other medications and food.
18. Teaching the proper care and application of any special dressings or skin treatments, (for example, dressings or treatments needed by patients with severe or widespread fungal infections, active and severe psoriasis or eczema, or due to skin deterioration due to radiation treatments.)

40.1.2.4 - Administration of Medications
(Rev. 1, 10-01-03)
A3-3118.1.B.4, HHA-205.1.B.4

Although drugs and biologicals are specifically excluded from coverage by the statute (§1861(m)(5) of the Act, the services of a nurse that are required to administer the medications safely and effectively may be covered if they are reasonable and necessary to the treatment of the illness or injury.

A. Injections

Intravenous, intramuscular, or subcutaneous injections and infusions, and hypodermoclysis or intravenous feedings require the skills of a licensed nurse to be performed (or taught) safely and effectively. Where these services are reasonable and necessary to treat the illness or injury, they may be covered. For these services to be reasonable and necessary, the medication being administered must be accepted as safe and effective treatment of the patient's illness or injury, and there must be a medical reason that the medication cannot be taken orally. Moreover, the frequency and duration of the administration of the medication must be within accepted standards of medical practice, or there must be a valid explanation regarding the extenuating circumstances to justify the need for the additional injections.

1. Vitamin B-12 injections are considered specific therapy only for the following conditions:

- Specified anemias: pernicious anemia, megaloblastic anemias, macrocytic anemias, fish tapeworm anemia;
- Specified gastrointestinal disorders: gastrectomy, malabsorption syndromes such as sprue and idiopathic steatorrhea, surgical and mechanical disorders such as resection of the small intestine, strictures, anastomosis and blind loop syndrome, and
- Certain neuropathies: posterolateral sclerosis, other neuropathies associated with pernicious anemia, during the acute phase or acute exacerbation of a neuropathy due to malnutrition and alcoholism.

For a patient with pernicious anemia caused by a B-12 deficiency, intramuscular or subcutaneous injection of vitamin B-12 at a dose of from 100 to 1000 micrograms no more frequently than once monthly is the accepted reasonable and necessary dosage schedule for maintenance treatment. More frequent injections would be appropriate in the initial or acute phase of the disease until it has been determined through laboratory tests that the patient can be sustained on a maintenance dose.

2. Insulin Injections

Insulin is customarily self-injected by patients or is injected by their families. However, where a patient is either physically or mentally unable to self-inject insulin and there is no other person who is able and willing to inject the patient, the injections would be considered a reasonable and necessary skilled nursing service.

EXAMPLE: A patient who requires an injection of insulin once per day for treatment of diabetes mellitus, also has multiple sclerosis with loss of muscle control in the arms and hands, occasional tremors, and vision loss that causes inability to fill syringes or self-inject insulin. If there weren't an able and willing caregiver to inject her insulin, skilled nursing care would be reasonable and necessary for the injection of the insulin.

The prefilling of syringes with insulin (or other medication that is self-injected) does not require the skills of a licensed nurse and, therefore, is not considered to be a skilled nursing service. If the patient needs someone only to prefill syringes (and therefore needs no skilled nursing care on an intermittent basis, physical therapy, or speech-language pathology services), the patient, therefore, does not qualify for any Medicare coverage of home health care. Prefilling of syringes for self-administration of insulin or other medications is considered to be assistance with medications that are ordinarily self-administered and is an appropriate home health aide service. (See §50.2.) However, where State law requires that a licensed nurse prefill syringes, a skilled nursing visit to prefill syringes is paid as a skilled nursing visit (if the patient otherwise needs skilled nursing care, physical therapy, or speech-language pathology services), but is not considered to be a skilled nursing service.

B. Oral Medications

The administration of oral medications by a nurse is not reasonable and necessary skilled nursing care except in the specific situation in which the complexity of the patient's condition, the nature of the drugs prescribed, and the number of drugs prescribed require the skills of a licensed nurse to detect and evaluate side effects or reactions. The medical record must document the specific circumstances that cause administration of an oral medication to require skilled observation and assessment.

C. Eye Drops and Topical Ointments

The administration of eye drops and topical ointments does not require the skills of a nurse. Therefore, even if the administration of eye drops or ointments is necessary to the treatment of an illness or injury and the patient cannot self-administer the drops, and there is no one available to administer them, the visits cannot be covered as a skilled nursing service. This section does not eliminate coverage for skilled nursing visits for observation and assessment of the patient's condition. (See §40.2.1.)

EXAMPLE 1: A physician has ordered skilled nursing visits to administer eye drops and ointments for a patient with glaucoma. The administration of eye drops and ointments does not require the skills of a nurse. Therefore, the skilled nursing visits cannot be covered as skilled nursing care, notwithstanding the importance of the administration of the drops as ordered.

EXAMPLE 2: A physician has ordered skilled nursing visits for a patient with a reddened area under the breast. The physician instructs the patient to wash, rinse, and dry the area daily and apply vitamin A and D ointment. Skilled nursing care is not needed to provide this treatment and related services safely and effectively.

40.1.2.5 - Tube Feedings
(Rev. 1, 10-01-03)
A3-3118.1.B.5, HHA-205.1.B.5

Nasogastric tube, and percutaneous tube feedings (including gastrostomy and jejunostomy tubes), and replacement, adjustment, stabilization. and suctioning of the tubes are skilled nursing services, and if the feedings are required to treat the patient's illness or injury, the feedings and replacement or adjustment of the tubes would be covered as skilled nursing services.

40.1.2.6 - Nasopharyngeal and Tracheostomy Aspiration
(Rev. 1, 10-01-03)
A3-4118.1.B.6, HHA-205.1.B.6

Nasopharyngeal and tracheostomy aspiration are skilled nursing services and, if required to treat the patient's illness or injury, would be covered as skilled nursing services.

40.1.2.7 - Catheters
(Rev. 1, 10-01-03)
A3-3118.1.B.7, HHA-205.1.B.7

Insertion and sterile irrigation and replacement of catheters, care of a suprapubic catheter, and in selected patients, urethral catheters, are considered to be skilled nursing services. Where the catheter is necessitated by a permanent or temporary loss of bladder control, skilled nursing services that are provided at a frequency appropriate to the type of catheter in use would be considered reasonable and necessary. Absent complications, Foley catheters generally require skilled care once approximately every 30 days and silicone catheters generally require skilled care once every 60–90 days and this frequency of service would be considered reasonable and necessary. However, where there are complications that require more frequent skilled care related to the catheter, such care would, with adequate documentation, be covered.

EXAMPLE: A patient who has a Foley catheter due to loss of bladder control because of multiple sclerosis has a history of frequent plugging of the catheter and urinary tract infections. The physician has ordered skilled nursing visits once per month to change the catheter, and has left a "PRN" order for up to three additional visits per month for skilled observation and evaluation and/or catheter changes if the patient or caregiver reports signs and symptoms of a urinary tract infection or a plugged catheter. During the certification period, the patient's family contacts the HHA because the patient has an elevated temperature, abdominal pain, and scant urine output. The nurse visits the patient and determines that the catheter is plugged and there are symptoms of a urinary tract infection. The nurse changes the catheter and contacts the physician to report findings and discuss treatment. The skilled nursing visit to change the catheter and to evaluate the patient would be reasonable and necessary to the treatment of the illness or injury.

40.1.2.8 - Wound Care
(Rev. 1, 10-01-03)
A3-3118.1.B.8, HHA-205.1.B.8

Care of wounds (including, but not limited to, ulcers, burns, pressure sores, open surgical sites, fistulas, tube sites, and tumor erosion sites) when the skills of a licensed nurse are needed to provide safely and effectively the services necessary to treat the illness or injury, is considered to be a skilled nursing service. For skilled nursing care to be reasonable and necessary to treat a wound, the size, depth, nature of drainage (color, odor, consistency, and quantity), and condition and appearance of the skin surrounding the wound must be documented in the clinical findings so that an assessment of the need for skilled nursing care can be made. Coverage or denial of skilled nursing visits for wound care may not be based solely on the stage classification of the wound, but rather must be based on all of the documented clinical findings. Moreover, the plan of care must contain the specific instructions for the treatment of the wound. Where the physician has ordered appropriate active treatment (e.g. sterile or complex dressings, administration of prescription medications, etc.) of wounds with the following characteristics, the skills of a licensed nurse are usually reasonable and necessary:

- Open wounds which are draining purulent or colored exudate or have a foul odor present or for which the patient is receiving antibiotic therapy;
- Wounds with a drain or T-tube with requires shortening or movement of such drains;
- Wounds which require irrigation or instillation of a sterile cleansing or medicated solution into several layers of tissue and skin and/or packing with sterile gauze;
- Recently debrided ulcers;
- Pressure sores (decubitus ulcers) with the following characteristics:
  - o There is partial tissue loss with signs of infection such as foul odor or purulent drainage; or
  - o There is full thickness tissue loss that involves exposure of fat or invasion of other tissue such as muscle or bone.

NOTE: Wounds or ulcers that show redness, edema, and induration, at times with epidermal blistering or desquamation do not ordinarily require skilled nursing care.

- Wounds with exposed internal vessels or a mass that may have a proclivity for hemorrhage when a dressing is changed (e.g., post radical neck surgery, cancer of the vulva);

- Open wounds or widespread skin complications following radiation therapy, or which result from immune deficiencies or vascular insufficiencies;
- Post-operative wounds where there are complications such as infection or allergic reaction or where there is an underlying disease that has a reasonable potential to adversely affect healing (e.g., diabetes);
- Third degree burns, and second degree burns where the size of the burn or presence of complications causes skilled nursing care to be needed;
- Skin conditions that require application of nitrogen mustard or other chemotherapeutic medication that present a significant risk to the patient;
- Other open or complex wounds that require treatment that can only be provided safely and effectively by a licensed nurse.

EXAMPLE 1: A patient has a second-degree burn with full thickness skin damage on the back. The wound is cleansed, followed by an application of Sulfamylon. While the wound requires skilled monitoring for signs and symptoms of infection or complications, the dressing change requires skilled nursing services.

EXAMPLE 2: A patient experiences a decubitus ulcer where the full thickness tissue loss extends through the dermis to involve subcutaneous tissue. The wound involves necrotic tissue with a physician's order to apply a covering of a debriding ointment following vigorous irrigation. The wound is then packed loosely with wet to dry dressings or continuous moist dressing and covered with dry sterile gauze. Skilled nursing care is necessary for a proper treatment and understanding of cellular adherence and/or exudate or tissue healing or necrosis.

NOTE: This section relates to the direct, hands-on skilled nursing care provided to patients with wounds, including any necessary dressing changes on those wounds. While a wound might not require this skilled nursing care, the wound may still require skilled monitoring for signs and symptoms of infection or complication (See §40.1.2.1) or skilled teaching of wound care to the patient or the patient's family. (See §40.1.2.3.)

40.1.2.9 - Ostomy Care
(Rev. 1, 10-01-03)
A3-3118.1.B.9, HHA-205.1.B.9

Ostomy care during the post-operative period and in the presence of associated complications where the need for skilled nursing care is clearly documented is a skilled nursing service. Teaching ostomy care remains skilled nursing care regardless of the presence of complications.

40.1.2.10 - Heat Treatments
(Rev. 1, 10-01-03)
A3-3118.1.B.10, HHA-205.1.B.10

Heat treatments that have been specifically ordered by a physician as part of active treatment of an illness or injury and require observation by a licensed nurse to adequately evaluate the patient's progress would be considered a skilled nursing service.

40.1.2.11 - Medical Gases
(Rev. 1, 10-01-03)
A3-3118.1.B.11, HHA-205.1.B.11

Initial phases of a regimen involving the administration of medical gases that are necessary to the treatment of the patient's illness or injury, would require skilled nursing care for skilled observation and evaluation of the patient's reaction to the gases, and to teach the patient and family when and how to properly manage the administration of the gases.

40.1.2.12 - Rehabilitation Nursing
(Rev. 1, 10-01-03)
A3-3118.1.B.12, HHA-205.1.B.12

Rehabilitation nursing procedures, including the related teaching and adaptive aspects of nursing that are part of active treatment (e.g., the institution and supervision of bowel and bladder training programs) would constitute skilled nursing services.

40.1.2.13 - Venipuncture
(Rev. 1, 10-01-03)
A3-3118.1.B.13, HHA-205.1.B.13

Effective February 5, 1998, venipuncture for the purposes of obtaining a blood sample can no longer be the sole reason for Medicare home health eligibility. However, if a beneficiary qualifies for home health eligibility based on a skilled need other than solely venipuncture (e.g., eligibility based on the skilled nursing service of wound care and meets all other Medicare home health eligibility criteria), medically reasonable and necessary venipuncture coverage may continue during the 60-day episode under a home health plan of care.

Sections 1814(a)(2)(C) and 1835(a)(2)(A) of the Act specifically exclude venipuncture, as a basis for qualifying for Medicare home health services if this is the sole skilled service the beneficiary requires. However, the Medicare home health benefit will continue to pay for a blood draw if the beneficiary has a need for another qualified skilled service and meets all home health eligibility criteria. This specific requirement applies to home health services furnished on or after February 5, 1998.

For venipuncture to be reasonable and necessary:

1. The physician order for the venipuncture for a laboratory test should be associated with a specific symptom or diagnosis, or the documentation should clarify the need for the test when it is not diagnosis/illness specific. In addition, the treatment must be recognized (in the Physician's Desk Reference, or other authoritative source) as being reasonable and necessary to the treatment of the illness or injury for venipuncture and monitoring the treatment must also be reasonable and necessary.
2. The frequency of testing should be consistent with accepted standards of medical practice for continued monitoring of a diagnosis, medical problem, or treatment regimen. Even where the laboratory results are consistently stable, periodic venipuncture may be reasonable and necessary because of the nature of the treatment.

Examples of reasonable and necessary venipuncture for stabilized patients include, but are not limited to those described below.

a. Captopril may cause side effects such as leukopenia and agranulocytosis and it is standard medical practice to monitor the white blood cell count and differential count on a routine basis (every three months) when the results are stable and the patient is asymptomatic.

b. In monitoring phenytoin (e.g., Dilantin) administration, the difference between a therapeutic and a toxic level of phenytoin in the blood is very slight and it is therefore appropriate to monitor the level on a routine basis (every three months) when the results are stable and the patient is asymptomatic.

c. Venipuncture for fasting blood sugar (FBS)

- An unstable insulin dependent or noninsulin dependent diabetic would require FBS more frequently than once per month if ordered by the physician.
- Where there is a new diagnosis or where there has been a recent exacerbation, but the patient is not unstable, monitoring once per month would be reasonable and necessary.
- A stable insulin or noninsulin dependent diabetic would require monitoring every 2–3 months.

d. Venipuncture for prothrombin

- Where the documentation shows that the dosage is being adjusted, monitoring would be reasonable and necessary as ordered by the physician.

- Where the results are stable within the therapeutic ranges, monthly monitoring would be reasonable and necessary.
- Where the results are stable within nontherapeutic ranges, there must be documentation of other factors which would indicate why continued monitoring is reasonable and necessary.

EXAMPLE: A patient with coronary artery disease was hospitalized with atrial fibrillation and subsequently discharged to the HHA with orders for anticoagulation therapy. Monthly venipuncture as indicated are necessary to report prothrombin (protime) levels to the physician, notwithstanding that the patient's prothrombin time tests indicate essential stability.

40.1.2.14 - Student Nurse Visits
(Rev. 1, 10-01-03)
A3-3118.1.B.14, HHA-205.1.B.14

Visits made by a student nurse may be covered as skilled nursing care when the HHA participates in training programs that utilize student nurses enrolled in a school of nursing to perform skilled nursing services in a home setting. To be covered, the services must be reasonable and necessary skilled nursing care and must be performed under the general supervision of a registered or licensed nurse. The supervising nurse need not accompany the student nurse on each visit.

40.1.2.15 - Psychiatric Evaluation, Therapy, and Teaching
(Rev. 1, 10-01-03)
A3-3118.1.B.15, HHA-205.1.B.15

The evaluation, psychotherapy, and teaching needed by a patient suffering from a diagnosed psychiatric disorder that requires active treatment by a psychiatrically trained nurse and the costs of the psychiatric nurse's services may be covered as a skilled nursing service. Psychiatrically trained nurses are nurses who have special training and/or experience beyond the standard curriculum required for a registered nurse. The services of the psychiatric nurse are to be provided under a plan of care established and reviewed by a physician.

Because the law precludes agencies that primarily provide care and treatment of mental diseases from participating as HHAs, psychiatric nursing must be furnished by an agency that does not primarily provide care and treatment of mental diseases. If a substantial number of an HHA's patients attend partial hospitalization programs or receive outpatient mental health services, the intermediary will verify whether the patients meet the eligibility requirements specified in §30 and whether the HHA is primarily engaged in care and treatment of mental disease.

Services of a psychiatric nurse would not be considered reasonable and necessary to assess or monitor use of psychoactive drugs that are being used for nonpsychiatric diagnoses or to monitor the condition of a patient with a known psychiatric illness who is on treatment but is considered stable. A person on treatment would be considered stable if their symptoms were absent or minimal or if symptoms were present but were relatively stable and did not create a significant disruption in the patient's normal living situation.

EXAMPLE 1: A patient is homebound for medical conditions, but has a psychiatric condition for which he has been receiving medication. The patient's psychiatric condition has not required a change in medication or hospitalization for over two years. During a visit by the nurse, the patient's spouse indicates that the patient is awake and pacing most of the night and has begun ruminating about perceived failures in life. The nurse observes that the patient does not exhibit an appropriate level of hygiene and is dressed inappropriately for the season. The nurse comments to the patient about her observations and tries to solicit information about the patient's general medical condition and mental status. The nurse advises the physician about the patient's general medical condition and the new symptoms and changes in the patient's behavior. The physician orders the nurse to check blood levels of medication used to treat the patient's medical and psychiatric conditions. The physician then orders the psychiatric nursing service to evaluate the patient's mental health and communicate with the physician about whether additional intervention to deal with the patient's symptoms and behaviors is warranted.

EXAMPLE 2: A patient is homebound after discharge following hip replacement surgery and is receiving skilled therapy services for range of motion exercise and gait training. In the past, the patient had been diagnosed with clinical depression and was successfully stabilized on medication. There has been no change in her symptoms. The fact that the patient is taking an antidepressant does not indicate a need for psychiatric nursing services.

EXAMPLE 3: A patient was discharged after two weeks in a psychiatric hospital with a new diagnosis of major depression. The patient remains withdrawn; in bed most of the day, and refusing to leave home. The patient has a depressed affect and continues to have thoughts of suicide, but is not considered to be suicidal. Psychiatric nursing is necessary for supportive interventions until antidepressant blood levels are reached and the suicidal thoughts are diminished further, to monitor suicide ideation, ensure medication compliance and patient safety, perform suicidal assessment, and teach crisis management and symptom management to family members.

40.1.3 - Intermittent Skilled Nursing Care
(Rev. 1, 10-01-03)
A3.3118.1.C, HHA-205.1.C

The law, at §1861(m) of the Act defines intermittent, for the purposes of §§1814(a)(2) and 1835(a)(2)(A), as skilled nursing care that is either provided or needed on fewer than 7 days each week, or less than 8 hours each day for periods of 21 days or less (with extensions in exceptional circumstances when the need for additional care is finite and predictable.)

To meet the requirement for "intermittent" skilled nursing care, a patient must have a medically predictable recurring need for skilled nursing services. In most instances, this definition will be met if a patient requires a skilled nursing service at least once every 60 days. The exception to the intermittent requirement is daily skilled nursing services for diabetics unable to administer their insulin (when there is no able and willing caregiver).

Since the need for "intermittent" skilled nursing care makes the patient eligible for other covered home health services, the intermediary should evaluate each claim involving skilled nursing services furnished less frequently than once every 60 days. In such cases, payment should be made only if documentation justifies a recurring need for reasonable, necessary, and medically predictable skilled nursing services. The following are examples of the need for infrequent, yet intermittent, skilled nursing services:

1. The patient with an indwelling **silicone** catheter who generally needs a catheter change only at 90-day intervals;

2. The patient who experiences a fecal impaction (i.e., loss of bowel tone, restrictive mobility, and a breakdown in good health habits) and must receive care to manually relieve the impaction. Although these impactions are likely to recur, it is not possible to pinpoint a specific timeframe; or

3. The blind diabetic who self-injects insulin may have a medically predictable recurring need for a skilled nursing visit at least every 90 days. These visits, for example, would be to observe and determine the need for changes in the level and type of care which have been prescribed thus supplementing the physician's contacts with the patient.

There is a possibility that a physician may order a skilled visit less frequently than once every 60 days for an eligible beneficiary if there exists an extraordinary circumstance of anticipated patient need that is documented in the patient's plan of care in accordance with 42 CFR 409.43(b). A skilled visit frequency of less than once every 60 days would only be covered if it is specifically ordered by a physician in the patient's plan of care and is considered to be a reasonable, necessary, and medically predictable skilled need for the patient in the individual circumstance.

Where the need for "intermittent" skilled nursing visits is medically predictable but a situation arises after the first visit making additional visits unnecessary, e.g., the patient is institutionalized or dies, the one visit would be paid at the wage-adjusted LUPA amount for that discipline type. However, a one-time order; e.g., to give gamma globulin following exposure to hepatitis, would not be considered a need for "intermittent" skilled nursing care since a recurrence of the problem that would require this service is not medically predictable.

Although most patients require services no more frequently than several times a week, Medicare will pay for part-time (as defined in §50.7) medically reasonable and necessary skilled nursing care seven days a week for a short period of time (two to three weeks). There may also be a few cases involving unusual circumstances where the patient's prognosis indicates the medical need for daily skilled services will extend beyond three weeks. As soon as the patient's physician makes this judgment, which usually should be made before the end of the 3-week period, the HHA must forward medical documentation justifying the need for such additional services and include an estimate of how much longer daily skilled services will be required.

A person expected to need more or less full-time skilled nursing care over an extended period of time, i.e., a patient who requires institutionalization, would usually not qualify for home health benefits.

40.2 - Skilled Therapy Services

(Rev. 1, 10-01-03)
A3-3118.2, HHA-205.2

40.2.1 - General Principles Governing Reasonable and Necessary Physical Therapy, Speech-Language Pathology Services, and Occupational Therapy

(Rev. 1, 10-01-03)
A3-3118.2.A, HHA-205.2.A

The service of a physical therapist, speech-language pathologist, or occupational therapist is a skilled therapy service if the inherent complexity of the service is such that it can be performed safely and/or effectively only by or under the general supervision of a skilled therapist. To be covered, the skilled services must also be reasonable and necessary to the treatment of the patient's illness or injury or to the restoration or maintenance of function affected by the patient's illness or injury. It is necessary to determine whether individual therapy services are skilled and whether, in view of the patient's overall condition, skilled management of the services provided is needed although many or all of the specific services needed to treat the illness or injury do not require the skills of a therapist.

The development, implementation, management, and evaluation of a patient care plan based on the physician's orders constitute skilled therapy services when, because of the patient's condition, those activities require the involvement of a skilled therapist to meet the patient's needs, promote recovery, and ensure medical safety. Where the skills of a therapist are needed to manage and periodically reevaluate the appropriateness of a maintenance program because of an identified danger to the patient, such services would be covered, even if the skills of a therapist were not needed to carry out the activities performed as part of the maintenance program.

While a patient's particular medical condition is a valid factor in deciding if skilled therapy services are needed, a patient's diagnosis or prognosis should never be the sole factor in deciding that a service is or is not skilled. The key issue is whether the skills of a therapist are needed to treat the illness or injury, or whether the services can be carried out by nonskilled personnel.

A service that is ordinarily considered nonskilled could be considered a skilled therapy service in cases in which there is clear documentation that, because of special medical complications, skilled rehabilitation personnel are required to perform or supervise the service or to observe the patient. However, the importance of a particular service to a patient or the frequency with which it must be performed does not, by itself, make a nonskilled service into a skilled service.

The skilled therapy services must be reasonable and necessary to the treatment of the patient's illness or injury within the context of the patient's unique medical condition. To be considered reasonable and necessary for the treatment of the illness or injury:

a. The services must be consistent with the nature and severity of the illness or injury, the patient's particular medical needs, including the requirement that the amount, frequency, and duration of the services must be reasonable;

b. The services must be considered, under accepted standards of medical practice, to be specific, safe, and effective treatment for the patient's condition;
c. The services must be provided with the expectation, based on the assessment made by the physician of the patient's rehabilitation potential, that the condition of the patient will improve materially in a reasonable and generally predictable period of time; or the services are necessary to the establishment of a safe and effective maintenance program. Services involving activities for the general welfare of any patient, e.g., general exercises to promote overall fitness or flexibility and activities to provide diversion or general motivation, do not constitute skilled therapy. Nonskilled individuals without the supervision of a therapist can perform those services;
d. Services of skilled therapists for the purpose of teaching the patient or the patient's family or caregivers necessary techniques, exercises or precautions are covered to the extent that they are reasonable and necessary to treat illness or injury. However, visits made by skilled therapists to a patient's home solely to train other HHA staff (e.g., home health aides) are not billable as visits since the HHA is responsible for ensuring that its staff is properly trained to perform any service it furnishes. The cost of a skilled therapist's visit for the purpose of training HHA staff is an administrative cost to the agency;

6

EXAMPLE: A patient with a diagnosis of multiple sclerosis has recently been discharged from the hospital following an exacerbation of her condition that has left her wheelchair bound and, for the first time, without any expectation of achieving ambulation again. The physician has ordered physical therapy to select the proper wheelchair for her long-term use, to teach safe use of the wheelchair and safe transfer techniques to the patient and the family. Physical therapy would be reasonable and necessary to evaluate the patient's overall needs, make the selection of the proper wheelchair, and teach the patient and/or family safe use of the wheelchair and proper transfer techniques.

e. The amount, frequency, and duration of the services must be reasonable.

40.2.2 - Application of the Principles to Physical Therapy Services
(Rev. 1, 10-01-03)
A3-3118.2.B, HHA-205.2.B

The following discussion of skilled physical therapy services applies the principles in §40.2 to specific physical therapy services about which questions are most frequently raised.

A. Assessment

The skills of a physical therapist to assess and periodically reassess a patient's rehabilitation needs and potential or to develop and/or implement a physical therapy program are covered when they are reasonable and necessary because of the patient's condition. Skilled rehabilitation services concurrent with the management of a patient's care plan include objective tests and measurements such as, but not limited to, range of motion, strength, balance, coordination, endurance, or functional ability.

B. Therapeutic Exercises

Therapeutic exercises which must be performed by or under the supervision of the qualified physical therapist to ensure the safety of the beneficiary and the effectiveness of the treatment, due either to the type of exercise employed or to the condition of the patient, constitute skilled physical therapy.

C. Gait Training

Gait evaluation and training furnished a patient whose ability to walk has been impaired by neurological, muscular or skeletal abnormality require the skills of a qualified physical therapist and constitute skilled physical therapy and are considered reasonable and necessary if they can be expected to improve materially the patient's ability to walk. Gait evaluation and training which is furnished to a patient whose ability to walk has been impaired by a condition other than a neurological, muscular, or skeletal abnormality would nevertheless be covered where physical therapy is reasonable and necessary to restore the lost function.

EXAMPLE 1: A physician has ordered gait evaluation and training for a patient whose gait has been materially impaired by scar tissue resulting from burns. Physical therapy services to evaluate the beneficiary's gait, establish a gait training program, and provide the skilled services necessary to implement the program would be covered.

EXAMPLE 2: A patient who has had a total hip replacement is ambulatory but demonstrates weakness and is unable to climb stairs safely. Physical therapy would be reasonable and necessary to teach the patient to climb and descend stairs safely.

Repetitive exercises to improve gait or to maintain strength and endurance and assistive walking are appropriately provided by nonskilled persons and ordinarily do not require the skills of a physical therapist. Where such services are performed by a physical therapist as part of the initial design and establishment of a safe and effective maintenance program, the services would, to the extent that they are reasonable and necessary, be covered.

EXAMPLE 3: A patient who has received gait training has reached their maximum restoration potential, and the physical therapist is teaching the patient and family how to perform safely the activities that are a part of the maintenance program. The visits by the physical therapist to demonstrate and teach the activities (which by themselves do not require the skills of a therapist) would be covered since they are needed to establish the program.

D. Range of Motion

Only a qualified physical therapist may perform range of motion tests and, therefore, such tests are skilled physical therapy.

Range of motion exercises constitute skilled physical therapy only if they are part of an active treatment for a specific disease state, illness, or injury that has resulted in a loss or restriction of mobility (as evidenced by physical therapy notes showing the degree of motion lost and the degree to be restored). Nonskilled individuals may provide range of motion exercises unrelated to the restoration of a specific loss of function often safely and effectively. Passive exercises to maintain range of motion in paralyzed extremities that can be carried out by nonskilled persons do not constitute skilled physical therapy.

However, as indicated in §40.2, where there is clear documentation that, because of special medical complications (e.g., susceptible to pathological bone fractures), the skills of a therapist are needed to provide services which ordinarily do not need the skills of a therapist, and then the services would be covered.

E. Maintenance Therapy

Where repetitive services that are required to maintain function involve the use of complex and sophisticated procedures, the judgment and skill of a physical therapist might be required for the safe and effective rendition of such services. If the judgment and skill of a physical therapist is required to safely and effectively treat the illness or injury, the services would be covered as physical therapy services.

EXAMPLE 4: Where there is an unhealed, unstable fracture that requires regular exercise to maintain function until the fracture heals, the skills of a physical therapist would be needed to ensure that the fractured extremity is maintained in proper position and alignment during maintenance range of motion exercises.

Establishment of a maintenance program is a skilled physical therapy service where the specialized knowledge and judgment of a qualified physical therapist is required for the program to be safely carried out and the treatment of the physician to be achieved.

EXAMPLE 5: A Parkinson's patient or a patient with rheumatoid arthritis who has not been under a restorative physical therapy program may require the services of a physical therapist to determine what type of exercises are required to maintain the patient's present level of function. The initial evaluation of the patient's needs, the designing of a maintenance program appropriate to their capacity and tolerance and the treatment objectives of the physician, the instruction of the patient, family or caregivers to carry out the program safely and effectively and such reevaluations as may be required by the patient's condition, would constitute skilled physical therapy.

While a patient is under a restorative physical therapy program, the physical therapist should regularly reevaluate the patient's condition and adjust any exercise program the patient is expected to carry out alone or with the aid of supportive personnel to maintain the function being restored. Consequently, by the time it is determined that no further restoration is possible (i.e., by the end of the last restorative session) the physical therapist will already have designed the maintenance program required and instructed the patient or caregivers in carrying out the program.

F. Ultrasound, Shortwave, and Microwave Diathermy Treatments

These treatments must always be performed by or under the supervision of a qualified physical therapist and are skilled therapy.

G. Hot Packs, Infra-Red Treatments, Paraffin Baths and Whirlpool Baths

Heat treatments and baths of this type ordinarily do not require the skills of a qualified physical therapist. However, the skills, knowledge, and judgment of a qualified physical therapist might be required in the giving of such treatments or baths in a particular case, e.g., where the patient's condition is complicated by circulatory deficiency, areas of desensitization, open wounds, fractures, or other complications.

H. Wound Care Provided Within Scope of State Practice Acts

If wound care falls within the auspice of a physical therapist's State Practice Act, then the physical therapist may provide the specific type of wound care services defined in the State Practice Act. Such visits in this specific situation can be billed as physical therapy visits and count toward the therapy threshold item in the case-mix methodology.

40.2.3 - Application of the General Principles to Speech-Language Pathology Services

(Rev. 1, 10-01-03)
A3-3118.2.C, HHA-205.2.C

The following discussion of skilled speech-language pathology services applies the principles to specific speech-language pathology services about which questions are most frequently raised.

1. The skills of a speech-language pathologist are required for the assessment of a patient's rehabilitation needs (including the causal factors and the severity of the speech and language disorders), and rehabilitation potential. Reevaluation would be considered reasonable and necessary only if the patient exhibited:

- A change in functional speech or motivation;
- Clearing of confusion; or
- The remission of some other medical condition that previously contraindicated speech-language pathology services.

Where a patient is undergoing restorative speech-language pathology services, routine reevaluations are considered to be a part of the therapy and cannot be billed as a separate visit.

2. The services of a speech-language pathologist would be covered if they are needed as a result of an illness or injury and are directed towards specific speech/voice production.

3. Speech-language pathology would be covered where the service can only be provided by a speech-language pathologist and where it is reasonably expected that the service will materially improve the patient's ability to independently carry out any one or combination of communicative activities of daily living in a manner that is measurably at a higher level of attainment than that prior to the initiation of the services.

4. The services of a speech-language pathologist to establish a hierarchy of speech-voice-language communication tasks and cueing that directs a patient toward speech-language communication goals in the plan of care would be covered speech-language pathology.

5. The services of a speech-language pathologist to train the patient, family, or other caregivers to augment the speech-language communication, treatment, or to establish an effective maintenance program would be covered speech-language pathology services.

6. The services of a speech-language pathologist to assist patients with aphasia in rehabilitation of speech and language skills are covered when needed by a patient.

7. The services of a speech-language pathologist to assist patients with voice disorders to develop proper control of the vocal and respiratory systems for correct voice production are covered when needed by a patient.

40.2.4 - Application of the General Principles to Occupational Therapy
(Rev. 1, 10-01-03)
A3-3118.2.D, HHA-205.2.D

The following discussion of skilled occupational therapy services applies the principles to specific occupational therapy services about which questions are most frequently raised.

40.2.4.1 - Assessment
(Rev. 1, 10-01-03)
A3-3118.2.D.1, HHA-205.2.D.1

The skills of an occupational therapist to assess and reassess a patient's rehabilitation needs and potential or to develop and/or implement an occupational therapy program are covered when they are reasonable and necessary because of the patient's condition.

40.2.4.2 - Planning, Implementing, and Supervision of Therapeutic Programs
(Rev. 1, 10-01-03)
A3-3118.2.D.2, HHA-205.2.D.2

The planning, implementing, and supervision of therapeutic programs including, but not limited to those listed below are skilled occupational therapy services, and if reasonable and necessary to the treatment of the patient's illness or injury would be covered.

A. Selecting and Teaching Task Oriented Therapeutic Activities Designed to Restore Physical Function.

EXAMPLE: Use of woodworking activities on an inclined table to restore shoulder, elbow, and wrist range of motion lost as a result of burns.

B. Planning, Implementing, and Supervising Therapeutic Tasks and Activities Designed to Restore Sensory-Integrative Function.

EXAMPLE: Providing motor and tactile activities to increase sensory output and improve response for a stroke patient with functional loss resulting in a distorted body image.

C. Planning, Implementing, and Supervising of Individualized Therapeutic Activity Programs as Part of an Overall "Active Treatment" Program for a Patient With a Diagnosed Psychiatric Illness.

EXAMPLE: Use of sewing activities that require following a pattern to reduce confusion and restore reality orientation in a schizophrenic patient.

D. Teaching Compensatory Techniques to Improve the Level of Independence in the Activities of Daily Living.

EXAMPLE: Teaching a patient who has lost use of an arm how to pare potatoes and chop vegetables with one hand.

EXAMPLE: Teaching a stroke patient new techniques to enable them to perform feeding, dressing, and other activities of daily living as independently as possible.

E. The Designing, Fabricating, and Fitting of Orthotic and Self-Help Devices.

EXAMPLE: Construction of a device which would enable a patient to hold a utensil and feed themselves independently.

EXAMPLE: Construction of a hand splint for a patient with rheumatoid arthritis to maintain the hand in a functional position.

F. Vocational and Prevocational Assessment and Training

Vocational and prevocational assessment and training that is directed toward the restoration of function in the activities of daily living lost due to illness or injury would be covered. Where vocational or prevocational assessment and training is related solely to specific employment opportunities, work skills, or work settings, such services would not be covered because they would not be directed toward the treatment of an illness or injury.

40.2.4.3 - Illustration of Covered Services
(Rev. 1, 10-01-03)
A3-3118.2.D.3, HHA-205.2.D.3

EXAMPLE 1: A physician orders occupational therapy for a patient who is recovering from a fractured hip and who needs to be taught compensatory and safety techniques with regard to lower extremity dressing, hygiene, toileting, and bathing. The occupational therapist will establish goals for the patient's rehabilitation (to be approved by the physician), and will undertake teaching techniques necessary for the patient to reach the goals. Occupational therapy services would be covered at a duration and intensity appropriate to the severity of the impairment and the patient's response to treatment.

EXAMPLE 2: A physician has ordered occupational therapy for a patient who is recovering from a CVA. The patient has decreased range of motion, strength, and sensation in both the upper and lower extremities on the right side. In addition, the patient has perceptual and cognitive deficits resulting from the CVA. The patient's condition has resulted in decreased function in activities of daily living (specifically bathing, dressing, grooming, hygiene, and toileting). The loss of function requires assistive devices to enable the patient to compensate for the loss of function and maximize safety and independence. The patient also needs equipment such as himi-slings to prevent shoulder subluxation and a hand splint to prevent joint contracture and deformity in the right hand. The services of an occupational therapist would be necessary to:

- Assess the patient's needs;
- Develop goals (to be approved by the physician);
- Manufacture or adapt the needed equipment to the patient's use;
- Teach compensatory techniques;
- Strengthen the patient as necessary to permit use of compensatory techniques; and

- Provide activities that are directed towards meeting the goals governing increased perceptual and cognitive function.

Occupational therapy services would be covered at a duration and intensity appropriate to the severity of the impairment and the patient's response to treatment.

50 - Coverage of Other Home Health Services
(Rev. 1, 10-01-03)
A3-3119, HHA-206

50.1 - Skilled Nursing, Physical Therapy, Speech-Language Pathology Services, and Occupational Therapy
(Rev. 1, 10-01-03)
A3-3119.1, HHA-206.1

Where the patient meets the qualifying criteria in §30, Medicare covers skilled nursing services that meet the requirements of §§40.1 and 50.7, physical therapy that meets the requirements of §40.2, speech-language pathology services that meet the requirements of §40.2, and occupational therapy that meets the requirements of §40.2.

Home health coverage is not available for services furnished to a qualified patient who is no longer in need of one of the qualifying skilled services specified in §30. Therefore, dependent services furnished after the final qualifying skilled service are not covered under the home health benefit, except when the dependent service was followed by a qualifying skilled service as a result of the unexpected inpatient admission or death of the patient or due to some other unanticipated event.

50.2 - Home Health Aide Services
(Rev. 1, 10-01-03)
A3-3119.2, HHA-206.2

For home health aide services to be covered:

- The patient must meet the qualifying criteria as specified in §30;
- The services provided by the home health aide must be part-time or intermittent as discussed in §50.7;
- The services must meet the definition of home health aide services of this section; and
- The services must be reasonable and necessary to the treatment of the patient's illness or injury.

NOTE: A home health aide must be certified consistent with the competency evaluation requirements.

The reason for the visits by the home health aide must be to provide hands-on personal care of the patient or services needed to maintain the patient's health or to facilitate treatment of the patient's illness or injury.

The physician's order should indicate the frequency of the home health aide services required by the patient. These services may include but are not limited to:

A. Personal Care

Personal care means:

1. Bathing, dressing, grooming, caring for hair, nail, and oral hygiene which are needed to facilitate treatment or to prevent deterioration of the patient's health, changing the bed linens of an incontinent patient, shaving, deodorant application, skin care with lotions and/or powder, foot care, and ear care; and
2. Feeding, assistance with elimination (including enemas unless the skills of a licensed nurse are required due to the patient's condition, routine catheter care and routine colostomy care), assistance with ambulation, changing position in bed, assistance with transfers.

EXAMPLE 1: A physician has ordered home health aide visits to assist the patient in personal care because the patient is recovering from a stroke and continues to have significant right side weakness that causes the patient to be unable to bathe, dress or perform hair and oral care. The plan of care established by the HHA nurse sets forth the specific tasks with which the patient needs assistance. Home health aide visits at an appropriate frequency would be reasonable and necessary to assist in these tasks.

EXAMPLE 2: A physician ordered four home health aide visits per week for personal care for a multiple sclerosis patient who is unable to perform these functions because of increasing debilitation. The home health aide gave the patient a bath twice per week and washed hair on the other two visits each week. Only two visits are reasonable and necessary since the services could have been provided in the course of two visits.

EXAMPLE 3: A physician ordered seven home health aide visits per week for personal care for a bed-bound, incontinent patient. All visits are reasonable and necessary because the patient has extensive personal care needs.

EXAMPLE 4: A patient with a well established colostomy forgets to change the bag regularly and has difficulty changing the bag. Home health aide services at an appropriate frequency to change the bag would be considered reasonable and necessary to the treatment of the illness or injury.

B. Simple Dressing Changes That Do Not Require the Skills of a Licensed Nurse

EXAMPLE 5: A patient who is confined to the bed has developed a small reddened area on the buttocks. The physician has ordered home health aide visits for more frequent repositioning, bathing and the application of a topical ointment and a gauze 4x4. Home health aide visits at an appropriate frequency would be reasonable and necessary.

C. Assistance With Medications Which Are Ordinarily Self-Administered and Do Not Require the Skills of a Licensed Nurse to Be Provided Safely and Effectively

NOTE: Prefilling of insulin syringes is ordinarily performed by the diabetic as part of the self-administration of the insulin and, unlike the injection of the insulin, does not require the skill of a licensed nurse to be performed properly. Therefore, if HHA staff performs the prefilling of insulin syringes, it is considered to be a home health aide service. However, where State law precludes the provision of this service by other than a licensed nurse or physician, Medicare will make payment for this service, when covered, as though it were a skilled nursing service. Where the patient needs only prefilling of insulin syringes and does not need skilled nursing care on an intermittent basis, physical therapy, speech-language pathology services, or have a continuing need for occupational therapy, then Medicare cannot cover any home health services to the patient (even if State law requires that the insulin syringes be filled by a licensed nurse).

Home health aide services are those services ordered in the plan of care that the aide is permitted to perform under State law. Medicare coverage of the administration of insulin by a home health aide will depend on whether or not the agency is in compliance with all Federal and State laws and regulations related to this task. However, when the task of insulin administration has been delegated to the home health aide, the task must be considered and billed as a Medicare home health aide service. By a State allowing the delegation of insulin administration to home health aides, the State has extended the role of aides, not equated aide services with the services of a registered nurse.

D. Assistance With Activities Which Are Directly Supportive of Skilled Therapy Services but Do Not Require the Skills of a Therapist to Be Safely and Effectively Performed Such as Routine Maintenance Exercises and

Repetitive Practice of Functional Communication Skills to Support Speech-Language Pathology Services

E. Provision of Services Incidental to Personal Care Services not Care of Prosthetic and Orthotic Devices

When a home health aide visits a patient to provide a health related service as discussed above, the home health aide may also perform some incidental services which do not meet the definition of a home health aide service (e.g., light cleaning, preparation of a meal, taking out the trash, shopping, etc.). However, the purpose of a home health aide visit may not be to provide these incidental services since they are not health related services, but rather are necessary household tasks that must be performed by anyone to maintain a home.

EXAMPLE 1: A home health aide visits a recovering stroke patient whose right side weakness and poor endurance cause her to be able to leave the bed and chair only with extreme difficulty. The physician has ordered physical therapy and speech-language pathology services for the patient and home health aide services three or four times per week for personal care, assistance with ambulation as mobility increases, and assistance with repetitive speech exercises as her impaired speech improves. The home health aide also provides incidental household services such as preparation of meals, light cleaning and taking out the trash. The patient lives with an elderly frail sister who is disabled and who cannot perform either the personal care or the incidental tasks. The home health aide visits at a frequency appropriate to the performance of the health related services would be covered, notwithstanding the incidental provision of noncovered services (i.e., the household services) in the course of the visits.

EXAMPLE 2: A physician orders home health aide visits three times per week. The only services provided are light housecleaning, meal preparation and trash removal. The home health aide visits cannot be covered, notwithstanding their importance to the patient, because the services provided do not meet Medicare's definition of "home health aide services."

50.3 - Medical Social Services
(Rev. 1, 10-01-03)
A3-3119.3, HHA-206.3

Medical social services that are provided by a qualified medical social worker or a social work assistant under the supervision of a qualified medical social worker may be covered as home health services where the beneficiary meets the qualifying criteria specified in §30, and:

1. The services of these professionals are necessary to resolve social or emotional problems that are or are expected to be an impediment to the effective treatment of the patient's medical condition or rate of recovery; and

2. The plan of care indicates how the services which are required necessitate the skills of a qualified social worker or a social work assistant under the supervision of a qualified medical social worker to be performed safely and effectively.

Where both of these requirements for coverage are met, services of these professionals which may be covered include, but are not limited to:

1. Assessment of the social and emotional factors related to the patient's illness, need for care, response to treatment and adjustment to care;

2. Assessment of the relationship of the patient's medical and nursing requirements to the patient's home situation, financial resources and availability of community resources;

3. Appropriate action to obtain available community resources to assist in resolving the patient's problem (**NOTE:** Medicare does not cover the services of a medical social worker to complete or assist in the

completion of an application for Medicaid because Federal regulations require the State to provide assistance in completing the application to anyone who chooses to apply for Medicaid.);

4. Counseling services that are required by the patient; and

5. Medical social services furnished to the patient's family member or caregiver on a short-term basis when the HHA can demonstrate that a brief intervention (that is, two or three visits) by a medical social worker is necessary to remove a clear and direct impediment to the effective treatment of the patient's medical condition or to the patient's rate of recovery. To be considered "clear and direct," the behavior or actions of the family member or caregiver must plainly obstruct, contravene, or prevent the patient's medical treatment or rate of recovery. Medical social services to address general problems that do not clearly and directly impede treatment or recovery as well as long-term social services furnished to family members, such as ongoing alcohol counseling, are not covered.

NOTE: Participating in the development of the plan of care, preparing clinical and progress notes, participating in discharge planning and in-service programs, and acting as a consultant to other agency personnel are appropriate administrative costs to the HHA.

6

EXAMPLE 1: The physician has ordered a medical social worker assessment of a diabetic patient who has recently become insulin dependent and is not yet stabilized. The nurse, who is providing skilled observation and evaluation to try to restabilize the patient notices during her visits that the supplies left in the home for the patient's use appear to be frequently missing, and the patient is not compliant with the regimen although she refuses to discuss the matter. The assessment by a medical social worker would be reasonable and necessary to determine if there are underlying social or emotional problems impeding the patient's treatment.

EXAMPLE 2: A physician ordered an assessment by a medical social worker for a multiple sclerosis patient who was unable to move anything but her head and who had an indwelling catheter. The patient had experienced recurring urinary tract infections and multiple infected ulcers. The physician ordered medical social services after the HHA indicated to him that the home was not well cared for, the patient appeared to be neglected much of the time, and the relationship between the patient and family was very poor. The physician and HHA were concerned that social problems created by family caregivers were impeding the treatment of the recurring infections and ulcers. The assessment and follow-up for counseling both the patient and the family by a medical social worker were reasonable and necessary.

EXAMPLE 3: A physician is aware that a patient with atherosclerosis and hypertension is not taking medications as ordered and adhering to dietary restrictions because he is unable to afford the medication and is unable to cook. The physician orders several visits by a medical social worker to assist in resolving these problems. The visits by the medical social worker to review the patient's financial status, discuss options, and make appropriate contacts with social services agencies or other community resources to arrange for medications and meals would be a reasonable and necessary medical social service.

EXAMPLE 4: A physician has ordered counseling by a medical social worker for a patient with cirrhosis of the liver who has recently been discharged from a 28-day inpatient alcohol treatment program to her home which she shares with an alcoholic and neglectful adult child. The physician has ordered counseling several times per week to assist the patient in remaining free of alcohol and in dealing with the adult child. The services of the medical social worker would be covered until the patient's social situation ceased to impact on her recovery and/or treatment.

EXAMPLE 5: A physician has ordered medical social services for a patient who is worried about his financial arrangements and payment for medical care. The services ordered are to arrange Medicaid if possible and resolve unpaid medical bills. There is no evidence that the patient's concerns are adversely impacting recovery or treatment of his illness or injury. Medical social services cannot be covered.

EXAMPLE 6: A physician has ordered medical social services for a patient of extremely limited income who has incurred large unpaid hospital and other medical bills following a significant illness. The patient's recovery is adversely affected because the patient is not maintaining a proper therapeutic diet, and cannot leave the home to acquire the medication necessary to treat their illness. The medical social worker reviews the patient's financial status, arranges meal service to resolve the dietary problem, arranges for home delivered medications, gathers the information necessary for application to Medicaid to acquire coverage for the medications the patient needs, files the application on behalf of the patient, and follows up repeatedly with the Medicaid State agency.

The medical social services that are necessary to review the financial status of the patient, arrange for meal service and delivery of medications to the home, and arrange for the Medicaid State agency to assist the patient with the application for Medicaid are covered. The services related to the assistance in filing the application for Medicaid and the follow-up on the application are not covered since they must be provided by the State agency free of charge, and hence the patient has no obligation to pay for such assistance.

EXAMPLE 7: A physician has ordered medical social services for an insulin dependent diabetic whose blood sugar is elevated because she has run out of syringes and missed her insulin dose for two days. Upon making the assessment visit, the medical social worker learns that the patient's daughter, who is also an insulin dependent diabetic, has come to live with the patient because she is out of work. The daughter is now financially dependent on the patient for all of her financial needs and has been using the patient's insulin syringes. The social worker assesses the patient's financial resources and determines that they are adequate to support the patient and meet her own medical needs, but are not sufficient to support the daughter. She also counsels the daughter and helps her access community resources. These visits would be covered, but only to the extent that the services are necessary to prevent interference with the patient's treatment plan.

EXAMPLE 8: A wife is caring for her husband who is an Alzheimer's patient. The nurse learns that the wife has not been giving the patient his medication correctly and seems distracted and forgetful about various aspects of the patient's care. In a conversation with the nurse, the wife relates that she is feeling depressed and overwhelmed by the patient's illness. The nurse contacts the patient's physician who orders a social work evaluation. In her assessment visit, the social worker learns that the patient's wife is so distraught over her situation that she cannot provide adequate care to the patient. While there, the social worker counsels the wife and assists her with referrals to a support group and her private physician for evaluation of her depression. The services would be covered.

EXAMPLE 9: The parent of a dependent disabled child has been discharged from the hospital following a hip replacement. Although arrangements for care of the disabled child during the hospitalization were made, the child has returned to the home. During a visit to the patient, the nurse observes that the patient is transferring the child from bed to a wheelchair. In an effort to avoid impeding the patient's recovery, the nurse contacts the patient's physician to order a visit by a social worker to mobilize family members or otherwise arrange for temporary care of the disabled child. The services would be covered.

50.4 - Medical Supplies (Except for Drugs and Biologicals Other Than Covered Osteoporosis Drugs) and the Use of Durable Medical Equipment

(Rev.26, Issued 11-05-04, Effective: 01-01-05, Implementation: 04-04-05)

50.4.1 - Medical Supplies
(Rev. 1, 10-01-03)
A3-3119.4.A, HHA-206.4.A

Medical supplies are items that, due to their therapeutic or diagnostic characteristics, are essential in enabling HHA personnel to conduct home visits or to carry out effectively the care the physician has ordered for the treatment or diagnosis of the patient's illness or injury. All supplies which would have been covered under the cost-based reimbursement system are bundled under home health PPS. Payment for the cost of supplies has been incorporated into the per visit and episode payment rates. Supplies fit into two categories. They are classified as:

- **Routine** - because they are used in small quantities for patients during the usual course of most home visits; or
- **Nonroutine** - because they are needed to treat a patient's specific illness or injury in accordance with the physician's plan of care and meet further conditions discussed in more detail below.

All HHAs are expected to separately identify in their records the cost of medical and surgical supplies that are not routinely furnished in conjunction with patient care visits and the use of which are directly identifiable to an individual patient.

50.4.1.1 - The Law, Routine and Nonroutine Medical Supplies, and the Patient's Plan of Care
(Rev. 1, 10-01-03)
A3-3119.4A.2, HHA-206.4A3, 4, 5

A. The Law

The Medicare law governing the home health PPS is specific to the type of items and services bundled to the HHA and the time the services are bundled. Medical supplies are bundled while the patient is under a home health plan of care. If a patient is admitted for a condition which is related to a chronic condition that requires a medical supply (e.g., ostomy patient) the HHA is required to provide the medical supply while the patient is under a home health plan of care during an open episode. The physician orders in the plan of care must reflect all nonroutine medical supplies provided and used while the patient is under a home health plan of care during an open 60-day episode. The consolidated billing requirement is not superseded by the exclusion of certain medical supplies from the plan of care and then distinguishing between medical supplies that are related and unrelated to the plan of care. Failure to include medical supplies on the plan of care does not relieve HHAs from the obligation to comply with the consolidated billing requirements. The comprehensive nature of the current patient assessment and plan of care requirements looks at the totality of patient needs. However, there could be a circumstance where a physician could be uncomfortable with writing orders for a preexisting condition unrelated to the reason for home health care. In those circumstances, PRN orders for such supplies may be used in the plan of care by a physician.

Thus, all medical supplies are bundled while the patient is under a home health plan of care during an open 60-day episode. This includes, but is not limited to, the above listed medical supplies as well as the Part B items provided in the final PPS rule. The latter item lists are subsequently updated in accordance with the current process governing the deletion, replacement and revision of Medicare Part B codes. Parenteral and enteral nutrition, prosthetics, orthotics, DME and DME supplies are not considered medical supplies and therefore not subject to bundling while the patient is under a home health plan of care during an open episode. However, §1834(h)(4)(c) of the Act specifically excludes from the term "orthotics and prosthetics" medical supplies including catheters, catheter supplies, ostomy bags and supplies related to ostomy care furnished by an HHA under §1861(m) of the Act. Therefore, these items are bundled while a patient is under a home health plan of care.

B. Relationship Between Patient Choice and Veterans Benefits

For veterans, both Medicare and Veteran's Administration (VA) benefits are primary. Therefore, the beneficiary who is a veteran has some choices in cases where the benefits overlap. The beneficiary, however, must select one or the other program as primary when obtaining active care. If the VA is selected as primary for home health care, then Medicare becomes a secondary payer. An HHA must provide the medical supplies a Medicare beneficiary needs no matter the payer; it is not obligated to provide medical supplies that are not needed. If a patient has medical supplies provided by the VA because of the patient's preference, then the HHA must not duplicate the supplies under Medicare. The beneficiary's choice is controlling. The HHA may not require the beneficiary to obtain or use medical supplies covered by the primary payer from any other source, including the VA.

C. Medical Supplies Purchased by the Patient Prior to the Start of Care

A patient may have acquired medical supplies prior to his/her Medicare home health start of care date. If a patient prefers to use his or her own medical supplies after having been offered appropriate supplies by the HHA and it is determined by the HHA that the patient's medical supplies are clinically appropriate, then the patient's choice is controlling. The HHA is not required to duplicate the medical supplies if the patient elects to use his or her own medical supplies. However, if the patient prefers to have the HHA provide medical supplies while the patient is under a Medicare home health plan of care during an open episode, then the HHA must provide the medical supplies. The HHA may not require that the patient obtain or use medical supplies from any other source. Given the possibility of subsequent misunderstandings arising between the HHA and the patient on this issue, the HHA should document the beneficiary's decision to decline HHA furnished medical supplies and use their own resources.

50.4.1.2 - Routine Supplies (Nonreportable)
(Rev. 1, 10-01-03)
A3-3119.4.A.1, HHA-206.4.A.1

Routine supplies are supplies that are customarily used in small quantities during the course of most home care visits. They are usually included in the staff's supplies and not designated for a specific patient. These supplies are included in the cost per visit of home health care services. Routine supplies would not include those supplies that are specifically ordered by the physician or are essential to HHA personnel in order to effectuate the plan of care.

Examples of supplies which are usually considered routine include, but are not limited to:

A. Dressings and Skin Care

- Swabs, alcohol preps, and skin prep pads;
- Tape removal pads;
- Cotton balls;
- Adhesive and paper tape;
- Nonsterile applicators; and
- 4 x 4s.

B. Infection Control Protection

- Nonsterile gloves;
- Aprons;
- Masks; and
- Gowns.

C. Blood Drawing Supplies

- Specimen containers.

D. Incontinence Supplies

- Incontinence briefs and Chux covered in the normal course of a visit. For example, if a home health aide in the course of a bathing visit to a patient determines the patient requires an incontinence brief change, the incontinence brief in this example would be covered as a routine medical supply

E. Other

- Thermometers; and
- Tongue depressors.

There are occasions when the supplies listed in the above examples would be considered nonroutine and thus would be considered a billable supply, i.e., if they are required in quantity, for recurring need, and are included in the plan of care. Examples include, but are not limited to, tape, and 4x4s for major dressings.

50.4.1.3 - Nonroutine Supplies (Reportable)
(Rev. 1, 10-01-03)
A3-3119.4.A.2, HHA-206.4.A.2

Nonroutine supplies are identified by the following conditions:

1. The HHA follows a consistent charging practice for Medicare and other patients receiving the item;
2. The item is directly identifiable to an individual patient;
3. The cost of the item can be identified and accumulated in a separate cost center; and
4. The item is furnished at the direction of the patient's physician and is specifically identified in the plan of care.

All nonroutine supplies must be specifically ordered by the physician or the physician's order for services must require the use of the specific supplies to be effectively furnished.

The charge for nonroutine supplies is excluded from the per visit costs.

Examples of supplies that can be considered nonroutine include, but are not limited to:

1. Dressings/Wound Care
- Sterile dressings;
- Sterile gauze and toppers;
- Kling and Kerlix rolls;
- Telfa pads;
- Eye pads;
- Sterile solutions, ointments;
- Sterile applicators; and
- Sterile gloves.
2. I.V. Supplies
3. Ostomy Supplies
4. Catheters and Catheter Supplies
- Foley catheters; and
- Drainage bags, irrigation trays.
5. Enemas and Douches
6. Syringes and Needles

7. Home Testing

- Blood glucose monitoring strips; and
- Urine monitoring strips.

Consider other items that are often used by persons who are not ill or injured to be medical supplies only where:

- The item is recognized as having the capacity to serve a therapeutic or diagnostic purpose in a specific situation; and
- The item is required as a part of the actual physician-prescribed treatment of a patient's existing illness or injury.

For example, items that generally serve a routine hygienic purpose, e.g., soaps and shampoos and items that generally serve as skin conditioners, e.g., baby lotion, baby oil, skin softeners, powders, lotions, are not considered medical supplies unless the particular item is recognized as serving a specific therapeutic purpose in the physician's prescribed treatment of the patient's existing skin (scalp) disease or injury.

Limited amounts of medical supplies may be left in the home between visits where repeated applications are required and rendered by the patient or other caregivers. Those items must be part of the plan of care in which the home health staff is actively involved. For example, the patient is independent in insulin injections but the nurse visits once a day to change wound dressings. The wound dressings/irrigation solution may be left in the home between visits. Supplies such as needles, syringes, and catheters that require administration by a nurse should not be left in the home between visits.

50.4.2 - Durable Medical Equipment
(Rev. 1, 10-01-03)
A3-3119.4.B, HHA-206.4.B

Durable medical equipment which meets the requirements of the Medicare Benefit Policy Manuals, Chapter 6, "Hospital Services Covered Under Part B," §80, and Chapter 15, "Covered Medical and Other Health Services" §110, is covered under the home health benefit with the beneficiary responsible for payment of a 20 percent coinsurance.

50.4.3 - Covered Osteoporosis Drugs
(Rev. 26, Issued 11-05-04, Effective: 01-01-05, Implementation: 04-04-05)

Sections 1861(m) and 1861(kk) of the Act provide for coverage of FDA approved injectable drugs for the treatment of osteoporosis. These drugs are expected to be provided by an HHA to female beneficiaries who are currently receiving services under an open home health plan of care, who meet existing coverage criteria for the home health benefit and who meet the criteria listed below. These drugs are covered on a cost basis when provided by an HHA under the circumstances listed below.

The home health visit (i.e., the skilled nurse's visit) to administer the drug is covered under all fee-for-service Medicare (Part A or Part B) home health coverage rules (see section 30 above). Coverage of the drug is limited to female beneficiaries who meet each of the following criteria:

- The individual is eligible for Medicare Part B coverage of home health services (the nursing visit to perform the injection may be the individual's qualifying service);
- The individual sustained a bone fracture that a physician certifies was related to post-menopausal osteoporosis; and
- The individual's physician certifies that she is unable to learn the skills needed to self-administer the drug or is otherwise physically or mentally incapable of administering the drug, and that her family or caregivers are unable or unwilling to administer the drug.

This drug is considered part of the home health benefit under Part B. Therefore, Part B deductible and coinsurance apply regardless of whether home health visits for the administration of the drug are covered under Part A or Part B.

For instructions on billing for covered osteoporosis drugs, see Pub. 100-04, Medicare Claims Processing Manual, chapter 10, section 90.1.

50.5 - Services of Interns and Residents
(Rev. 1, 10-01-03)
A3-3119.5, HHA-206.5

Home health services include the medical services of interns and residents-in-training under an approved hospital teaching program if the services are ordered by the physician who is responsible for the plan of care and the HHA is affiliated with or is under common control of a hospital furnishing the medical services. Approved means:

- 113.Approved by the Accreditation Council for Graduate Medical Education;
- 114.In the case of an osteopathic hospital, approved by the Committee on Hospitals of the Bureau of Professional Education of the American Osteopathic Association;
- 115.In the case of an intern or resident-in-training in the field of dentistry, approved by the Council on Dental Education of the American Dental Association; or
- 116.In the case of an intern or resident-in-training in the field of podiatry, approved by the Council on Podiatric Education of the American Podiatric Association.

50.6 - Outpatient Services
(Rev. 1, 10-01-03)
A3-3119.6, HHA-206.6

Outpatient services include any of the items or services described above which are provided under arrangements on an outpatient basis at a hospital, skilled nursing facility, rehabilitation center, or outpatient department affiliated with a medical school, and (1) which require equipment which cannot readily be made available at the patient's place of residence, or (2) which are furnished while the patient is at the facility to receive the services described in (1). The hospital, skilled nursing facility, or outpatient department affiliated with a medical school must all be qualified providers of services. However, there are special provisions for the use of the facilities of rehabilitation centers. The cost of transporting an individual to a facility cannot be reimbursed as home health services.

50.7 - Part-Time or Intermittent Home Health Aide and Skilled Nursing Services
(Rev. 1, 10-01-03)
A3-3119.7, HHA-206.7, A3-3119.7A, HHA-206.7A, A3-3119.7.B, HHA-206.7.B

Where a patient is eligible for coverage of home health services, Medicare covers either part-time or intermittent home health aide services or skilled nursing services subject to the limits below. The law at §1861(m) of the Act clarified: "the term "part-time or intermittent services" means skilled nursing and home health aide services furnished any number of days per week as long as they are furnished (combined) less than 8 hours each day and 28 or fewer hours each week (or, subject to review on a case-by-case basis as to the need for care, less than 8 hours each day and 35 or fewer hours each week).

50.7.1 - Impact on Care Provided in Excess of "Intermittent" or "Part- Time" Care
(Rev. 1, 10-01-03)
A3-3119.7.C, HHA-206.7.C

Home health aide and/or skilled nursing care, in excess of the amounts of care that meet the definition of part-time or intermittent, may be provided to a home care patient or purchased by other payers without bearing on whether the home health aide and skilled nursing care meets the Medicare definitions of part-time or intermittent.

EXAMPLE: A patient needs skilled nursing care monthly for a catheter change and the home health agency also renders needed daily home health aide services 24 hours per day that will be needed for a long and indefinite period of time. The HHA bills Medicare for the skilled nursing and home health aide services which were provided before the 35th hour of service each week, and bills the beneficiary (or another payer) for the remainder of the care. If the intermediary determines that the 35 hours of care are reasonable and necessary, Medicare would cover the 35 hours of skilled nursing and home health aide visits.

50.7.2 - Application of this Policy Revision
(Rev. 1, 10-01-03)
A3-3119.7.D, HHA-206.7.D

6

Additional care covered by other payers discussed in §50.7.1 does not affect Medicare coverage when the conditions listed below apply. A patient must meet the criteria for Medicare coverage of home health services, before this policy revision becomes applicable to skilled nursing services and/or home health aide services. The definition of "intermittent" with respect to the need for skilled nursing care where the patient qualifies for coverage based on the need for "skilled nursing care on an intermittent basis" remains unchanged. Specifically:

1. This policy revision always applies to home health aide services when the patient qualifies for coverage;
2. This policy revision applies to skilled nursing care only when the patient needs physical therapy or speech-language pathology services or continued occupational therapy, and also needs skilled nursing care; and
3. If the patient needs skilled nursing care but does not need physical therapy or speech-language pathology services or occupational therapy, the patient must still meet the longstanding and unchanged definition of "intermittent" skilled nursing care in order to qualify for coverage of any home health services.

60 - Special Conditions for Coverage of Home Health Services Under Hospital Insurance (Part A) and Supplementary Medical Insurance (Part B)
(Rev. 1, 10-01-03)
A3-3122, HHA-212

60.1 - Post-Institutional Home Health Services Furnished During A Home Health Benefit Period—Beneficiaries Enrolled in Part A and Part B
(Rev. 1, 10-01-03)
A3-3122.1, HHA-212.1, A3-3122.1, HHA-212.2, PMs A-97-12, A-97-16, A-98-49

Section 1812(a)(3) of the Act provides post-institutional home health services for individuals enrolled in Part A and Part B and home health services for individuals who are eligible for Part A only. For beneficiaries who are enrolled in Part A and Part B, Part A finances post-institutional home health services furnished during a home health spell of illness for up to 100 visits during a spell of illness.

Part A finances up to 100 visits furnished during a home health spell of illness if the following criteria are met:

- Beneficiaries are enrolled in Part A and Part B and qualify to receive the Medicare home health benefit;
- Beneficiaries must have at least a three consecutive day stay in a hospital or rural primary care hospital; and
- Home health services must be initiated and the first covered home health visit must be rendered within 14 days of discharge from a 3 consecutive day stay in a hospital or rural primary care hospital or within 14 days of discharge from a skilled nursing facility in which the individual was provided post-hospital extended care services. If the first home health

visit is not initiated within 14 days of discharge, then home health services are financed under Part B.

After an individual exhausts 100 visits of Part A post-institutional home health services, Part B finances the balance of the home health spell of illness. A home health spell of illness is a period of consecutive days beginning with the first day not included in a previous home health spell of illness on which the individual is furnished post-institutional home health services which occurs in a month the individual is entitled to Part A. The home health spell of illness ends with the close of the first period of 60 consecutive days in which the individual is neither an inpatient of a hospital or rural primary care hospital nor an inpatient of a skilled nursing facility (in which the individual was furnished post-hospital extended care services) nor provided home health services.

EXAMPLE 1: An individual is enrolled in Part A and Part B, qualifies for the Medicare home health benefit, has a three consecutive day stay in a hospital, and is discharged on May 1. On May 5, the individual receives the first skilled nursing visit under the plan of care. Therefore, post-institutional home health services have been initiated within 14 days of discharge. The individual is later hospitalized on June 2. Prior to the June 2 hospitalization, the individual received 12 home health visits. The individual stays in the hospital for four consecutive days, is discharged and receives home health services. That individual continues the May 5 home health spell of illness and would have 88 visits left under that home health spell of illness under Part A. That individual could not start another home health spell of illness (100 visits under Part A) until a 60-day consecutive period in which the individual was not an inpatient of a hospital, rural primary care hospital, an inpatient of a skilled nursing facility (in which the individual was furnished post-hospital extended care services), or provided home health services had passed.

EXAMPLE 2: An individual is enrolled in Part A and Part B, qualifies for the Medicare home health benefit, has a three consecutive day stay in a hospital, and home health is initiated within 14 days of discharge. The individual exhausts the 100 visits under Part A post-institutional home health services, continues to need home health services, and receives home health services under Part B. The individual is then hospitalized for 4 consecutive days. The individual is again discharged and receives home health services. The individual cannot begin a new home health spell of illness because 60 days did not pass in which the individual was not an inpatient of a hospital or rural primary care hospital or an inpatient of a skilled nursing facility in which the individual was furnished post-hospital extended care services. The individual would be discharged and Part B would continue to finance the home health services.

60.2 - Beneficiaries Who Are Enrolled in Part A and Part B, but Do Not Meet Threshold for Post-Institutional Home Health Services
(Rev. 1, 10-01-03)
A3-3122.1, HHA-212.3

If beneficiaries are enrolled in Part A and Part B and are eligible for the Medicare home health benefit, but do not meet the three consecutive day stay requirement or the 14 day initiation of care requirement, then all of their home health services would be financed under Part B. For example, this situation would include, but is not limited to, beneficiaries enrolled in Part A and Part B who are coming from the community to a home health agency in need of home health services or who stay less than three consecutive days in a hospital and are discharged. Any home health services received after discharge would be financed under Part B.

60.3 - Beneficiaries Who Are Part A Only or Part B Only
(Rev. 1, 10-01-03)
A3-3122.1, HHA-212.4

If a beneficiary is enrolled **only** in Part A and qualifies for the Medicare home health benefit, then all of the home health services are financed under Part A. The 100-visit limit does **not** apply to beneficiaries who are only enrolled in Part A. If a beneficiary is enrolled **only** in Part B and qualifies for the Medicare home health benefit, then all of the home health services are financed under Part B. There is no 100-visit limit under Part B. The new definition of post-institutional home health services provided during a home health spell of illness **only** applies to those beneficiaries who are enrolled in **both** Part A and Part B and qualify for the Medicare home health benefit.

60.4 - Coinsurance, Copayments, and Deductibles
(Rev. 1, 10-01-03)
A3-3122.1, HHA-212.5

There is no coinsurance, copayment, or deductible for home health services and supplies other than the following:

- Coinsurance required for durable medical equipment (DME) covered as a home health service and
- Deductible and coinsurance for the osteoporosis drug, which is part of the home health benefit only paid under Part B.

The coinsurance liability of the beneficiary for DME and osteoporosis drug furnished as a home health service is 20 percent of the fee schedule amount for the services.

70 - Duration of Home Health Services
(Rev. 1, 10-01-03)
A3-3123, HHA-215, A3-3123.1, HHA-215.1

70.1 - Number of Home Health Visits Under Supplementary Medical Insurance (Part B)
(Rev. 1, 10-01-03)
A3-3123.2, HHA-215.2

To the extent that all coverage requirements are met, payment may be made on behalf of eligible beneficiaries under Part B for an unlimited number of covered home health visits. The determination of Part A or Part B Trust Fund financing and coverage is made in accordance with the financing shift required by the BBA described above in §60.

70.2 - Counting Visits Under the Hospital and Medical Plans
(Rev. 1, 10-01-03)
A3-3124, HHA-218, A3-3124.1, HHA-218.1, A3-3124.2, HHA-218.2, A3-3124.3, HHA-218.3

The number of visits are counted in the same way whether paid under the hospital (Part A) or supplemental medical (Part B) Medicare trust funds.

A. Visit Defined

A visit is an episode of personal contact with the patient by staff of the HHA, or others under arrangements with the HHA, for the purpose of providing a covered home health service. Though visits are provided under the HH benefit as part of episodes, and episodes are unlimited, each visit must be uniquely billed as a separate line item on a Medicare HH claim, and data on visit charges is still used in formulating payment rates.

B. Counting Visits

Generally, one visit may be covered each time an HHA employee, or someone providing home health services under arrangements with the HHA, enters the patient's home and provides a covered service to a patient who meets the criteria in §30.

If the HHA furnishes services in an outpatient facility under arrangements with the facility, one visit may be covered for each type of service provided.

If two individuals are needed to provide a service, two visits may be covered. If two individuals are present, but only one is needed to provide the care, only one visit may be covered.

A visit is initiated with the delivery of covered home health services and ends at the conclusion of delivery of covered home health services. In those circumstances in which all reasonable and necessary home health services cannot be provided in the course of a single visit, HHA staff or others providing services under arrangements with the HHA may remain at the patient's home between visits (e.g., to provide noncovered services). However, if all covered services could be provided in the course of one visit, only one visit may be covered.

EXAMPLES:

1. If an occupational therapist and an occupational therapy assistant visit the patient together to provide therapy and the therapist is there to supervise the assistant, one visit is counted.
2. If a nurse visits the patient in the morning to dress a wound and later must return to replace a catheter, two visits are counted.
3. If the therapist visits the patient for treatment in the morning and the patient is later visited by the assistant for additional treatment, two visits are counted.
4. If an individual is taken to a hospital to receive outpatient therapy that could not be furnished in their own home (e.g., hydrotherapy) and, while at the hospital receives speech-language pathology services and other services, two or more visits would be charged.
5. Many home health agencies provide home health aide services on an hourly basis (ranging from 1 to 8 hours a day). However, in order to allocate visits properly against a patient's maximum allowable visits, home health aide services are to be counted in terms of visits. Thus, regardless of the number of continuous hours a home health aide spends in a patient's home on any given day, one "visit" is counted for each such day. If, in a rare situation, a home health aide visits a patient for an hour or two in the morning, and again for an hour or two in the afternoon, two visits are counted.

C. Evaluation Visits

The HHAs are required by regulations to have written policies concerning the acceptance of patients by the agency. These include consideration of the physical facilities available in the patient's place of residence, the homebound status, and the attitudes of family members for the purpose of evaluating the feasibility of meeting the patient's medical needs in the home health setting. When personnel of the agency make such an initial evaluation visit, the cost of the visit is considered an administrative cost of the agency and is not chargeable as a visit since at this point the patient has not been accepted for care. If, however, during the course of this initial evaluation visit, the patient is determined suitable for home health care by the agency, and is also furnished the first skilled service as ordered under the physician's plan of care, the visit would become the first billable visit in the 60-day episode.

The intermediary will cover an observation and evaluation (or reevaluation) visit made by a nurse (see §40.1.2.1 for a further discussion of skilled nursing observation and evaluation visits) or other appropriate personnel, ordered by the physician for the purpose of evaluating the patient's condition and continuing need for skilled services, as a skilled visit.

A supervisory visit made by a nurse or other appropriate personnel (as required by the conditions of participation) to evaluate the specific personal care needs of the patient or to review the manner in which the personal care needs of the patient are being met by the aide is an administrative function, not a skilled visit.

80 - Specific Exclusions From Coverage as Home Health Services
(Rev. 1, 10-01-03)
A3-3125, HHA-230.A

In addition to the general exclusions from coverage under health insurance listed in the Medicare Benefit Policy Manual, Chapter 16, "General Exclusions from Coverage," the following are also excluded from coverage as home health services:

80.1 - Drugs and Biologicals
(Rev. 1, 10-01-03)
A3-3125.A, HHA-230.A

Drugs and biologicals are excluded from payment under the Medicare home health benefit.

A drug is any chemical compound that may be used on or administered to humans or animals as an aid in the diagnosis, treatment, prevention of disease or other condition, for the relief of pain or suffering, or to control or improve any physiological pathologic condition.

A biological is any medicinal preparation made from living organisms and their products including, but not limited to, serums, vaccines, antigens, and antitoxins. The one drug exception is the osteoporosis drug, which is part of the home health benefit, and home health agencies may provide services such as vaccines outside the home health benefit.

80.2 - Transportation
(Rev. 1, 10-01-03)
A3-3125.B, HHA-230.B

The transportation of a patient, whether to receive covered care or for other purposes, is excluded from home health coverage. Costs of transportation of equipment, materials, supplies, or staff may be allowable as administrative costs, but no separate payment is made.

80.3 - Services That Would Not Be Covered as Inpatient Services
(Rev. 1, 10-01-03)
A3-3125C, HHA-230.C

Services that would not be covered if furnished as inpatient hospital services are excluded from home health coverage.

80.4 - Housekeeping Services
(Rev. 1, 10-01-03)
A3-3125D, HHA-230D

Services for which the sole purpose is to enable the patient to continue residing in their home (e.g., cooking, shopping, Meals on Wheels, cleaning, laundry) are excluded from home health coverage.

80.5 - Services Covered Under End Stage Renal Disease (ESRD) Program
(Rev. 1, 10-01-03)
A3-3125.E, HHA-230.E

Services that are covered under the ESRD program and are contained in the composite rate reimbursement methodology, including any service furnished to an ESRD beneficiary that is directly related to that individual's dialysis, are excluded from coverage under the Medicare home health benefit. However, to the extent a service is not directly related to a patient's dialysis, e.g., a nursing visit to furnish wound care for an abandoned shunt site, and other requirements for coverage are met, the visit would be covered. Within these restrictions, beneficiaries may simultaneously receive items and services under the ESRD program at home at the same time as receiving services under the home health benefit not related to ESRD.

80.6 - Prosthetic Devices
(Rev. 1, 10-01-03)
A3-3125F, HHA-230F

Prosthetic items are excluded from home health coverage. However, catheters, catheter supplies, ostomy bags, and supplies related to ostomy care are not considered prosthetic devices if furnished under a home health plan of care and are not subject to this exclusion from coverage but are bundled while a patient is under a HH plan of care.

80.7 - Medical Social Services Furnished to Family Members
(Rev. 1, 10-01-03)
A3-3125G, HHA-230G

Except as provided in §50.3, medical social services furnished solely to members of the patient's family and that are not incidental to covered medical social services being furnished to the patient are not covered.

80.8 - Respiratory Care Services
(Rev. 1, 10-01-03)
A3-3125.H, HHA-230.H

If a respiratory therapist is used to furnish overall training or consultative advice to HHA staff and incidentally furnishes respiratory therapy services to patients in their homes, the costs of the respiratory therapist's services are allowable only as administrative costs to the HHA. Visits by a respiratory therapist to a patient's home are not separately billable during a HH episode when a HH plan of care is in effect. However, respiratory therapy services furnished as part of a plan of care other than a home health plan of care by a licensed nurse or physical therapist and that constitute skilled care may be covered and separately billed as skilled visits when the beneficiary is not in a home health episode. Note that Medicare billing does not recognize respiratory therapy as a separate discipline, but rather sees the services in accordance with the revenue code used on the claims (i.e. 042x).

80.9 - Dietary and Nutrition Personnel
(Rev. 1, 10-01-03)
A3-3125.I, HHA-230.I

If dieticians or nutritionists are used to furnish overall training or consultative advice to HHA staff and incidentally furnish dietetic or nutritional services to patients in their homes, the costs of these professional services are allowable only as administrative costs. Visits by a dietician or nutritionist to a patient's home are not separately billable.

90 - Medical and Other Health Services Furnished by Home Health Agencies
(Rev. 37, Issued: 08-12-05; Effective/Implementation: 09-12-05)

Payment may be made by intermediaries to a home health agency which furnishes either directly or under arrangements with others the following "medical and other health services" to beneficiaries with Part B coverage in accordance with Part B billing and payment rules other than when a home health plan of care is in effect.

1. Surgical dressings (for a patient who is not under a home health plan of care), and splints, casts, and other devices used for reduction of fractures and dislocations;

2. Prosthetic (Except for items excluded from the term "orthotics and prosthetics" in accordance with §1834(h)(4)(C) of the Act for patients who are under a home health plan of care);

3. Leg, arm, back, and neck braces, trusses, and artificial legs, arms, and eyes and adjustments to these items when ordered by a physician. (See the Medicare Benefit Policy Manual, Chapter 15);

4. Outpatient physical therapy, outpatient occupational therapy, and outpatient speech-language pathology services (for a patient not under a home health plan of care). (See the Medicare Benefit Policy Manual, Chapter 15); and

5. Rental and purchase of durable medical equipment. (See the Medicare Benefit Policy Manual, Chapter 15.) If a beneficiary meets all of the criteria for coverage of home health services and the HHA is providing home health care under the Hospital Insurance Program (Part A), any DME provided and billed to the intermediary by the HHA to that patient must also be provided under Part A. Where the patient meets the criteria for coverage of home health services and the HHA is providing the home

health care under the Supplementary Medical Insurance Program (Part B) because the patient is not eligible for Part A, the DME provided by the HHA may, at the beneficiary's option, be furnished under the Part B home health benefit or as a medical and other health service. Irrespective of how the DME is furnished, the beneficiary is responsible for a 20 percent coinsurance.

6. Ambulance service. (See the Medicare Benefit Policy Manual, Chapter 10, Ambulance Services)

7. Hepatitis B Vaccine. Hepatitis B vaccine and its administration are covered under Part B for patients who are at high or intermediate risk of contracting hepatitis B. High risk groups currently identified include: end-stage renal disease (ESRD) patients, hemophiliacs who receive factor VIII or IX concentrates, clients of institutions for the mentally retarded, persons who live in the same household as an hepatitis B virus carrier, homosexual men, illicit injectable drug users. Intermediate risk groups currently identified include staff in institutions for the mentally retarded, workers in health care professions who have frequent contact with blood or blood-derived body fluids during routine work. Persons in the above listed groups would not be considered at high or intermediate risk of contracting hepatitis B, however, if there is laboratory evidence positive for antibodies to hepatitis B. ESRD patients are routinely tested for hepatitis B antibodies as part of their continuing monitoring and therapy. The vaccine may be administered, upon the order of a doctor of medicine or osteopathy, by home health agencies.

8. Hemophilia clotting factors. Blood clotting factors for hemophilia patients competent to use such factors to control bleeding without medical or other supervision and items related to the administration of such factors are covered under Part B.

10. Pneumococcal and influenza vaccines. See Medicare Benefit Policy Manual, Chapter 15, "Covered Medical and Other Health Services," §50.4.2 "Immunizations."

11. Splints, casts. See the Medicare Benefit Policy Manual, Chapter 15, "Covered Medical and Other Health Services."

Antigens. See the Medicare Benefit Policy Manual, Chapter 15, "Covered Medical and Other Health Services."

100 - Physician Certification for Medical and Other Health Services Furnished by Home Health Agency (HHA)
(Rev. 1, 10-01-03)
A3-3128, HHA-224

A physician must certify that the medical and other health services covered by medical insurance which were provided by (or under arrangements made by) the HHA were medically required. This certification needs to be made only once where the patient may require over a period of time the furnishing of the same item or service related to one diagnosis. There is no requirement that the certification be entered on any specific form or handled in any specific way as long as the approach adopted by the HHA permits the intermediary to determine that the certification requirement is, in fact, met. A written physician's order designating the services required would also be an acceptable certification.

110 - Use of Telehealth in Delivery of Home Health Services
(Rev. 1, 10-01-03)
PM A-01-02, HHA-201.13

Section 1895(e) of the Act governs the home health prospective payment system (PPS) and provides that telehealth services are outside the scope of the Medicare home health benefit and home health PPS.

This provision does not provide coverage or payment for Medicare home health services provided via a telecommunications system. The law does not permit the substitution or use of a telecommunications system to provide any covered home health services paid under the home health PPS, or any covered home health service paid outside of the home health PPS. As stated in 42 CFR 409.48(c), a visit is an episode of personal contact with the beneficiary by staff of the home health agency (HHA), or others under arrangements with the HHA for the purposes of providing a covered service. The provision clarifies that there is nothing to preclude an HHA from adopting telemedicine or other technologies that they believe promote efficiencies, but that those technologies will not be specifically recognized or reimbursed by Medicare under the home health benefit. This provision does not waive the current statutory requirement for a physician certification of a home health plan of care under current §§1814(a)(2)(C) or 1835(a)(2)(A) of the Act.

PART SEVEN

NANDA-I–APPROVED NURSING DIAGNOSES

7

NANDA-I is the abbreviation for North American Nursing Diagnosis Association-International, the official name of this nursing diagnosis association.

2007-2008 NANDA-I NURSING DIAGNOSES

Activity intolerance
Risk for **Activity** intolerance
Ineffective **Airway** clearance
Latex **Allergy** response
Risk for latex **Allergy** response
Anxiety
Death **Anxiety**
Risk for **Aspiration**
Risk for impaired parent/child **Attachment**
Autonomic dysreflexia
Risk for **Autonomic** dysreflexia
Risk-prone health **Behavior**
Disturbed **Body** image
Risk for imbalanced **Body** temperature
Bowel incontinence
Effective **Breastfeeding**
Ineffective **Breastfeeding**
Interrupted **Breastfeeding**
Ineffective **Breathing** pattern
Decreased **Cardiac** output
Caregiver role strain
Risk for **Caregiver** role strain
Readiness for enhanced **Comfort**
Impaired verbal **Communication**
Readiness for enhanced **Communication**
Decisional **Conflict**
Parental role **Conflict**
Acute **Confusion**
Chronic **Confusion**
Risk for acute **Confusion**
Constipation
Perceived **Constipation**
Risk for **Constipation**
Contamination
Risk for **Contamination**
Compromised family **Coping**
Defensive **Coping**
Disabled family **Coping**
Ineffective **Coping**
Ineffective community **Coping**
Readiness for enhanced **Coping**
Readiness for enhanced community **Coping**
Readiness for enhanced family **Coping**
Risk for sudden infant **Death** syndrome
Readiness for enhanced **Decision** making
Ineffective **Denial**
Impaired **Dentition**
Risk for delayed **Development**
Diarrhea
Risk for compromised human **Dignity**

Moral **Distress**
Risk for **Disuse** syndrome
Deficient **Diversional** activity
Disturbed **Energy** field
Impaired **Environmental** interpretation syndrome
Adult **Failure** to thrive
Risk for **Falls**
Dysfunctional **Family** processes: alcoholism
Interrupted **Family** processes
Readiness for enhanced **Family** processes
Fatigue
Fear
Readiness for enhanced **Fluid** balance
Deficient **Fluid** volume
Excess **Fluid** volume
Risk for deficient **Fluid** volume
Risk for imbalanced **Fluid** volume
Impaired **Gas** exchange
Risk for unstable blood **Glucose**
Grieving
Complicated **Grieving**
Risk for complicated **Grieving**
Delayed **Growth** and development
Risk for disproportionate **Growth**
Ineffective **Health** maintenance
Health-seeking behaviors (specify)
Impaired **Home** maintenance
Readiness for enhanced **Hope**
Hopelessness
Hyperthermia
Hypothermia
Disturbed personal **Identity**
Readiness for enhanced **Immunization** status
Functional urinary **Incontinence**
Overflow urinary **Incontinence**
Reflex urinary **Incontinence**
Stress urinary **Incontinence**
Total urinary **Incontinence**
Urge urinary **Incontinence**
Risk for urge urinary **Incontinence**
Disorganized **Infant** behavior
Risk for disorganized **Infant** behavior
Readiness for enhanced organized **Infant** behavior
Ineffective **Infant** feeding pattern
Risk for **Infection**
Risk for **Injury**
Risk for perioperative positioning **Injury**

7

Insomnia
Decreased **Intracranial** adaptive capacity
Deficient **Knowledge** (specify)
Readiness for enhanced **Knowledge**
Sedentary **Lifestyle**
Risk for impaired **Liver** function
Risk for **Loneliness**
Impaired **Memory**
Impaired bed **Mobility**
Impaired physical **Mobility**
Impaired wheelchair **Mobility**
Nausea
Unilateral **Neglect**
Noncompliance
Imbalanced **Nutrition:** less than body requirements
Imbalanced **Nutrition**: more than body requirements
Readiness for enhanced **Nutrition**
Risk for imbalanced **Nutrition**: more than body requirements
Impaired **Oral** mucous membrane
Acute **Pain**
Chronic **Pain**
Readiness for enhanced **Parenting**
Impaired **Parenting**
Risk for impaired **Parenting**
Risk for **Peripheral** neurovascular dysfunction
Risk for **Poisoning**
Post-trauma syndrome
Risk for **Post-trauma** syndrome
Readiness for enhanced **Power**
Powerlessness
Risk for **Powerlessness**
Ineffective **Protection**
Rape-trauma syndrome
Rape-trauma syndrome compound reaction
Rape-trauma syndrome silent reaction
Impaired **Religiosity**
Readiness for enhanced **Religiosity**
Risk for impaired **Religiosity**
Relocation stress syndrome
Risk for **Relocation stress** syndrome
Ineffective **Role** performance
Readiness for enhanced **Self-care**
Bathing/hygiene **Self-care** deficit
Dressing/grooming **Self-care** deficit
Feeding **Self-Care** deficit
Toileting **Self-care** deficit
Readiness for enhanced **Self-concept**

Chronic low **Self-esteem**
Situational low **Self-esteem**
Risk for situational low **Self-esteem**
Self-mutilation
Risk for **Self-mutilation**
Disturbed **Sensory** perception
Sexual dysfunction
Ineffective **Sexuality** patterns
Impaired **Skin** integrity
Risk for impaired **Skin** integrity
Sleep deprivation
Readiness for enhanced **Sleep**
Impaired **Social** interaction
Social isolation
Chronic **Sorrow**
Spiritual distress
Risk for **Spiritual** distress
Readiness for enhanced **Spiritual** well-being
Stress overload
Risk for **Suffocation**
Risk for **Suicide**
Delayed **Surgical** recovery
Impaired **Swallowing**
Effective **Therapeutic** regimen management
Ineffective **Therapeutic** regimen management
Ineffective community **Therapeutic** regimen management
Ineffective family **Therapeutic** regimen management
Readiness for enhanced **Therapeutic** regimen management
Ineffective **Thermoregulation**
Disturbed **Thought** processes
Impaired **Tissue** integrity
Ineffective **Tissue** perfusion
Impaired **Transfer** ability
Risk for **Trauma**
Impaired **Urinary** elimination
Readiness for enhanced **Urinary** elimination
Urinary retention
Impaired spontaneous **Ventilation**
Dysfunctional **Ventilatory** weaning response
Risk for other-directed **Violence**
Risk for self-directed **Violence**
Impaired **Walking**
Wandering

North American Nursing Diagnosis Association-International: Nursing diagnoses: definitions and classification 2007–2008, Philadelphia, 2007, NANDA.

PART EIGHT

HOME CARE DEFINITIONS AND ABBREVIATIONS

8

KEY HOME HEALTHCARE DEFINITIONS

485: See Plan of Care (POC).

487: See Plan of Care (POC).

488: See Additional Documentation Requests (ADRs).

ABN: See Home Health Advance Beneficiary Notice.

Abuse: The Centers for Medicare and Medicaid Services define *abuse* as incidents or practices by organizations that, although not usually considered fraudulent, are inconsistent with accepted sound medical, business, or fiscal practices, and that directly or indirectly create unnecessary costs for the Medicare program. Improper reimbursement or reimbursement of services that do not meet professionally recognized standards or that are not medically necessary are examples of abuse.

Access: The availability of healthcare and the ability of an individual to receive services such as home care or hospice, including factors related to cost, location, and transportation.

Accreditation: A rigorous process that examines various components of home care, hospice, or other site operations and clinical practice. The achievement of accreditation designates that the organization has gone through the accreditation process and meets predetermined standards as measured by on-site survey team members.

Activities of Daily Living (ADLs): Basic, usually self-care directed activities that are performed daily. These activities include personal hygiene tasks such as bathing, grooming, dressing, eating/feeding, and obtaining and preparing food. Other ADLs include toileting and transferring activities. These activities are important indicators because they demonstrate the patient's functional status or healthcare needs relative to the patient's level of functional independence.

Additional Documentation Requests (ADRs or 488s): Requests by a carrier or intermediary for additional documentation regarding a particular Medicare claim when a coverage or coding determination cannot be made from the information that has been provided on that claim. Agencies have 30 days to respond to ADRs, also known as 488s.

Admission—Start of Care (SOC): First billable visit made by the home health clinician.

Advance Directive(s): A legal document that allows an individual to give directions about future medical care or to designate another person(s) to make such medical decisions if he/she has lost his/her decision-making abilities. Advance directives may include living wills, durable powers of attorney for healthcare, and similar documents relaying the patient's wishes. The Patient Self-Determination Act of 1990 mandates that certain healthcare providers query patients, at the time of admission to the agency or facility, about advance directives and whether they need assistance in generating an advance directive(s) document.

Advocacy: A role assumed by a healthcare professional designed to maximize patient self-determination through education, support, and affirmation of patient healthcare decisions.

Agency for Healthcare Research and Quality (AHRQ): An agency of the U.S. Department of Health and Human Services (DHHS) that supports research projects and facilitates the development of clinical practice guidelines related to the delivery of healthcare services.

Assessment: The systematic review and analysis of data from a multitude of sources that assist in the identification of needs, abilities, and available resources.

Assistive Devices: Equipment designed to improve or increase a patient's ability to perform a movement or activity. Examples of assistive devices are wheelchairs, walkers, canes, reachers, adaptive eating utensils, splints, electrolarynx, and communication boards/picture boards.

Balanced Budget Act of 1997: The passed legislation that made numerous changes and budget cuts to the Medicare program, including the implementation of a prospective payment system (PPS) for home care.

Benchmark: A systematic process to measure or quantify; a standard for comparing two similar types of products and services to identify areas for improvement in an organization.

Beneficiary: A Medicare patient or the consumer of Medicare care or services.

Capitation: A set dollar amount established to cover the cost of healthcare services delivered to an individual. The amount is based on the number of members in the plan, not the amount of services used.

Care Coordination: The process utilized by the multidisciplinary clinical team and the patient and/or caregivers in the development of a viable, realistic, outcome-based plan of care. Care coordination may be formalized in a care planning conference or be informal between two or more individuals and documented in the clinical record.

Care Plan: A plan of action for care that is developed, delivered, and evaluated by a nurse, therapist, or other team member of a home care or hospice organization. This may also be called the *plan of care (POC),* and the format varies among organizations.

Caregiver: Anyone who provides care or services to or for a patient.

Case Management: Supervision of the care given to a specific patient or caseload population to ensure allocation of appropriate resources to achieve optimal outcomes. In home healthcare, this is often a care model in which the nurse or therapist case manager supervises, renders skilled care, and/or collaborates with other ordered professional services. Communication among the services and disciplines involved in the care must be documented in the clinical record. In care conferences, input is given to the case manager to assist the interdisciplinary team in reaching the patient's goals.

Case (Care) Manager: One person who is responsible for the overall care of the patient and for the use of resources for that care. The case (care) manager may be a nurse, social worker, or therapist, and is the primary person responsible for developing patient care outcomes for her or his case load. A case manager is accountable for meeting outcomes within an appropriate length of stay, effective use of resources, and pre-established standards, and collaborates with other team members and the patient to accomplish those outcomes.

Case Mix: The distribution of different types of patients seen at a healthcare setting; a collection of case types.

Case-Mix Adjustment: A methodology to ensure that agencies are not penalized for serving a mix of patients whose care needs are more expensive than those of the group on which the predetermined payment rate is based, and to eliminate the incentive for agencies to reject patients who may require unusual or higher resources utilization (e.g., visits, services).

Case-Mix Report: A graphic or tabular document that provides average values for patient attributes at start of care. Comparative data are provided for either (1) agency case mix for a prior time period, (2) case mix for a reference sample of patients from other agencies, or (3) both of the above.

Centers for Medicare & Medicaid Services (CMS): Formerly the Health Care Financing Administration or HCFA, CMS is an agency of the United States government under the Department of Health and Human Services (DHHS) that is responsible for the Medicare and Medicaid programs. The agency provides direction that includes various requirements, policies, payment for services, and many other operational aspects of the programs. CMS sets the coverage policy and payment and other guidelines and directs the activities of government contractors (e.g., carriers and fiscal intermediaries).

Certified OASIS Specialist-Clinical (COS-C): The COS-C is awarded upon successful completion of a voluntary certificate examination that home care providers take to demonstrate and establish their expertise and commitment to OASIS data accuracy. The examination is administered by the OASIS Certificate and Competency Board, Inc. (OCCB).

Certification: Organizations desiring to participate in the Medicare program must meet participation conditions for certification (the Medicare Conditions of Participation [COPs]). State agencies (such as the Department of Health) certify to the Department of Health and Human Services (DHHS) that the home care, hospice, or other types of organizations satisfy, and continue to satisfy, healthcare quality requirements for participation in the Medicare program.

Certification Period (see also Episode): A 60-day period of time in the Medicare Home Health program; home care agencies usually obtain orders and provide care for a certification period.

Certified Diabetes Educator (CDE): Diabetes educators are educated and licensed healthcare professionals including registered nurses, registered dietitians, and pharmacists, who possess distinct and specialized knowledge in diabetes self-management education. The examination for this credential is administered by the National Certification Board for Diabetes Educators.

Certified Home Health Agency (HHA): A Medicare-certified organization that provides care to patients in their homes. The agency may or may not be licensed, depending on state requirements, but must have a survey or a special review to accept Medicare patients.

Chronic: A slow or persistent illness or health problem that must be cared for throughout life. Examples include diabetes, glaucoma, heart failure, and some chronic lung conditions.

Claims Denials: Payment for services is refused by the insuring organization. This may be due to the frequency of service, providing a non-covered service, use of an invalid procedure code, lack of physician signature, failure to document homebound status of a patient, and many others.

Classification System: A system of categorizing elements of similar groups using pre-established criteria.

Client: One who receives care. Also called the *patient, customer,* or *consumer* of healthcare services or products. An individual, customer, consumer, or patient who receives care or services.

Clinical (Critical) Path(way) (CP): Also known as *care path* or *clinical guideline*, a structured plan for care, often categorized by diagnosis or patient problem, that defines specific care interventions, team members, and other information across a time line. Clinical management tools that organize, sequence, and time the major interventions of nursing staff, therapists, and other health professions for a particular case or type of condition. The pathways describe a standard of practice and are, in essence, a clinical "budget" for allocating resources.

Clinical Record: The documentation that chronicles the patient's stay throughout the course of care while on the home care or hospice organization's service roster. The importance of the home care clinical record is that it is the one source of specific clinical information and entries used to make payment (or denial) determinations and to facilitate regulatory compliance (e.g., Medicare certification or coverage compliance reviews), and that it is the source for communication among team members to help assure the safe provision of patient-centered care.

Coinsurance: The amount or percentage of the cost of services that consumers may be required to pay under a cost-sharing agreement with their insurance plan or program. It may also be called a co-payment.

Collaboration: The active process of working together and valuing another's input toward reaching patient goals. In healthcare, collaboration is a joint effort by staff from many disciplines who together plan the care processes, which leads to improved patient care.

Competency: The quantifiable ability of an individual to perform a task based on established criteria.

Conditions of Participation (CoPs): The framework and standards used to survey home care, hospice, or other Part A organizations. Organizations must be in compliance with these standards or face sanctions and penalties and risk losing their Medicare certification. The ongoing demonstration of compliance with the COPs is the challenge for the entire team. Many of the conditions are related to care and planning and clinical information, such as forms, that are housed in the home care clinical record.

Continuum of Care: The array of healthcare services available to an individual based on the assessed need of the patient and provided at the most appropriate level.

Cost Containment: Measures or requirements established by organizations involved in the delivery of healthcare to control increases in utilization or expenditures.

Criteria: Established standards against which performance or any other measure is judged.

Daily Care: Medicare defines daily care as care delivered 7 days a week. Patients who receive daily care must have a realistic, projected end date. *This means that the home care nurse needs a projected endpoint for daily visits. Patients who need daily nursing care for an unspecified amount of time or indefinitely do not receive coverage under Medicare.* The *only* exception to an endpoint for daily care is insulin injections under certain circumstances. Ask your supervisor for clarification.

Department of Health and Human Services (DHHS): Also known as Health and Human Services (HHS), oversees the Centers for Medicare and Medicaid Services (CMS) and the Medicare (federal) and Medicaid (state) programs.

Diagnostic-Related Groups (DRGs): A code of classifying patient illnesses according to principal diagnosis and treatment requirements. Under Medicare, each DRG has its own price (weight) that a hospital is paid regardless of the actual cost of treatment.

Discharge: Two types of discharge may occur: discipline-specific discharge and agency discharge.

Episode (see also Certification Period): Also known as the certification period (60 days) or the time a patient is under care within 60 days.

Evaluation Visit (Assessment Visit): This is the first or initial home visit to determine whether the patient meets the HHA's criteria for admission. It is often the first skilled visit, made when the nurse or therapist already has specific physician's orders and is providing a skilled service to the patient.

Fee For Service (FFS): A health plan in which beneficiaries choose their healthcare provider and the health plan pays the provider's charge for services. This type of plan usually includes some element of utilization review or prior approval by the plan for certain, if not all, services.

Fiscal Intermediary (FI): Regional Home Health Intermediaries (RHHIs) are the insurance companies who function as specialized fiscal intermediaries and contract with CMS to process claims and make payment determinations on all home care and hospice claims.

Fraud: Medicare defines fraud as making false statements or representations of material facts in order to obtain some benefit or payment for which no entitlement would otherwise exist. Fraud is the intentional deception or misrepresentation to the government, including incorrect reporting of diagnoses or procedures to maximize benefits, billing for beneficiaries who do not qualify for benefits (e.g., beneficiaries who are not homebound) and falsifying records to meet or continue to meet the Medicare Conditions of Participation.

Functional Limitation: A restriction or impairment in the ability to perform a motion or activity in an efficient, independent, safe, or typical manner.

Goals: The endpoint of care or the desired results for care of an action or series of actions an individual or organization might strive for. For example, if the goal is to provide safe mobility, everything done should support that goal. Team members work together to achieve patient goals. A goal is different from an objective in that a goal is more broad-based. Objectives are more quantifiable and specific and are derived from a goal statement.

Health and Human Services (HHS): Oversees the Centers for Medicare and Medicaid Services (CMS) and the Medicare (federal) and Medicaid (state) programs.

Home Care/Home Health: The provision of a range of health services, products, supplies, and equipment to patients in their homes. Medicare currently reimburses skilled nursing, speech-language pathology, physical and occupational therapy, medical social work, and home health aide services.

Home Exercise Program (HEP): A series of activities, exercises, and/or tasks designed to achieve desired therapeutic and functional outcomes. The home exercise program is designed to be carried out by the patient, possibly with the assistance of a caregiver, on a regular and predetermined basis, to supplement the skilled treatment plan, or in an effort to extend or maintain therapeutic benefit after discontinuation of skilled services.

Home Health Advance Beneficiary Notice (HHABN or ABN): Since 2002, HHABNs (CMS-R-296) have been required by Medicare home health agencies to inform Medicare beneficiaries about possible non-covered items and/or services provided by the HHA and to alert beneficiaries that they may be liable for payment. The HHABN allows HHAs to collect payment for these services from Medicare beneficiaries based on section 1879 of the Social Security Act (SSA).

Home Health Agency (HHA) (see also Certified Home Health Agency): An organization that provides care to patients in their homes. The agency may or may not be licensed, depending on state requirements. Medicare-certified agencies must have a survey or a special review to accept Medicare patients.

Home Health Resource Group (HHRG): A score based on the OASIS documentation that uses a case-mix classification system reflecting the severity of the patient's condition for each of three domains—clinical, functional, and service utilization—and also relies on the position of the episode within a sequence of adjacent Medicare payment episodes, as well as the number of rehabilitation therapy visits.

Homebound: Synonymous with *confined primarily to the home as a result of medical reasons,* the term connotes that it is a "considerable and taxing effort" and a "normal inability" to leave the home. Please refer to Part Seven for specific descriptions and examples of homebound as listed in the HHA manual.

Hospice Care: A special way of caring for patients with a life threatening illness or a limited life expectancy. Hospice team members provide care for patients and their family members and try to make every remaining day the best that it can be. Hospice team members may include specially trained hospice volunteers, bereavement counselors, certified nursing assistants (CNAs) or hospice aides, spiritual counselors, nurses, therapists, and social workers. Hospice is a philosophy, not a place; most hospice care is provided at home but can be provided in any setting, such as in a skilled nursing facility, an inpatient hospice unit, or a community hospice home. Services are provided to patients with a documented life-limiting illness for whom the focus changes from curative intervention to palliative care. The service implies patient knowledge and acceptance of disease prognosis and life expectancy. Medicare coverage includes nursing care, medical social services, physician services, counseling services, medical supplies, home health aide and homemaker services, and physical, occupational, and speech-language pathology therapy services. Other important hospice services include volunteer support, spiritual support, and bereavement counseling.

ICD-9-CM Code: A coding methodology developed to identify specific clinical diagnoses for the purpose of data collection and payment. DRGs are assigned an ICD-9 code. OASIS items M0190, M0210, M0230, M0240, and M0246 are also based on ICD-9 codes.

Instrumental Activities of Daily Living (IADLs): Instrumental activities of daily living, such as shopping, cooking, transportation, financial management, homemaking, and home maintenance, are activities necessary for independent living in the community. They represent a higher level of functioning that the ADLs, which are necessary for self-care.

Interdisciplinary: An approach to clinical care requiring representation from various disciplines (i.e., occupational therapy, nursing, speech-language pathology, physical therapy, social work, etc.) to work collaboratively within a holistic and integrated treatment plan.

Interdisciplinary Team (IDT): The IDT is a key component of hospice care; it is the hospice and palliative care team members responsible for the patient's plan of care and may include: clinicians, social workers, physicians (including hospice medical directors), dietitians, bereavement counselors, spiritual counselors, chaplains, volunteers, physical therapists, occupational therapists, speech-language pathologists, home health aides, homemakers, pharmacists, and others, depending on the hospice's unique mission and population served.

Intermittent: Medicare defines intermittent as a maximum of 28 hours per week of skilled nursing and home health aide care combined. The 28-hour maximum can be increased to 35 hours if the documentation indicates that the condition requires additional care that is medically necessary. The services can be provided for up to 6 days a week. When nursing is the qualifying service for Medicare home health, intermittent also means a need and plan to provide more than 1 skilled nursing visit.

International Normalized Ratio (INR): The International Normalized Ratio is a mathematical "correction" of the results of the one-stage prothrombin time (PT). It is a common scale that standardizes PT ratio determinations worldwide.

Intervention: Nursing or therapy actions that help move the patient toward desired outcomes.

Length of Stay (LOS): The number of hospital or home care days for each patient. Each patient's hospitalization or home care stay is subject to review to determine the appropriateness of the length of stay (ALOS = average length of stay).

Licensure: A legal right granted by a government agency complying with state statute allowing an individual (e.g., registered nurse, licensed vocational nurse, physical therapist, etc.) and/or an organization (e.g., hospital, skilled nursing facility, home health agency, etc.) the ability to practice or operate in a certain specialty or geographic area.

Local Coverage Determination (LCD): An administrative and educational tool to specify under what clinical circumstances a service is reasonable and necessary; each contractor is allowed by CMS to implement local coverage determinations (LCDs).

Long-Term Care: A variety of health services provided to individuals with physical or mental disabilities needing assistance on a continuing basis. These services can be provided in a multitude of settings (e.g., homes, subacute skilled nursing facilities, retirement facilities, assistive living centers, intermediate care facilities, senior day services, etc.).

Low Utilization Payment Adjustment (LUPA): The payment adjustment that occurs when a patient is provided with a relatively small number of visits in a given episode. LUPAs change the Medicare payment from an episode payment to payment per visit; thus, LUPAs decrease the agency's payment for low utilization patients.

Managed Care: Care that is organized to achieve specific patient outcomes within fiscally responsible time frames (length of stay) using resources that are appropriate in amount and sequenced to the specific case type and population of the individual patient. Care is structured by case management care plans and clinical paths that are based on knowledge by case type regarding usual length of stay, critical events and their timing, anticipated outcomes, and resource utilization.

Management and Evaluation (M&E) of the Plan of Care (POC): M&E is a covered Medicare service for homebound patients needing complex intervention and care coordination and is called various things, including skilled management, skilled planning and assessment, skilled management and planning, and case management.

Medicaid: A state-administered program available only to certain low-income individuals and families who fit into an eligibility group that is recognized by federal and state law. Each state sets its own guidelines regarding eligibility and services; eligibility for children is based on the child's status, not the parent's.

Medicare: A federal program for people who are over age 65 years or disabled or who have end-stage renal disease (ESRD) or Amyotrophic Lateral Sclerosis (ALS or Lou Gehrig's disease). Medicare is complex but has two main parts, Part A and Part B, which cover different services, such as physician visits, inpatient hospitalization, home care, and hospice. Part D provides partial coverage for prescription medications. Medicare is a medical insurance program, and, like all insurance programs, it has exclusions, eligibility, and coverage rules.

Medicare Managed Care: An alternative insurance product for Medicare beneficiaries that allows commercial insurers to contract with the CMS to provide similar Medicare-covered services. These are also called "Medicare advantage plans." Providers must have a contract with such insurers to provide beneficiary care.

Medication Reconciliation: The process of obtaining, maintaining, and communicating to the patient and the next provider of service, a complete, accurate, and detailed list of all prescription and non-prescription drugs and appropriate tests to maintain optimal medication safety throughout care.

Modalities: Any physical agent applied to produce therapeutic changes to biologic tissue and include, but are not limited to, thermal, acoustic, light, mechanical, or electric energy. Examples include TENS units and ultrasound therapy.

OASIS (*O*utcome and *AS*sessment *I*nformation *S*et): A set of data items developed largely for the purpose of measuring (and risk adjusting) patient outcomes in home healthcare. OASIS items include sociodemographic, physiologic, mental/behavioral/emotional health status, functional status, and service utilization information. Since the OASIS is used for measuring outcomes, most data items are obtained at start of care and follow-up time points (i.e., every 60 days, recertification, and discharge). The OASIS is part of a comprehensive assessment.

Occupational Safety and Health Administration (OSHA): Clinicians have heard much in recent years about the need for the practice of universal precautions. The Labor Department's OSHA released its final rule to prevent occupational transmission of blood borne pathogens and infections. Employers must create infection control policies that support universal precautions. In addition, nurses, home health aides, therapists, and other staff members must be educated about the policy. In practice, this means that hepatitis B immunizations are available when the job requires exposure to blood or other potentially infectious body fluids. The HHA must also provide infection control and personal protective equipment (PPE) and supplies. This includes antimicrobial soap, alcohol-based hand cleansers, gloves, face masks or other protective shields, aprons that are fluid proof, gowns, and other needed protection. These should be provided by the agency, free of charge to the home care staff. There are also guidelines on blood or other body fluid transport, blood spill clean up, and the safe disposal of infectious waste.

Office of the Inspector General (OIG): By law, the OIG's mission is to protect the integrity of the DHHS programs and the health and welfare of beneficiaries served by these programs. This is done through a nationwide program of audits, investigations, surveys, inspections, sanctions, and fraud alerts. The Inspector General informs the Secretary of Health and Human Services of program and management problems, and recommends legislative, regulatory, and operational approaches to correct them.

Outcome (Clinical): Change in patient health status between two or more time points. Outcomes are changes that are intrinsic to the patient and can be positive, negative, or neutral changes in health status.

Outcome Enhancement: The second phase of OBQI, consisting of selecting target outcomes(s), investigating to determine key care behaviors that influenced the target outcome(s), and developing and implementing a plan of action to remedy substandard care practices or to reinforce exemplary care practices.

Outcome Measure: A quantification of a change in health status between two or more time points. In OBQI, outcome measures are computed using OASIS data from start of care and from subsequent time points or discharge. Two common types of outcome measures used in OBQI pertain to improvement in or stabilization of a specific health status attribute.

Outcome Report: A graphic or tabular document that compares an agency's patient outcomes for a given time period to either (1) analogous agency-level outcomes for a prior time period, (2) outcomes for a reference sample of patients from other agencies, or (3) both of the above. An outcome report contains information on selected outcome measures for all patients in the agency or for patients with specific conditions.

Outcome-Based Quality Improvement (OBQI): A two-stage quality improvement approach, premised on the principle that patient outcomes are central to continuous quality improvement. The first stage begins with collecting uniform patient health status data and culminates with an outcome report that reflects agency performance by comparing the agency's outcomes to those of a reference group of patients (which could be patients from a prior period at the same agency). The second stage (or the outcome enhancement stage) consists of selecting target outcomes for follow up. It entails conducting an investigation to determine key care behaviors that influence these target outcomes, culminating with the development and implementation of a plan of action to remedy substandard care practices or reinforce exemplary care practices. The effects of implementing the plan of action are evaluated in the next outcome report.

Outlier: Additional reimbursement from Medicare to a full episode payment in cases where costs of services delivered far exceed the HHRG episode payment. The outlier payment helps the HHA recoup some of the high cost of the care.

Palliative Care: The active total care of patients whose disease is not responsive to curative treatment. The goal of palliative care is to achieve the best quality of life for very ill patients. It is medically directed care with interdisciplinary care plan development and implementation, coordination with community services, family involvement, and use of volunteers.

Partial Episode Payment (PEP): A reduced episode payment that may be made based on the number of service days in an episode (always less than 60 days, employed in cases of transfers to another agency or discharges with readmissions to the same agency or another agency).

Patient Safety Organization: the U.S. Department of Health and Human Services (HHS) plans to establish "patient safety organizations." These organizations create the structure for health care providers, such as HHAs, to report patient safety events with the goal of identifying ways to make patients/care safer.

Payer: The insurance company financially responsible for the services or care provided to patients. Examples include Medicare or other insurance companies.

Performance Measure: Quantifiable standards or measurements to determine how successful a healthcare provider has been in meeting established outcomes or goals of care.

Personal Emergency Response Systems (PERS): PERS are a unique technology that links the frail or elderly with community resources, neighbors, or a friend at the push of a button or through voice-activated mechanisms. Although there are different types, all are telephone-service dependent. PERS may be appropriate for single patients returning home after surgery, patients who live alone or spend many hours at home alone, or for patients at risk from falls. PERS signal for help at the push of a button, which is worn by the PERS subscriber. For the system to be effective, the emergency device must be worn at all times. Home care and hospice nurses are in a unique position to identify this safety need in the community setting, so a referral can be initiated.

Plan of Care (POC): Formerly known as the CMS-485, the POC is a plan of action for care that is developed, implemented, and evaluated by home care clinicians (see also *Care Plan).* Most agencies still use the CMS-485 form for the POC. The CMS-485 form has 28 fields, and includes information on the agency, patient demographics, diagnoses, allergies, functional status, medications, goals, prognoses, and orders for services, treatments, and interventions. Field 28 indicates that reporting false information on the form is a federal offense, punishable by fine and/or imprisonment. If an Addendum or Medical Update to the POC is needed, the CMS-487 form is completed.

Point of Service Clinical Documentation: Refers to technology that enables clinicians to use laptop, hand-held, or other types of portable computers to collect patient information, and record clinical documentation.

Once entered, data is then transferred (or uploaded) to a central computer system that houses a master database. Information that will be needed for upcoming visits may also be downloaded to the computer device prior to the visits.

Pricer: Software modules in Medicare claims processing systems, specific to certain benefits, used in pricing claims, most often under prospective payment systems.

Procedures: The application of clinical skills and/or services by a nurse or therapist for improved function or other assessed need (e.g., wound care). This can be achieved through hands-on care, training or exercise, and must include active interventions between the nurse and patient, or the therapist and patient.

Progressive Corrective Action (PCA): The targeting or directing of medical review efforts by the Medicare contractor to identify providers who may be providing inappropriate or non-covered care. Often this review takes place long after the care has been provided; hence a paid claim is not necessarily a covered claim. *This is why the documentation must be accurate and complete and support covered care.*

Prospective Payment System (PPS): The third-party payment system that establishes certain payment rates for services regardless of the actual cost of care provided.

Prothrombin Time (PT/INR): Laboratory measurements of the time (in seconds) required for blood to clot.

Quality: A degree of excellence that is defined both externally (e.g., regulatory and accrediting bodies, etc.) and internally for/by an organization; the achievement of outcomes that provides patient health, well-being and satisfaction.

Quality Assessment/Improvement (QA/QI): The measurement or assessment of care that is provided to an individual or group.

Quality Improvement (QI): The implementation of an organized, continuous, data-driven evaluation and systems change process that focuses on patient rights, outcomes of care; patient, physician and provider satisfaction; and performance improvement.

Quality Indicator: A specific, valid, and reliable measure of access, care outcomes, or satisfaction, or a measure of a process of care that has been empirically shown to be predictive of access, care outcomes, or satisfaction.

Regional Home Health Intermediary: An insurance company functioning as a specialized fiscal intermediary who contracts with CMS to process claims and make payment determinations about home care and hospice claims from across the country. Each RHHI is allowed to implement local coverage determinations (LCDs).

Recertification/Recertification OASIS: A patient with ongoing home care needs must be recertified every 60 days in the Medicare program with a new POC. A Recertification OASIS as part of the comprehensive assessment must also be performed between day 56 and 60 of the prior episode.

Rehabilitative Services (Rehabilitative Care): In HHC, this includes the services of PT, OT, and S-LP therapy, all of which should be restorative in focus. When any of these services are indicated, based on patient need, diagnosis, and patient rehabilitation potential status, there must be sufficient documentation of communication among all services. This multidisciplinary case conferencing or care coordination should be reflected in the progress notes at least every 4 to 6 weeks.

Resource Utilization: The use of assets; the kinds and number of items (e.g., nursing hours, visits, supplies, etc.) used in performing patient care.

Resumption of Care (ROC)/Resumption of Care OASIS: A patient receiving home health services who is hospitalized during the episode and requires home health services past discharge must have the POC updated as needed and a Resumption of Care OASIS as part of the comprehensive assessment must also be performed. Depending on *when* the discharge occurs, the patient *may* have to be discharged from the home health agency and readmitted.

Risk Adjustment: The process of minimizing the effects of risk-factor differences when comparing outcome findings between two groups of patients. Two common risk adjustment methods are grouping/stratification and (multivariate) statistical procedures.

Risk Factor: A patient condition or circumstance that (negatively) influences the likelihood of a patient attaining the outcome.

Sentinel Event: A significant or serious patient event or outcome that needs to be evaluated immediately for gaps in quality and safe care. Sentinel events are commonly legal and risk management concerns.

Significant Change in Condition (SCIC): When a patient experiences a major decline or improvement in status during an episode of care, a SCIC (RFA-5) should be completed even though the data is no longer used to adjust the episode case-mix.

Standard: A level of performance or set of conditions considered acceptable by some authority or by the individual or individuals engaged in performing or maintaining the set of conditions in question.

Start of Care (SOC)/Start of Care OASIS: The Start of Care is the patient admission and first billable visit. The Start of Care OASIS as part of the comprehensive assessment must be completed within the first five days or as agency policy dictates.

Supervisory Visit: Supervisory visits are a requirement of the Medicare home health program. LPNs, HHAs, and therapy aides (LPTAs, COTAs) must be supervised by RNs or therapists. According to the Medicare COPs, HHAs must be supervised at least once every 14 days by an RN, PT, or OT. Supervisory visits include assuring that the HHA's POC is still appropriate or advancing the POC to meet the patient's progress toward self-management. It also includes assuring the HHA is following the POC and that the patient is satisfied with the care provided.

Some states do not allow LPNs or therapy assistants to make home health visits, and states have different standards for supervisory visit frequency. All must be supervised and also defined by agency policy where states do not define.

Telehealth: Telehealth is an emerging electronic telecommunication technology to deliver health services to the patient at the point of care. The Institute of Medicine defines it as "the use of electronic information and communications technologies to provide and support healthcare when distance separates participants."

Timeline: Identifies when an event or a series of events should occur, following a pre-established and agreed-upon framework for those events to happen or specific outcomes to be achieved.

Transfer: The process or moving of a person from one surface or location to another. Examples of transfers include moving from supine to sit, moving from a wheelchair to a bed, getting into and out of a tub, or getting into or out of a car.

Transfer OASIS: Completed when patient is transferred to another facility (hospital, nursing home, etc.).

UB-04: The claim or bill form, in either paper or electronic version, used by most institutional healthcare providers. It is published by CMS as the UB-04 Form 1450, but the standard itself is maintained by a non-governmental body: The National Uniform Billing Committee, an entity under the American Hospital Association in Chicago.

Utilization Management: A program established by healthcare providers to assess efficiency and quality of patient care based on established criteria.

Validity: The amount or degree to which an observed or measured outcome or event correlates with the criteria or event it was intended to measure.

Variance: The difference between what is expected and what actually happens. Variances are differentiated by system (internal or external), practitioner, and patient.

KEY HOME HEALTHCARE ABBREVIATIONS

The following abbreviations are among those most commonly used in the practice of home care. Please refer to your agency's own designated list of approved abbreviations for daily use in documentation.

ABN Advance beneficiary notice
ACE Acute care episode
ACHC The Accreditation Commission for Health Care
ad lib As desired
ADLs Activities of daily living
ADR Additional documentation request or additional development request; also adverse drug reaction
AHRQ Agency for Healthcare Research and Quality
AIDS Acquired immune deficiency syndrome
AKA Above knee amputation
ALS Amyotrophic lateral sclerosis (Lou Gehrig's disease)
AMB Ambulatory
AMI Acute myocardial infarction
AOTA American Occupational Therapy Association
APHA American Public Health Association
APRN, BC Advanced Practice Registered Nurse, Board Certified; formerly CNS
APTA American Physical Therapy Association
ASHA American Speech-Language-Hearing Association
ASCVD Arteriosclerotic cardiovascular disease
ASD Atrial septal defect
ASHD Arteriosclerotic heart disease
BBA Balanced Budget Act of 1997
BBRA Balanced Budget Refinement Act of 1999
BIPA Benefits Improvement and Protection Act of 2000
BKA Below knee amputation

BM	Bowel movement
BP	Blood pressure
BPH	Benign prostatic hypertrophy
BRP	Bathroom privileges
BS	Blood sugar
CA	Cancer
CAH	Critical access hospital
CABG	Coronary artery bypass graft
CAHPS	Consumer Assessment of Healthcare Providers and Systems
CAM	Complementary and alternative medicine
CAPD	Continuous ambulatory peritoneal dialysis
CBC	Complete blood count
CBO	Congressional Budget Office
CCN	CMS certification number
CDC	Centers for Disease Control and Prevention
CDE	Certified diabetes educator
CEA	Carcinoembryonic antigen
CERT	Certification
CFS	Clinical Function Severity
CHAP	Community Health Accreditation Program
CHIP	Children's Health Insurance Program
CMI	Case mix index
CMN	Certificate of medical necessity
CMS	Centers for Medicare & Medicaid Services
CMW	Case-mix weight
CNS	Clinical nurse specialist
CON	Certificate of need
COPD	Chronic obstructive pulmonary disease
COPS	(Medicare) Conditions of Participation
COS-C	Certificate OASIS Specialist - Clinical
COTA	Certified Occupational Therapy Assistant
CPM	Continuous or constant passive motion
CPR	Cardiopulmonary resuscitation
CPT	Current procedural terminology
C/S	Cesarean section
CVA	Cerebral vascular accident
CXR	Chest x-ray

DHHS	Department of Health and Human Services
DJD	Degenerative joint disease
DM	Diabetes mellitus
DME	Durable medical equipment
DMERC	Durable medical equipment regional carrier
DOE	Dyspnea on exertion
DRG	Diagnostic-related group
DX	Diagnosis
ECG/EKG	Electrocardiogram
ED	Emergency department
EDC	Estimated date of confinement
EN	Enteral nutrition
EOB	Explanation of benefits
EOL	End-of-life
EOMB	Explanation of Medicare benefits
ER	Emergency room
ESRD	End-stage renal disease
FBS	Fasting blood sugar
FC	Final claim
FFS	Fee for service
FHR	Fetal heart rate
FI	Fiscal intermediary
FMR	Focused medical review
FX	Fracture
FY	Fiscal year
GAO	Government Accounting Office
GI	Gastrointestinal
HAART	Highly active antiretroviral therapy
HAVEN	Home assessment validation and entry
HCPCS	CMS Common Procedure Coding System
HEP	Home exercise program
HF	Heart failure
HHA	Home health agency or Home health aide
HHABN	Home Health Advance Beneficiary Notice
HHC	Home healthcare
HHRG	Home health resource group
HHS	Health and Human Services (Department of)
HICN	Health insurance claim number

HIM	Health Insurance Manual
HIPPA	Health Insurance Portability and Accountability Act
HIPPS	Health Insurance Prospective Payment System
HIQI	Health Insurance Query for HHAs
HME	Home medical equipment
HMO	Health maintenance organization
HVGS	High voltage galvanic stimulation
IADLs	Instrumental activities of daily living
ICD-9-CM	International Classification of Diseases-9th Revision-Clinical Modification
IDDM	Insulin-dependent diabetes mellitus
IG	Inspector general
IM	Intramuscular
INR	International normalized ratio
IOM	Institute of Medicine
IPPB	Intermittent positive pressure breathing
IV	Intravenous
JCAHO	Joint Commission on Accreditation of Healthcare Organizations
LCD	Local Coverage Determination
LE	Lower extremity
LLE	Left lower extremity
LLL	Left lower lung
LPTA	Licensed Physical Therapy Assistant
LUE	Left upper extremity
LUPA	Low utilization payment adjustment
MAC	Medicare administrative contractor
MedPAC	Medicare Payment Advisory Commission
MI	Myocardial infarction
MOW	Meals on Wheels
MR	Medical review
MSA	Metropolitan statistical area
MSP	Medicare secondary payer
MSS	Medical social services
MSW	Medical Social Worker
NCSB	Neurological, cognitive, sensory, and behavioral variables

NHP	Nursing home placement
NIDDM	Non-insulin-dependent diabetes mellitus
NIH	National Institutes of Health
NIOSH	National Institute of Occupational Safety and Health
NOA	Notice of admission
NPI	National Provider Identifier
NRS	Non-routine supplies
O_2	Oxygen
OASIS	*O*utcome and *AS*sessment *I*nformation *S*et
OBQI	Outcome-based quality improvement
OBQM	Outcome-based quality monitoring
OBS	Organic brain syndrome
OIG	Office of Inspector General
ORIF	Open reduction internal fixation
ORT	Operation Restore Trust
OSHA	Occupational Safety and Health Administration
OT	Occupational therapy or Occupational therapist
OTA	Occupational Therapy Assistant
PACE	Program of all-inclusive care for the elderly
PCA	Patient-controlled analgesia; also Progressive Corrective Action
PEN	Parenteral and enteral nutrition
PEP	Partial episode payment
PICC (line)	Peripherally inserted central catheter
PKU	Phenylketonuria
PM	Program memoranda
PN	Parenteral nutrition
P/O(s)	Prosthetics and orthotics
PO	By mouth (orally)
POC	Plan of care
POT	Plan of treatment
PPO	Preferred provider organization
PPS	Prospective payment system
PRE	Progressive resistive exercises
PRN	As needed
PSO	Patient safety organizations (PSOs)

PT	Physical therapy or physical therapist
PTA	Physical therapist assistant
PU	Pressure ulcer
PVD	Peripheral vascular disease
QI	Quality improvement
RA	Remittance advice
RAP	Request for anticipated payment
RHHI	Regional Home Health Intermediary
RLE	Right lower extremity
RLL	Right lower lung
ROC	Resumption of care
ROM	Range of motion
ROVER	RHHI OASIS verification
RT	Respiratory therapy or Respiratory therapist
RUE	Right uppcr extremity
Rx	Prescription
SCI	Spinal cord injury
SCIC	Significant change in condition
SE	Side effects
S-LP	Speech-language pathology or speech-language pathologist
SNF	Skilled nursing facility
SNV	Skilled nursing visit
SOB	Shortness of breath
SOC	Start of care
S/P	Status post
SQ	Subcutaneous
SX	Symptoms
TENS	Transcutaneous electrical nerve stimulation
THR	Total hip replacement
TIA	Transient ischemic attack
Title XVIII	The Medicare section of the Social Security Act
Title XIX	The Medicaid section of the Social Security Act
Title XX	The Social Services section of the Social Security Act
TKR	Total knee replacement
TO	Telephone order

TOB	Type of bill
TPN	Total parenteral nutrition
TPR	Temperature, pulse, and respiration
TUR	Transurethral resection
TURP	Transurethral resection of prostate
TX	Treatment
UA/C&S	Urinalysis/culture and sensitivity
UE	Upper extremity
UPIN	Unique physician identification number
UPN	Universal product numbers
URI	Upper respiratory infection
UTI	Urinary tract infection
VA	Veteran administration
VAD	Vascular access device
VO	Verbal order
WIC	Women, Infants, and Children Program
WNL	Within normal limits
WOCN	Wound Ostomy Certified Nurse
www	World Wide Web

DO NOT USE ABBREVIATIONS

Affirmed by The Joint Commission in May 2005, this list was created as part of the requirements for meeting National Patient Safety Goal Requirement 2B (Standardize a list of abbreviations, acronyms and symbols that are not to be used throughout the organization). Home care organizations may add to this list, so it is important to know what your organization considers "Do Not Use Abbreviations." For further information, visit www.jointcommission.org.

THE JOINT COMMISSION'S OFFICIAL "DO NOT USE" LIST

Do Not Use	Potential Problem	Use Instead
U (Unit)	Mistaken for "O" (zero), the number "4" (four) or "cc"	Write "unit"
IU (International Unit	Mistaken for IV (intravenous) or the number 10 (ten)	Write "international unit"
Q.D., QD, q.d., qd (daily) Q.O.D., QOD, q.o.d., qod (every other day)	Mistaken for each other Period after the Q mistaken for "I" and the "O" mistaken for "I"	Write "daily" Write "every other day"
Trailing zero (X.0 mg) Lack of leading zero (.X mg)	Decimal point is missed	Write X mg Write 0.X mg
MS $MS0_4$ and $MgSO_4$	Can mean morphine sulfate or magnesium sulfate	Write "morphine sulfate" Write "magnesium sulfate"

Source: The Joint Commission, Oakbrook Terrace, IL.

In addition, The Joint Commission has added additional abbreviations, acronyms, and symbols which are problematic for possible future inclusion in the Official "Do Not Use" List. These are listed in the following table.

Do Not Use	Potential Problem	Use Instead
> (greater than) < (less than)	Misinterpreted as the number "7" (seven) or the letter "L" Confused for one another	Write "greater than" Write "less than"
Abbreviations for the drug names	Misinterpreted due to similar abbreviations for multiple drugs	Write drug names in full
Apothecary units	Unfamiliar to many practitioners Confused with metric units	Use metric units
@	Mistaken for the number "2" two	Write "at"
cc	Mistaken for U (units) when poorly written	Write "ml" or milliliters"
ug	Mistaken for mg (milligrams) resulting in one thousand-fold overdose	Write "mcg" or "micrograms"

Source: The Joint Commission, Oakbrook Terrace, IL.

PART NINE

GUIDELINES FOR HOME MEDICAL EQUIPMENT AND SUPPLY CONSIDERATIONS

9

The home medical equipment (HME; also known as durable medical equipment or DME) industry provides equipment, supplies, and services to consumers for higher degrees of independence, function, and quality of life. The scope of services provided by HME providers includes communication intake/referral information with physicians, selecting appropriate equipment, evaluating the home and setting up the equipment, educating patients and their caregivers on how to use the equipment properly, servicing the equipment as needed (24 hours a day), cleaning and disinfecting the equipment when it is retrieved from the patient, and completing payer claims paperwork for patients. HME companies can be accredited, but all must be service oriented and responsive to meeting the needs of clinicians, home care and hospice organizations, and patients' unique needs.

Under Part B, Medicare assists in the purchase of some medical equipment and also rents some equipment. Medicare helps pay for equipment if the item meets the following requirements: it is prescribed or ordered by a physician, is medically necessary, and addresses a medical need. Medicare pays 80% of the Medicare-approved charge, and the patient or secondary insurance is responsible for the remaining 20% (co-payment portion) of the bill.

Medicare DME regional carriers have medical coverage policies and documentation requirements. Physicians must provide and sign a certificate of medical necessity, which proves to Medicare that the equipment should be covered for medical reasons. In some cases a physician prescription is required before delivery of certain pieces of HME or DME.

The most common equipment for patients in the home setting is listed in the following section. Please consult the Centers for Medicare and Medicaid Services carrier's manual or equipment company representative for any specific coverage or documentation requirements because Medicare makes ongoing changes to coverage of equipment and supplies. Most private insurers also have an equipment benefit; the specific rules and coverage depend on the insurance program. Physicians' orders are needed for all of these items. The equipment and supplies used by patients should be documented in item #14 of the plan of care.

The term *covered* means that generally, with appropriate certification from the physician and documented need of the patient, the item would be covered for some reimbursement.

Equipment	Indications/Guidelines
Alternating pressure pad and pump (covered)	Patient is bedridden and has (or is prone to) pressure ulcers
Apnea monitor (covered)	For coverage of equipment, physician documentation needs to show high-risk history that necessitates monitoring
Bathtub lifts/seat safety rails (not covered)	Convenience or comfort item, although may be an appropriate safety item
Bedpan (covered)	Bedridden patient
Bedside commode (covered)	Impaired ambulation, patient confined to room or bed
Blood glucose monitor machine (covered)	Diabetes mellitus
Cane (covered)	Impaired ambulation condition
Commode (covered)	Patient confined to room or bed
Continuous passive motion (CPM) devices (covered)	For patients who have had a total knee replacement
Crutches (covered)	Impaired ambulation
Electric hospital bed with rails (covered)	Condition requires frequent change in position, usually cardiac, lung processes, or spinal cord injuries may be covered; if the patient can operate the controls,

Equipment	Indications/Guidelines
	some payers see this as a convenience item for the caregiver (NOTE: Overbed table usually not covered, can be rented privately)
Food pumps, enteral feedings (patient dependent)	Diagnosis dependent, usually via gastrostomy (G-tube) or feeding tubes
Gel flotation pads and mattresses (covered)	Patient is bedridden and has (or is prone to) pressure ulcers
Geriatric chair (covered)	Medical need justified by diagnosis in lieu of a wheelchair
High-tech specialty beds including low air-loss beds/mattresses, Clinitrons (patient dependent)	Supportive physician documentation of pressure ulcer in bedbound patient; refer to DME/HME representative for specific coverage and documentation requirements
Home phototherapy (covered)	Physician documentation supportive of increased bilirubin as documented by lab results
Hospital bed, non-electric, with rails (covered)	Patient usually confined to bed and chair; need for bed must be clearly evident in the documentation
Hospital bed, electric	See Electric hospital bed with rails
Hydraulic lift (covered)	Condition requires movement in chair/bedridden patient
Infusion pump (covered)	Ordered in conjunction with a course of treatment by

Equipment	Indications/Guidelines
	physician that is appropriate to patient diagnosis
Intermittent positive pressure breathing (IPPB) machine (covered)	Severely impaired respiratory status
Lamb's wool pads (covered)	Patient is usually confined to bed/chair and is prone to pressure ulcers
Mattress (covered)	Ordered in conjunction with hospital bed when meets those requirements
Nebulizer (covered)	Severely impaired respiratory status/system
Oxygen therapy (patient dependent, if meets diagnostic requirements of blood gas)	Covered conditions include most severe lung disease processes; for ranges of acceptable laboratory values, refer to specific requirements
Personal emergency response system (generally not covered)	Not seen as therapeutic, although often indicated for patients with history of falls or at risk for falls
Postural drainage board(s) (covered)	Impaired pulmonary status
Quadripod (Quad) cane (covered)	Impaired ambulation
Raised toilet seat (not covered) 3 in 1 commode (covered)	Seen as primarily a safety item, although frequently indicated for status post-hip surgery patients
Respiratory equipment (e.g., IPPB, oxygen, humidifiers, iron lung, ventilators)	Covered if patient's ability to breathe is impaired; pulse oximetry or other tests to support medical necessity may be requested

Equipment	Indications/Guidelines
Side rails	Not covered when attached to patient's own bed; covered when attached to hospital bed and patient qualifies for hospital bed
Suction machine (covered)	Based on diagnosis, clinical need, and physician documentation
Telephone alert systems (generally not covered)	Not seen as therapeutic in purpose, although often indicated for elderly patients at risk for falls
Transient electric nerve stimulation (TENS) unit (covered)	Extensive physician documentation of pain; usually for an orthopedic or neurological diagnosis
Traction equipment (covered)	Documentation of orthopedic impairment describing need for equipment by physician
Trapeze (covered)	Bed confinement, need for body position change, or respiratory condition
Ventilator (covered)	Based on diagnosis, may include neuromuscular diseases or respiratory failure
Walker (covered)	Impaired ambulation condition
Water pressure pads/mattress (covered)	Patient is usually confined to chair/bed and has (or is prone to) pressure ulcers
Wheelchair (covered)	Patient either bedbound or chairbound, needs specialty wheelchair (NOTE: Special sizes or features are based on physician documentation and patient condition)

PART TEN

DIRECTORY OF EVIDENCE-BASED AND OTHER RESOURCES

10

DIRECTORY OF EVIDENCE-BASED AND OTHER RESOURCES

Accreditation Programs

The Community Health Accreditation Program, Inc. (CHAP) (www.chapinc.org) was the first, non-profit accrediting body for community-based healthcare organizations in the United States. It began in 1965 as a joint venture between the American Public Health Association (APHA) and the National League for Nursing (NLN) based on the premise that accreditation was the mechanism for recognizing excellence in community health practice. CHAP was granted "deeming authority" by the Centers for Medicare and Medicaid Services (CMS) in 1992 for home health and in 1999 for hospice. In 2006 CMS granted CHAP full deeming authority for home medical equipment (HME). Therefore, instead of state surveys, CHAP and other entities with "deeming authority," have regulatory authorization to survey agencies providing home health and hospice services to determine whether they meet the Medicare Conditions of Participation (COPs).

The Joint Commission (www.jointcommission.org) was established in 1951 and is an independent, not-for-profit organization for standards-setting and accrediting in healthcare that focuses on improving the quality and safety of care. The Joint Commission's comprehensive accreditation process evaluates an organization's compliance with these standards and other accreditation requirements. Joint Commission accreditation is recognized nationwide as a symbol of quality that reflects an organization's commitment to meeting certain performance standards. To earn and maintain The Joint Commission's Gold Seal of Approval™, an organization must undergo an on-site survey by a Joint Commission survey team at least every three years.

The Accreditation Commission for Healthcare (www.ACHC.org) also provides accreditation services and seeks to improve healthcare quality by accrediting health programs that pass a rigorous, comprehensive review. For consumers and

10

employers, the seal is a reliable indicator that an organization is well-managed and delivers high quality care and service.

Administration

www.homecareinformation.net offers online education, including interdisciplinary orientation and care planning related to Medicare and other aspects of home health care presented by knowledgeable home care experts.

Book Resources:
Harris, MD: *The handbook of Home Health Care Administration,* ed 4, Sudbury, MA, 2005, Jones and Bartlett.

Aging (see Older Adults)

Alzheimer's Disease/Dementia

The Alzheimer's Association (www.alz.org or 800-272-3900) offers brochures and other resources for professionals and families that include information on getting the right diagnosis and a 24/7 helpline.

The American Hospice Foundation (www.americanhospice.org or 202-223-0204) offers a pamphlet entitled "Alzheimer's Disease and Hospice."

The National Institutes of Health (NIH) (http://nihseniorhealth.gov) offers information devoted to caring for older adults. Sections cover specific problems such as Alzheimer's disease and include facts on risk factors, symptoms, diagnosis, and treatment as well as select information on related diseases like dementia and senile dementia.

The National Institutes of Health National Institute on Aging's Alzheimer's Disease Education and Referral (ADEAR) Center (www.nia.nih.gov/Alzheimers or 800-438-4380) has information and booklets available to professionals, patients, and families on Alzheimer's disease. ADEAR offers two booklets from Duke University's Family Support Program for caregivers and families outlining struggles and solutions when dealing with anger in dementia patients: "Hit Pause—Helping Dementia Families Deal With Anger" for $3.00 and "Wait A Minute" for $2.00. In addition, ADEAR offers the Connections newsletter (www.nia.nih.gov/Alzheimers/ResearchInformation/Newsletter), which provides information about Alzheimer's disease and caregiving.

Book Resources:

Mace NL, Rabins PV: *The 36-hour day: a family guide to caring for people with Alzheimer disease, other dementias, and memory loss in later life*, ed 4, Baltimore, 2006, Johns Hopkins University Press.

McLay E, Young EP: *Mom's OK, she just forgets: the Alzheimer's journey from denial to acceptance, a handbook for families,* 2007, Amherst, MA, Prometheus Books.

Arthritis

The American Academy of Orthopaedic Surgeons (www.aaos.org) offers resources and information related to arthritis.

The Arthritis Foundation (www.arthritis.org or 800-283-7800) offers brochures that include "Meet Your Arthritis Health Care Team" and publish the *Arthritis Today* magazine that can be subscribed to through the website.

The National Institute of Arthritis and Musculoskeletal and Skin Diseases (www.niams.nih.gov or 877-226-4267) offers question-and-answer publications and resources on arthritis and rheumatic diseases.

www.Pain-Topics.org provides free evidence-based clinical news, information, research, and education on causes and effective treatment of many types of pain.

Associations for Home Care, Hospice and Home Care, Hospice Clinicians and Paraprofessionals

The American Association for Homecare (AAHomecare) (www.aahomecare.org) works to strengthen access to home care and represents healthcare providers, equipment manufacturers, and other organizations in the homecare community.

The National Association for Home Care and Hospice (www.nahc.org) is the nation's largest trade association representing the interests and concerns of home care agencies, hospices, home care aide organizations, and medical equipment suppliers.

The National Hospice and Palliative Care Organization (www.nhpco.org) provides resources and information for professionals and patients and families with hospice needs.

The National Private Duty Association (www.privatedutyhomecare.org) offers private duty home care providers education and best practices.

The Visiting Nurse Association (www.vnaa.org) represents VNAs and offers education and other resources. The peer-reviewed, interdisciplinary journal, *Home Healthcare Nurse,* is the official journal of the VNAA.

Certified Diabetes Educator

The American Association of Diabetes Educators (AADE) (www.diabeteseducator.org) is a multidisciplinary organization dedicated to integrating successful self-management as a key outcome in the care of people with diabetes and related conditions.

Dietitian

The American Dietetic Association (ADA) (www.eatright.org) is the largest organization of food and nutrition professionals and serves the public by promoting optimal nutrition, health, and well-being.

Home Health Nursing

The Home Healthcare Nurses Association (HHNA) (www.hhna.org) became an affiliate of the National Association for Home Care and Hospice in 1999. The peer-reviewed, interdisciplinary journal, *Home Healthcare Nurse,* is the official journal of the HHNA.

Hospice Nursing

The Hospice and Palliative Nurses Association (HPNA) (www.hpna.org) was established in 1986 and is the nation's largest and oldest professional nursing organization dedicated to promoting excellence in hospice and palliative nursing care.

Medical Social Worker

The National Association of Social Workers (NASW) (www.socialworkers.org) is the largest membership organization of professional social workers in the world and works to enhance professional growth and development, create and maintain professional standards, and advance sound social policies.

Occupational Therapist

The American Occupational Therapy Association (AOTA) (www.aota.org) is a professional organization committed to supporting the professional community through monitoring, responding to, and influencing healthcare, education, and community-related systems and the way that occupational therapy is integrated into the delivery of services within those systems.

Pharmacist

The American Pharmacists Association (APhA) (www.pharmacist.com) is the largest association of pharmacists in the United States and provides a forum for discussion, consensus building, and policy setting for the profession.

Physical Therapy

The American Physical Therapy Association (APTA) (www.apta.org) is a national professional organization to foster advancements in physical therapy practice, research, and education.

Physician (Home Care)

The American Academy of Home Care Physicians (AAHCP) (www.aahcp.org) began in 1988 and serves the needs of thousands of physicians and related professionals and agencies interested in improving care of patients in the home. Members include home care physicians—physicians who make house calls, care for homebound patients, act as home health agency medical directors, and refer patients to home care agencies. Specialties include internal medicine, family practice, pediatrics, geriatrics, psychiatry, emergency medicine, and others.

Psychiatric Nursing

The American Psychiatric Nurses Association (APNA) (www.apna.org) is a professional organization for those committed to the specialty practice of psychiatric mental health nursing, to health and wellness promotion through identification of mental health issues, to prevention of mental health problems, and to the care and treatment of persons with psychiatric disorders.

Respiratory Therapist

The American Association for Respiratory Care (AARC) (www.aarc.org) is the only professional society for respiratory therapists in hospitals, nursing homes, and home care, managers of respiratory and cardiopulmonary services, and educators who provide respiratory care training.

Speech-Language Pathologist

The American Speech-Language-Hearing Association (ASHA) (www.asha.org) is the professional, scientific, and credentialing association for speech-language pathologists, audiologists, and speech, language, and hearing scientists in the United States and internationally.

Spiritual Counselor/Chaplain

The Association of Professional Chaplains (www.professionalchaplains.org) is an interfaith professional pastoral care association of providers of pastoral care endorsed by faith groups to serve persons in physical, spiritual, or mental need in diverse settings throughout the world.

Wound, Ostomy, Continence Nursing

The Wound, Ostomy and Continence Nurses Society (WOCN) (www.wocn.org) was founded in 1968 and is a professional, international nursing society for experts in the care of patients with wound, ostomy, and incontinence, and supports its members by promoting educational, clinical, and research opportunities to advance the practice and guide the delivery of expert healthcare to individuals with wounds, ostomies, and incontinence.

Cancer (Adult)

The American Cancer Society (www.cancer.org or 800-ACS-2335 or 800-395-LOOK [800-395-5665]) has support groups such as "I Can Cope" and "Look Good … Feel Better" for women undergoing chemotherapy or radiation. It also offers resources and information on various cancers for patients, families, and professionals.

Cancer Care (www.cancercare.org or 800-813-HOPE [4673]) offers information for those dealing with cancer—patients, family members, friends, and health professionals providing care. It provides online support groups, fact sheets with titles that include "Prevention and Early Detection" and "Young Adults with Cancer," and fact sheets and publications in Spanish.

The City of Hope National Medical Center (www.cityofhope.org or 626-256-HOPE [626-256-4673]) offers information on adult and pediatric cancers of all kinds for patients and caregivers, families, and professionals. Information pages on each type of cancer include what the cancer is, what parts of the body the cancer effects and how, and what each stage of the cancer involves. It also has information on treatment and patient referral options for current trials and research.

The Intercultural Cancer Council (www.iccnetwork.org) provides fact sheets and information about minorities and cancer, underserved populations, and news, statistics, and links to other resources for healthcare professionals and patients alike. It also publishes a newsletter entitled *The Voice* that can be viewed or subscribed to through the website.

The National Cancer Institute (NCI) (www.cancer.gov or 800-4-CANCER [800-422-6237]) produces a newsletter entitled the *NCI Cancer Bulletin* with articles on research and training to reduce the suffering caused by cancer.

The National Coalition for Cancer Survivorship (NCCS) (www.canceradvocacy.org or 301-650-9127 or 888-650-9127) offers a free educational resource called the *Cancer Survivor Toolbox*. This includes topics on communication, negotiating, and concerns for older adults.

The Oncology Nursing Society (www.ons.org or 866-257-4ONS [866-257-4667]) has a "Breast Cancer Patient Resource Area" and links to organizations and journals to help patients.

Cancer.net (www.cancer.net or 703-797-1914) offers patient and clinician education materials.

Book Resources:

Cope DG, Reb AM, editors: *An evidence-based approach to the treatment of care of the older adult with cancer*, Pittsburgh, 2006, Oncology Nursing Society (www.ons.org or 866-257-4667). This book details commonly occurring cancers in aging patients, palliative care considerations, symptom management, alternative therapies, and other issues specifically for older adult patients.

Cancer (Child)

The Agency for Healthcare Research and Quality (AHRQ) (www.ahrq.gov or 800-358-9295) offers "Acute Pain Management in Infants, Children, and Adolescents: Operative or Medical Procedures and Trauma (Quick Reference Guide for Clinicians)" (AHCPR 92-0020).

The American Cancer Society (www.cancer.org or 800-227-2345) offers information and support groups for children and adolescents with cancer.

The Brain Tumor Society (www.tbts.org or 800-770-8287) has information on healthy eating habits and programs such as the Connection of Personal Experiences program for patient support.

Children's Hospice International (www.chionline.org or 800-242-4453) has information on children's hospice, palliative care, and end-of-life care services and how to locate a local program. Publications are available for families and professionals.

The City of Hope National Medical Center (www.cityofhope.org or 626-256-4673) offers information on adult and pediatric cancers of all kinds for patients and caregivers, families, and professionals. Information pages on each type of cancer include what the cancer is, what parts of the body the cancer effects and how, and what each stage of the cancer involves. Information is available on treatment, patient referral options, and current trials.

Compassionate Friends (www.compassionatefriends.org or 877-969-0010) is an organization that offers grief support for families after the death of a child. Chapters across the country hope to offer families an opportunity to work toward a positive resolution after the loss of a child of any age.

The Dougy Center for Grieving Children and Families (www.dougy.org or 866-775-5683) offers support for children, teenagers, and their families when dealing with the death of a loved one. Sections are specifically tailored for adults who want to help a grieving child, children, teens, and those working with students. Information is offered through the website and centers across the country.

The Make-A-Wish Foundation (www.wish.org or 800-722-WISH [9474]) fulfills special wishes for children with a life-threatening illness and their families.

SuperSibs (www.supersibs.org or 866-444-SIBS [7427]) offers support for siblings of children with cancer including scholarships, grief support, and resources for siblings and parents of children with cancer.

Cardiac

The Agency for Healthcare Research and Quality (AHRQ) (www.ahrq.gov or 800-358-9295 or 410-381-3150) offers free resources including a *Quick Reference Guide for Clinicians, Cardiac Rehabilitation, Clinical Practice*

Guideline No. 17 and the *Consumer Version*. Patient guides are available in English and Spanish.

The American Heart Association (www.americanheart.org or 800-AHA-USA1 [800-242-8721]) offers professional and patient resources that include the American College of Cardiology/American Heart Association Practice Guideline *Guidelines for the Management of Patients with Acute Myocardial Infarction*. Cardiac pharmacology and the long-term management of the patient to facilitate a return to prior levels of activity are discussed in depth. Other resources include "Know the Facts, Get the Stats," a guide to heart disease, stroke, and risks, "Heart Insight," a monthly publication for professionals and consumers, and *Answers by Heart*, patient information sheets on a variety of topics related to heart care. They are split up into three categories—cardiovascular conditions, treatments and tests, and lifestyle and risk reduction—and include titles such as "How Can I Live With Heart Failure?," "How Do I Manage My Medicines?," "How Can I Handle the Stress of Not Smoking?," "What Is High Blood Pressure Medicine?," and "How Do I Follow a Healthy Diet?"

Heart Failure Online (www.heartfailure.org) is available in both English and Spanish with information about the heart, specifics of heart failure, prevention and treatment information, a frequently asked questions page, and a glossary of heart-related terms.

The Heart Failure Society of America (www.abouthf.org or 651-642-1633) offers information on heart failure and cardiac care guidelines, including the New York Heart Association classification for the stages of heart failure, with symptoms that affect patients' daily activities and quality of life.

The National Heart, Lung, and Blood Institute (www.nhlbi.nih.gov or 301-592-8573) has information about heart failure (what it is, the signs and symptoms, treatment options, how it is diagnosed) and cardiac care that includes "Your Guide to Lowering Your Blood Pressure with DASH," which explains the DASH eating plan and how it can help control blood pressure, the "High Blood Cholesterol—What You Need to Know" brochure, and "Live Healthier,

Live Longer," which offers helpful tips and information for prevention and management of heart failure.

Centers for Medicare and Medicaid Services (CMS) (see Medicare)

Children (General)

The Muscular Dystrophy Association (www.mdausa.org or 800-752-1717) offers resources related to muscular dystrophy.

The United Cerebral Palsy (UCP) association (www.ucp.org) provides information and resources related to cerebral palsy and advocates for the rights of persons with any disability.

Clinical Guidelines (see Evidence-Based Clinical Guidelines)

Constipation Care (see Gastrointestinal)

Cultural Care

Culturally Competent Nursing Care: A Cornerstone of Caring is a free, 9-hour continuing education units course for nursing professionals from the U.S. Department of Health and Human Services' Office of Minority Health that has been endorsed by the American Nurses Association and can be accessed at www.thinkculturalhealth.org.

The National Institute of Diabetes and Digestive and Kidney Diseases (NIDDK) (www.niddk.nih.gov) has portals that feature Spanish health materials and resources. Full-time bilingual information specialists respond to requests for Spanish health materials from the NIDDK clearinghouses. The Spanish portals include

- www.diabetes-espanol.niddk.nih.gov for diabetes information
- www.digestive-espanol.niddk.nih.gov for digestive diseases information
- www.kidney-espanol.niddk.nih.gov for kidney and urologic diseases information

Dementia (see Alzheimer's Disease/Dementia)

Knowledge and Skills Needed for Dementia Care: A Guide for Direct Care Workers in Everyday Language helps direct-care workers determine whether they have the skills they need to deliver person-centered dementia care—and where to go for assistance if they need training. Includes an overview of the primary diseases that may cause dementia symptoms, top ten warning signs of Alzheimer's disease and other dementia-related diseases, a description of structures of the brain, and a glossary of words used in the text. Copies (pdf) of the new version may be downloaded for free from the Michigan Dementia Coalition website. Visit www.dementiacoalition.org or call (517) 324-7320.

Depression

The Agency for Healthcare Research and Quality (AHRQ) (www.ahrq.gov or 800-358-9295) has a patient guide entitled "Depression Is a Treatable Illness" (AHCPR Pub. No. 93-0053).

The American Psychiatric Nurses Association's website is www.apna.org.

The American Psychiatric Association (www.psych.org or 202-682-6220) provides information and resources for patients and families about symptoms and treatments for depression. It sponsors a mental health website (www.healthyminds.org) that offers mental health resources for professionals and consumers.

The Centers for Disease Control and Prevention (CDC) (www.cdc.gov) offers information on depression that includes "Preventing Suicide: Program Activities Guide," a booklet with information on the causes and risks related to suicide and on prevention.

The Depression and Bipolar Support Alliance (www.dbsalliance.org or 800-826-3632) offers information about depression, anxiety, bipolar disorder, and other mood-altering disorders that includes causes, signs, and treatment options.

The National Institute of Mental Health (www.nimh.nih.gov or 800-421-4211) has resources on depression and other mental health problems.

The Paralyzed Veterans of America (PVA) (www.pva.org or 800-424-8200) offers publications including "Depression Following Spinal Cord Injury" and a consumer guide entitled "Depression: What You Should Know" for mood disorders, including depression, with information on signs and treatments.

Diabetes (Adult)

The American Diabetes Association (ADA) (www.diabetes.org or 800-DIABETES [800-342-2383]) offers resources for patients, families, and professionals that include themed research summaries on topics such as "Blood Glucose Control" and "Attitudes Toward Insulin Therapy." It also offers information about "Diabetic Heart and Blood Vessel Disease" with articles that include "Lifestyle Changes Improve Artery Health."

The Centers for Disease Control and Prevention (CDC) (www.cdc.gov/diabetes or 800-CDC-INFO [800-232-4636]) offers a Public Health Resource page on diabetes with information on diabetes, eating right, and publications that include fact sheets and statistics in both English and Spanish.

The Diabetes Action Research and Education Foundation (www.diabetesaction.org or 202-333-4520) offers resources on the website that include healthy recipes, frequently asked questions, an "Ask the Diabetes Educator" page, and news updates on research and funding projects.

The Joslin Diabetes Center (www.joslin.org or 617-732-2400) has educational resources on managing diabetes, a "Diabetes Words and Phrases" page, research information, and professional education programs.

The National Amputation Foundation (www.nationalamputation.org or 516-887-3600) has information and support.

The National Diabetes Information Clearinghouse (www.diabetes.niddk.nih.gov or 301-654-3327) offers fact sheets, information packets, and professional publications.

The National Federation of the Blind (NFB) (www.nfb.org or 410-296-7760) publishes *Voice of the Diabetic* four times a year as a free service to those with diabetes, healthcare programs, and others. It is available on the web or in print.

Diabetes (Child)

The American Diabetes Association (ADA) (www.diabetes.org or 800-DIABETES [800-342-2383]) offers resources for patients, families, and professionals.

The Centers for Disease Control and Prevention (CDC) (www.cdc.gov/diabetes or 800-CDC-INFO [800-232-4636]) offers a Public Health Resource page on diabetes with information on diabetes, eating right, and publications that include fact sheets and statistics in English and Spanish.

The Diabetes Action Research and Education Foundation (www.diabetesaction.org or 202-333-4520) offers resources on the website that include healthy recipes, frequently asked questions, an "Ask the Diabetes Educator" page, and news updates on research and funding projects.

The Juvenile Diabetes Research Foundation International (www.jdrf.org or 800-223-1138) promotes education in diabetes and has an online support team.

The National Diabetes Information Clearinghouse (www.diabetes.niddk.nih.gov or 301-654-3327) offers fact sheets, information packets, and professional publications.

Book Resources:

American Association of Diabetic Educators: *The art and science of diabetes self-management*, Chicago, 2006, American Association of Diabetic Educators.

Dementia (see Alzheimer's Disease)

Disease Prevention (see Health Promotion/Disease Prevention/Wellness)

End-of-Life Care (see Hospice)

Evidence-Based Clinical Guidelines

The Agency for Healthcare Research and Quality (AHRQ) (www.ahrq.gov) has a congressional mandate to develop evidence-based clinical guidelines to improve the quality, safety, efficiency, and effectiveness of healthcare and encourage providers, consumers, and patients to use evidence-based information to make informed treatment choices/decisions.

Geriatrics At Your Fingertips—Online Edition (2007–2008) (www.geriatricsatyourfingertips.org) from the American Geriatrics Society offers current evidence-based assessment and intervention guidelines for a variety of geriatric issues (e.g., falls, anxiety, incontinence, malnutrition). Also included are the most utilized and up-to-date geriatric assessment instruments for a variety of conditions that include pain, mental status, and depression. The hard cover copy of the book can be ordered through the website.

The John A. Hartford Foundation Institute for Geriatric Nursing (www.hartfordign.org) has a series of geriatric assessment tools and provides information for nurses on geriatric topics, certifications, geriatric nursing news, and upcoming conferences.

The National Consensus Project (www.nationalconsensusproject.org) is an initiative to improve the delivery of palliative care and offers clinical practice guidelines for core components of clinical palliative care.

The National Quality Measures Clearinghouse™ (NQMC) (www.qualitymeasures.ahrq.gov), sponsored by the Agency for Healthcare Research and Quality, is a database for information on specific evidence-based healthcare quality measures and measure sets. Its mission is to provide practitioners and healthcare providers accessibility to detailed information on quality measures. You can subscribe to the weekly e-mail update service through the website.

The National Guideline Clearinghouse™ (NGC) (www.guideline.gov) was created by the Agency for Healthcare Research and Quality in partnership with the American Medical Association and the American Association of Health Plans—now America's Health Insurance Plans (AHIP)—to compile a comprehensive database of evidence-based clinical practice guidelines and related documents for physicians, nurses, and other health professionals. You can subscribe to the weekly e-mail update service through the website.

Book Resources:

Mezey M, Fulmer T, Abraham I, Zwicker D, editors: *Geriatric nursing protocols for best practice*, ed 2, New York, 2003, Springer Publishing Co.

Falls (see also Safety)

The American Occupational Therapy Association (AOTA) (www.aota.org) offers resources on fall prevention that include "Fall Prevention for People With Disabilities and Older Adults."

The Centers for Disease Control and Prevention (CDC) National Center for Injury Prevention and Control (www.cdc.gov/ncipc/duip/preventadultfalls.htm or 800-CDC-INFO [800-232-4636]) has resources and links on fall prevention that include a tool kit to prevent senior falls, "Check for Safety: A Home Fall Prevention Checklist for Older Adults," and "What You Can Do to Prevent Falls."

The Center for Healthy Aging (www.healthyagingprograms.org) offers a free e-newsletter, *Falls Free*, with updates on news, statistics, and links for falls prevention, and information on safety and falls prevention.

The National Council on Aging (www.ncoa.org or 202-479-1200) offers information on promoting a national fall action plan.

www.americangeriatrics.org offers resources.

www.neurology.org also offers fall-related materials.

Environmental Geriatrics (www.environmentalgeriatrics.com) offers resources for older adults and caregivers to ensure safety within the home and an article entitled "Falls and Hip Fractures Among Older Adults."

The Fall Prevention Center of Excellence (www.stopfalls.org or 213-740-1364) provides assessment tools, tool kits, resources, and references on fall prevention.

The Fall Prevention Project (www.temple.edu/older_adult) targets practitioners, educators, and students to help older adults avoid falls in the home.

"A Housing Safety Checklist" is a comprehensive list of safety precautions for all rooms of the house and outdoors to ensure safety and is available for free download from the North Carolina Cooperative Extension (www.ces.ncsu.edu).

The National Safety Council (www.nsc.org or 800-621-7619) offers information on fall prevention and safety that includes fact sheets such as "Designs on Building Safe Homes for the Elderly" and "Falls Pose a Serious Threat to the Elderly."

The New York State Office for the Aging (www.agingwell.state.ny.us) has created a list of "Home Safety Tips" for keeping homes safe and "user friendly" for seniors that includes information on mobility assistance and fire safety.

Gastrointestinal

The American College of Gastroenterology (www.gi.org) offers resources related to gastrointestinal health issues that include

- Your Doctor Has Ordered a Colonoscopy. What Questions Should You Ask?
- AGG Recommendations for Colorectal Cancer Screening—Patient Reference Cards
- Understanding Irritable Bowel Syndrome

The American Gastroenterological Association (www.gastro.org or 310-654-2055) offers information for caregivers and patients about the causes of constipation in adults and children, prevention misconceptions about constipation, and treatments.

The Crohn's and Colitis Foundation of America (www.ccfa.org or 800-932-2423 or 800-343-3637) offers resources for professionals and patients.

The National Digestive Diseases Information Clearinghouse (www.digestive.niddk.nih.gov or 800-891-5389) has information and resources on digestive problems such as constipation that are available in English and Spanish.

The National Institute of Health (NIH) Division of Nutrition Research Coordination (http://dnrc.nih.gov or 800-222-4225) has nutrition education materials available for patients and professionals for treatment and prevention of many diseases and problems related to the digestive system.

The Oley Foundation (www.oley.org or 800-776-OLEY) has support and information options that include a *Lifeline Letter* bi-monthly newsletter for people living with home parenteral and/or enteral nutrition and fact sheets such as "Questions New Tube Feeders Should Be Asking."

The Oral Cancer Foundation (www.oralcancerfoundation.org or 949-646-8000) has an information page on tube feeding that includes a section on "Care of the Patient."

Genitourinary

The American Urological Association (AUA) (www.auanet.org) has information on the website for patients and professionals and physician-created resources for pediatric and adult conditions on the urology health site (www.urologyhealth.org).

The National Association for Continence (NAFC) (www.nafc.org or 800-BLADDER [800-252-3337]) has information on incontinence that includes treatment options, explanations, and how to find help.

The National Federation of the Blind (NFB) (www.nfb.org or 410-296-7760) publishes *Voice of the Diabetic* four times a year as a free service to those with diabetes and others that includes healthcare programs and information on kidney disease. It is available on the web or in print.

The National Kidney and Urologic Diseases Information Clearinghouse (www.kidney.niddk.nih.gov or 800-891-5390) offers information on treatment, booklets such as the

"Kidney Failure Glossary," and other resources for patients and professionals. There is a new Spanish website at www.nkdep.nih.gov/espanol. A brochure is offered that highlights the risk factors commonly associated with renal failure, diabetes, and high blood pressure that specifically targets Hispanic and Latino populations at high risk of diabetes and hypertension.

The National Kidney Foundation (NKF) (www.kidney.org or 800-622-9010) provides services that include patient peer counseling, education, medication programs, transportation, and financial assistance. One useful patient education resource is "What You Should Know About Infectious Disease: A Guide for Hemodialysis Patients and Their Families." This 13-page booklet reviews infection control, vaccines, and information about infectious diseases. Also available are "It's Just Part of My Life," a booklet for young adults living with kidney disease and dialysis, and a newsletter entitled *Family Focus*.

The Paralyzed Veterans of America (PVA) (www.pva.org or 800-242-8200) offers resources that include "Bladder Management for Adults with Spinal Cord Injury: A Clinical Practice Guideline for Healthcare Professionals," "Preservation of Upper Limb Function Following Spinal Cord Injury," "Respiratory Management Following Spinal Cord Injury," and "Neurogenic Bowel Management in Adults with Spinal Cord Injury."

The Simon Foundation for Continence (www.simonfoundation.org or 800-23SIMON [800-237-4666]) offers information for patients and professionals on defining incontinence, diagnosis, prevention in all age groups, and educational resources that include books with titles such as *Managing Incontinence: A Guide to Living With Loss of Bladder Control*.

The Wound, Ostomy and Continence Nurses Society (www.wocn.org or 888-224-9626) offers fact sheets and patient guides for incontinence.

Guidelines (see Evidence-Based Clinical Guidelines)

Health Promotion/Disease Prevention/Wellness

The American Geriatrics Society Foundation for Health in Aging (www.healthinaging.org or 800-563-4916) has resources and information pages for consumers and providers.

The Centers for Disease Control and Prevention (CDC) Division for Adult and Community Health (DACH) (www.cdc.gov/nccdphp/dach) is charged with managing programs that provide cross-cutting chronic disease and health promotion expertise and support to the CDC's National Center for Chronic Disease Prevention and Health Promotion (NCCDPHP), states, communities, and other partners. DACH also manages several important and high-profile chronic disease prevention and control programs for specific chronic diseases, and is charged with assessing new and emerging chronic disease issues and launching new programs for NCCDPHP.

The Centers for Medicare and Medicaid Services (CMS) has updated preventive services brochures for healthcare professionals that include topics such as expanded benefits, diabetes-related services, cancer screenings, adult immunizations, bone mass measurements, glaucoma screenings, and smoking and tobacco-use cessation counseling services. To download and view brochures online, visit the Medicare Learning Network (MLN) Publications web page at www.cms.hhs.gov/MLNProducts/MPUB/list.asp and select the title of the brochure from the list. To order copies, visit the MLN Product Ordering Page at http://cms.meridianksi.com/kc/main/kc_frame.asp?kc_ident=kc0001&loc=5.

Choose to Move (www.choosetomove.com), created by the American Heart Association, is a 12-week program designed to help women incorporate healthy activity and eating habits into their daily routines.

The Food and Drug Administration has launched a new website "Consumer Health Information for You and Your Family" and an e-newsletter to keep consumers up-to-date with the latest health information (www.fda.gov).

Healthy People 2010 (www.healthypeople.gov) is a national initiative to provide a framework for prevention. It is a statement of national health objectives for 2010 designed to identify the most significant preventable threats to health and establish national goals to reduce these threats.

Immunizations: Medicare pays for certain immunizations and information and links to other important immunization websites, such as the Centers for Disease Control and Prevention, can be found at www.cms.hhs.gov/AdultImmunizations.

Preventive services/screening: Medicare pays for certain preventive services and information is available at www.medicare.gov/Health/Overview.asp. A concise guide, "Staying Healthy: Medicare's Preventive Services" (CMS Pub. No 10110), can be downloaded from this site or by calling 800-MEDICARE (800-633-4227).

Hospice/End-of Life Care/Palliative Care (see also Pain Management)

The Agency for Healthcare Research and Quality (AHRQ) (www.ahrq.gov or 800-335-9100) offers clinical practice guidelines on pain management.

The American Academy of Hospice and Palliative Medicine (www.aahpm.org) provides position statements and other resources regarding important issues in hospice and palliative care.

The American Hospice Foundation (www.americanhospice.org) offers free publications that include "Talking About Hospice: Tips for Nurses," "Providing Care at Home: Can I Do It?" Select publications are available in Spanish.

Americans for Better Care of the Dying (www.abcd-caring.org or 703-647-8505) provides resources on public policy and hospice and has useful links to other hospice resources.

The Center to Advance Palliative Care (www.getpalliativecare.org) has a new website that provides information for patients and families about what palliative care consists of, options for palliative care, and a page to help the patient and family decide if palliative care is the right choice. There are other information sheets that include "What should you know about palliative care."

Children's Hospice International (www.chionline.org or 800-242-4453) offers information about children's hospice, palliative care, and end-of-life care services, and how to locate a local program. There are publications available for families and professionals.

City of Hope Pain/Palliative Care Resource Center (www.cityofhope.org/prc) disseminates information and resources to assist others in improving the quality of pain management and end-of-life care. The site contains a variety of materials that include pain assessment tools, patient education materials, and end-of-life resources.

The Commission on Aging With Dignity (www.agingwithdignity.org or 800-594-7437) offers a living will, "Five Wishes," for $5.00 a copy. Five Wishes is a living will and a durable power of attorney for healthcare, valid in most states, and addresses an individual's medical wishes and personal, emotional, and spiritual needs. The project was supported by a grant from The Robert Wood Johnson Foundation.

Compassionate Friends (www.compassionatefriends.org or 877-969-0010) is an organization that offers grief support for families after the death of a child. Chapters across the country hope to offer families an opportunity to work towards a positive resolution after the loss of a child of any age.

The Dougy Center for Grieving Children and Families (www.dougy.org or 866-775-5683) offers support for children, teenagers, and their families when dealing with the death of a loved one. Sections are specifically tailored for adults who want to help a grieving child, children, teens, and those working with students. The information is available through the website and in centers across the country.

Dying Well (www.dyingwell.org) provides resources for people facing life-limiting illness, their families, and their professional caregivers.

The Hospice and Palliative Nurses Association (www.hpna.org or 412-787-9301) offers news and information on the site for caregivers that includes tip sheets on skin care, dementia, and recognizing pain, and patient teaching sheets on "Hospice and Palliative Care," "Managing Pain," "Managing Anxiety" and others.

The website www.hospice-america.org is a valuable resource and contains links to numerous sponsored listings related to hospice and other senior care.

The Hospice Foundation of America (www.hospicefoundation.org or 800-854-3402) has information on hospice goals and care, grieving, and publications and videos for families and professionals. Also on the website is an e-newsletter that features updates on news and events regarding hospice care in the United States.

The National Consensus Project (www.nationalconsensusproject.org) is an initiative to improve the delivery of palliative care and offers clinical practice guidelines for core components of clinical palliative care.

The National Hospice and Palliative Care Organization (www.nhpco.org or 703-243-5900) offers information for professionals, patients, and caregivers.

Pain Treatment Topics (www.pain-topics.org or 847-724-0862) provides evidence-based information and research on clinical treatment and better management of many pain conditions for consumers and professionals.

Palliative Care Matters (www.pallcare.info) is designed for professionals working in hospice.

Booklet Resources:

Barbara Karnes Books, Inc. offers informational booklets on the website that include "Gone From My Sight—The Dying Experience," "My Friend, I Care," and "A Time to Live."

All are available in English and Spanish; "Gone From My Sight" is also available in Russian, French, and Italian. They are $2.00 plus shipping and handling. Booklets are available through http://www.bkbooks.com or by writing to B.K. Books, P.O. Box 822139, Vancouver, WA 98682.

"Palliative Care: Complete Care Everyone Deserves": This 16-page booklet is produced by the National Alliance for Caregiving (NAC) and Friends and Relatives of Institutionalized Aged (FRIA) of New York. A free copy of the booklet can be obtained by sending an e-mail to info@caregiving.org. The booklet can also be downloaded through NAHC's website www.caregiving.org/care.pdf and FRIA's website www.fria.org.

Book Resources:

Heffner JE, Byock I: *Palliative and end-of-life pearls*, Philadelphia, 2002, Hanley & Belfus.

Kuebler KK, Berry PH, Heidrich DE: *Palliative and end-of-life care: clinical practice guidelines*, ed 2, Philadelphia, 2007, Saunders.

Marrelli TM: *Hospice and palliative care handbook: quality, compliance and reimbursement,* ed 2, St Louis, 2005, Mosby.

Matzo ML, Sherman DW: *Gerontologic palliative care nursing,* St Louis, 2003, Mosby.

Infection Control

The Association for Professionals in Infection Control (APIC) (www. apic.org or 202-789-1890) has information and resources regarding continuing education and professional practice standards for health care professionals.

The Centers for Disease Control and Prevention (CDC) (www.cdc.gov) offers handwashing guidelines from the *Morbidity and Mortality Weekly Report* (www.cdc.gov/mmwr/preview/mmwrhtml/rr5115a1.htm) and other resources related to infection control.

Book Resources:

McGoldrick, M: *Infection prevention and control program,* Saint Simons Island, GA, 2007, Home Health Systems (www.homecareandhospice.com)

Rhinehart E, McGoldrick M: *Infection Control in Home care and Hospice,* Sudbury, PA, 2006, Jones and Bartlett (www.homecareandhospice.com)

Medicare

The Centers for Medicare and Medicaid Services (CMS) Home Health Agency Center (www.cms.hhs.gov/center/hha.asp) has links to sites within CMS on home health agencies that include Billing/Payment, Policies/Regulations, Initiatives, OASIS, Conditions of Coverage and Conditions of Participation, CMS Manuals and Transmittals (including State Operations Manual and Interpretive Guidelines), Beneficiary Notices, Educational Resources, and Demonstrations/Research.

The Centers for Medicare and Medicaid Services (CMS) Hospice Center (http://www.cms.hhs.gov/center/hospice.asp) has links to sites within CMS on hospice agencies that include Billing/Payment, Policies/Regulations, Initiatives, Conditions of Coverage and Conditions of Participation, CMS Manuals and Transmittals (including State Operations Manual and Interpretive Guidelines), Beneficiary Notices, Educational Resources, and Demonstrations.

The Health Insurance Portability and Accountability Act of 1996 (HIPAA, Title II) (www.cms.hhs.gov/hipaageninfo) required the Department of Health and Human Services to establish national standards for electronic healthcare transactions and national identifiers for providers, health plans, and employers. This Centers for Medicare and Medicaid Services site has links to related information on HIPAA.

Medicare & You, 2008 Medicare Handbook, a handbook for those receiving Medicare benefits, can be downloaded at www.medicare.gov/publications/pubs/pdf/10050.pdf.

Medicare Learning Network (www.cms.hhs.gov/medlearn) is the site for official Centers for Medicare and Medicaid Services (CMS) national provider education products to promote national consistency of Medicare provider information developed for CMS initiatives.

Regional Home Health Intermediaries (RHHIs) websites and toll-free numbers for each state are found at the Centers for Medicare and Medicaid Services (CMS) Home Care website (www.cms.hhs.gov/center/hha.asp).

www.homecareinformation.net offers online education, including interdisciplinary orientation and care planning related to Medicare and other aspects of home health care presented by knowledgeable home care experts.

Medications

The Agency for Healthcare Research and Quality (www.ahrq.gov) offers a resource entitled "Your Medicine: Play It Safe" for consumers and includes handy forms to keep track of medication information (www.ahrq.gov/consumer/safemeds/safemeds.htm).

The U.S. Food and Safety Administration's Center for Drug Evaluation and Research (http://www.fda.gov/cder/drug/MedErrors/default.htm) has resources and links on drugs and medications errors.

The Institute for Safe Medication Practices (ISMP) (www.ismp.org) is devoted to medication error prevention and safe medication use and has numerous resources related to medication safety information. An important resource is a fact sheet on oral medications that should not be crushed (www.ismp.org/Tools/DoNotCrush.pdf).

The National Institute on Drug Abuse (www.nida.nih.gov) offers useful resources related to medication interactions and drug abuse in the older adult population.

www.palliativedrugs.com provides information for health professionals about the use of drugs in palliative care.

The U.S. Food and Drug Administration (www.otcsafety.org) has publications from the Council on Family Health that can be downloaded in English and Spanish and include "Medicines and You: A Guide for Older Adults" and "Drug Interactions: What You Should Know."

Article: Fick DM, Cooper JW, Wade WE, Waller JL, Maclean JR, Beers MH. Updating the Beers criteria for potentially inappropriate medication use in older adults: results of a US consensus panel of experts. *Arch Intern Med* 2003;163:2716–2724.

Memory Loss (see Alzheimer's Disease/Dementia)

Musculoskeletal

The American Academy of Orthopedic Surgeons (www.aaos.org) has an Orthopedic Connection page specifically for patients (www.orthoinfo.org) with information about patient-centered care for arthritis, osteoporosis, and joint replacement that includes the articles "Activities After a Hip Replacement" and "Keep Moving for Life."

The Amputee Coalition of America (ACA) (www.amputee-coalition.org or 888-267-5669) offers information about prosthetics, rehabilitation, and peer support group. A Spanish section provides information about the ACA, its programs, and the organization's most popular and informative articles. The ACA publishes *inMotion*, a bimonthly publication with news, resources, and support for those with amputated limbs.

The Arthritis Foundation (www.arthritis.org or 800-568-4045) has free brochures that include "Meet Your Arthritis Health Care Team." It publishes the *Arthritis Today* magazine that can be obtained through subscription at the website.

The Myasthenia Gravis Foundation of America (www.myasthenia.org or 800-541-5454) supplies information and offers patient support groups.

The National Amputation Foundation (www.nationalamputation.org or 516-887-3600) offers information and support for amputees and their families.

The National Institute on Aging (NIA) (www.nia.nih.gov or 800-222-2225) has information and resources on fracture prevention, causes, and recovery.

The National Institute of Arthritis and Musculoskeletal and Skin Diseases Information Clearinghouse (www.niams.nih.gov or 877-22-NIAMS [800-22-64267]) offers question-and-answer publications and other resources that include "Questions and Answers About Arthritis and Rheumatic Diseases."

The National Institute of Health Osteoporosis and Related Bone Diseases National Resource Center (www.niams.nih.gov/Health_Info/Bone/ or 1-800-624-BONE [800-624-2663]) offers information on health topics that include general bone health and Paget's disease.

The National Multiple Sclerosis Society (www.nationalmssociety.org or 800-FIGHT-MS [800-344-4867]) offers clinical bulletins on topics such as "Aging with MS," "Overview of Multiple Sclerosis," "Swallowing Disorders and Their Management," and brochures such as "Managing Specific Issues," "Staying Well," and "Newly Diagnosed."

The National Osteoporosis Foundation (www.nof.org or 202-223-2226) offers patient information that includes "Fall Prevention" and "Medications and Osteoporosis" and fact sheets such as "Bone Density" and "Bone Basics." It also offers professional resources and clinical guideline information.

The Parkinson's Disease Foundation (www.pdf.org or 800-457-6676) supplies information and offers patient support groups.

Neurologic (see also Alzheimer's Disease)

The American Stroke Association (www.strokeassociation.org or 888-4-STROKE [888-478-7653]) offers a free subscription to *Stroke CONNECTION Magazine* and other resources for patients and professionals.

The Amyotrophic Lateral Sclerosis Association (ALSA) (www.alsa.org or 818-880-9007) offers information on the symptoms, forms, genetics, and other facts about ALS, also called Lou Gehrig's disease. Information for patients, families, and caregivers includes pages on "Facts About Family Caregivers" and "Caregiving Tips and Hints."

The National Institute of Neurological Disorders and Stroke (www.ninds.nih.gov or 800-352-9424) has information pages that include "Stroke Rehabilitation Information" and "What You Need to Know About Stroke" on stroke treatment, prognosis, and research.

www.neurology.org offers fall and safety-related information.

Nutrition

5 A Day for Better Health (www.5aday.gov or 800-422-6237) offers information on the benefits of fruits and vegetables, using fruits and vegetables for weight management, and how fruits and vegetables can protect your health. There is also serving size information, recipes, and nutritional tips on what to eat throughout the day.

The Administration on Aging (www.aoa.gov or 305-348-1517) in partnership with the National Resource Center on Nutrition offers the Eat Better and Move More program, a 12-week nutrition and exercise plan that is part of the *You Can! Steps to Healthier Aging* campaign designed to help older adults live longer, healthier lives with simple meal and exercise strategies.

The American Diabetes Association (www.diabetes.org or 800-342-2383) offers themed research collections that include Diabetes Prevention, which explains topics such as "Pollutants in the Body Contribute to Diabetes Risk" and "Fatness, Fitness, and Lifestyle."

The American Dietetic Association (ADA) (www.eatright.org or 800-366-1655) offers nutrition fact sheets that include

"Step Up to Nutrition and Health" and professional and consumer resources.

Dietitian.com (www.dietitian.com) is a question-and-answer website with health topics that include diets, vitamins, and drug nutrient interaction.

FoodFit (www.foodfit.com) provides information on healthy eating, healthy cooking, fitness, healthy weight loss plans, and menu planners, an e-mail newsletter that offers fitness tips, recipes, and nutrition information.

The Food and Nutrition Information Center (http://fnic.nal.usda.gov or 301-504-5414) provides information for all age groups on healthy foods, food safety, and the amount of calories and nutrients in many food items and groups.

HealthyEating (http://healthyeating.net) offers news and resources on nutrition and fitness that include food guides and pyramids, vitamin and mineral indexes, and resource pages on topics such as diabetes, heart disease, and stroke.

The National Heart, Lung, and Blood Institute (www.nhlbi.nih.gov) offers nutritional resources that include "Your Guide to Lowering Your Blood Pressure with DASH," which explains the DASH eating plan and how it can help control blood pressure.

The National Institute of Health (NIH) Division of Nutrition Research Coordination (http://dnrc.nih.gov) offers nutrition education materials available for patients and professionals.

Nutrition.gov (www.nutrition.gov) is a division of the U.S. Food and Drug Administration offering a variety of information dealing with nutrition related to specific diseases and problems and facts on food safety. Also available is a *Maturity Health Matters* online newsletter with information for older adults, families, and caregivers.

The United States Department of Agriculture (USDA) (www.mypyramid.gov) offers the food pyramid resource, "My Pyramid," which includes suggested serving sizes, guidelines on keeping food fresh, and sources of essential vitamins.

OASIS (see also Quality)

The OASIS Downloads/Documentation webpage (www.qtso.com/hhadownload.html) includes the newest version of the OASIS, OASIS questions and answers, guides and manuals, and a link to the OASIS Outcome-Based Quality Improvement/Outcome-Based Quality Monitoring Manual. This information is also available from links on the Centers for Medicare and Medicaid Services (CMS) Home Health Agency Center site (www.cms.hhs.gov/center/hha.asp).

The Home Health Compare website (www.medicare.gov/hhcompare) contains information on home health agencies for consumers and allows comparison of agencies based on the latest quality measures.

The OASIS Certificate and Competency Board (www.oasiscertificate.org) is a non-profit organization to promote greater reliability in OASIS data through consistent application of guidelines provided by the Centers for Medicare and Medicaid Services (CMS). It also maintains up-to-date links to Centers for Medicare and Medicaid Services (CMS) and other OASIS resource websites.

OASIS ANSWERS, Inc. (www.oasisanswers.com) conducts training and other consulting services for clients at the state association, federal government, quality improvement organization, private industry, and individual provider levels.

OASIS NP (non-perishable) is a computerized, non-perishable train-the-trainer tool for agencies to ensure clinicians are proficient in performing the OASIS assessment. For more information, contact the National Association for Home Care & Hospice (www.nahc.org) via e-mail at OASISNP@nahc.org.

OASIS web-based training from the Centers for Medicare and Medicaid Services is located at www.oasistraining.org/oasis11/upfront/U1.asp.

Risk-adjusted Home Health Outcome Reports include risk-adjusted improvement, stabilization, and utilization outcome reports by state (www.cms.hhs.gov/OASIS/09a_hhareports.asp#TopOfPage)

Older Adults

The Administration on Aging (AoA) (www.aoa.gov or 305-348-1517) provides resources and information for older adults and their caregivers and operates the Center for Communication and Consumer Services (202-6619-0724). AoA, in partnership with the National Resource Center on Nutrition, offers the Eat Better and Move More program, a 12-week nutrition and exercise plan that is part of the *You Can! Steps to Healthier Aging* campaign designed to help older adults live longer, healthier lives with simple meal and exercise strategies.

The American Geriatrics Society Foundation for Health in Aging (www.healthinaging.org or 800-563-4916) has numerous resources and information pages available for consumers and providers.

The Arthritis Foundation (www.arthritis.org or 404-872-7100) offers resources for older adults.

BenefitsCheckUp (www.benefitscheckup.org) was developed by the National Council on Aging and assists seniors and their families in determining benefit eligibility for services in their areas.

The Centers for Disease Control and Prevention (www.cdc.gov/healthyliving) offers resources on healthy living for all age groups including older adults (www.cdc.gov/aging).

The Commission on Aging with Dignity (www.agingwithdignity.org or 800-594-7437) offers a living will, "Five Wishes," that can be ordered online and is valid in most states.

Elder Care Online (www.ec-online.net) is an internet community of caregivers for older adults that includes information on education and support for caregivers, safety advice, and resources.

The National Council on Aging (www.ncoa.org) offers many resources, such as information about safety and healthy aging.

Eldercare Locator (www.eldercare.gov or 800-677-1116) is a public service of the U.S. Administration on Aging and helps older adults and their caregivers find services in their areas.

FirstGov for Seniors (www.seniors.gov) offers a wide range of information on government services and provides information on a number of topics such as health, housing, and consumer protection for older Americans.

Geriatrics At Your Fingertips—Online Edition (2007–2008) (www.geriatricsatyourfingertips.org) from the American Geriatrics Society offers current evidence-based assessment and intervention guidelines for a variety of geriatric issues (e.g., falls, anxiety, incontinence, malnutrition). Also included are the most utilized and up-to-date geriatric assessment instruments for a variety of conditions that include pain, mental status, and depression. The hard cover copy of the book can be ordered through the website.

The John A. Hartford Foundation Institute for Geriatric Nursing (www.hartfordign.org) has a series of geriatric assessment tools available and provides information for nurses on geriatric topics, certifications, geriatric nursing news, and upcoming conferences. Visit www.ConsultGeriRN.org.

The National Academy of Elder Law Attorneys (NAELA) (www.naela.org) provides a national registry of attorneys specializing in elder law and a question-and-answer section on finding and working with an elder law attorney.

The National Association of Area Agencies on Aging (www.n4a.org or 202-872-0888) offers reports such as the "Maturing Americans Report" and information sheets that include "Background on Flu Shots" and publications such as "Making the Link: Connecting Caregivers with Services Through Physicians."

The National Center on Elder Abuse (NCEA) (www.ncea.aoa.gov/ncearoot/Main_Site/index.aspx) is directed by the U.S. Administration on Aging and helps ensure that older Americans live with dignity, integrity, independence, and without abuse, neglect, and exploitation. The NCEA is a resource for policy makers, social service and healthcare practitioners, the justice system, researchers, advocates, and families.

The National Eye Institute (NEI) (www.nei.nih.gov or 301-496-5248) offers brochures, posters, videos, and teaching resources and other information for professionals and patients with eye diseases or conditions and those at risk of developing eye diseases.

The National Family Caregiver Support Program (NFCSP), established as a result of the Older Americans Act Amendments of 2000, supports caregiver programs through area agencies on aging across the country. You can locate services in your community by calling the Eldercare Locator at 800-677-1116.

The National Family Caregivers Association (NFCA) (www.thefamilycaregiver.org or 800-896-3650) offers information and support through the website for caregivers with resources such as "Family Caregiving 101" and "A Home Healthcare Primer."

The National Institute on Aging (www.nia.nih.gov or 800-222-2225) offers research and health information resources for consumers and providers that include "Working With Your Older Patient: A Clinician's Handbook."

The National Institutes of Health (NIH) (www.nihseniorhealth.gov) has a website devoted to senior citizens with sections on specific problems, such as high blood pressure, Alzheimer's disease, and stroke that include facts on risk factors, prevention, symptoms, and treatment, and resources on exercise for older adults, sleeping well, and taking medicines. The site also provides information on depression with facts about depression, symptoms of depression, and treatment.

Seniors in a Gay Environment (SAGE) (www.sageusa.org or 212-741-2247) provides information and resources for older gay and lesbian adults.

Since You Care® guides can be downloaded and printed at www.maturemarketinstitute.com or by writing to maturemarketinstitute@metlife.com or MetLife Mature Market Institute, 57 Greens Farms Road, Westport, CT 06880. Guides include Alzheimer's Disease: Caregiving Challenges, Becoming An Effective Advocate for Care, Choosing An Assisted Living Facility, Community Services, Falls and Fall

Prevention, Family Caregiving, Final Arrangements, Hiring An Independent Caregiver, Hospice Care, Legal Matters, Long Distance Caregiving, Making The Nursing Home Choice, Medicare And Medicaid Programs—The Basics, Medications and the Older Adult, Preventing Elder Abuse, and Understanding Home Care Agency Options.

The U.S. Administration on Aging (AoA) (www.aoa.gov or 202-619-0724) is an agency of the U.S. Department of Health and Human Services that provides resources and information for older adults and their caregivers.

The U.S. Food and Drug Administration (www.cfhinfo.org) has publications from the Council on Family Health for download in English and Spanish that include *Medicines and You: A Guide for Older Adults* and *Drug Interactions: What You Should Know*.

Orientation

www.homecareinformation.net offers ongoing information and preventions.

Orthopedic (see Musculoskeletal)

Pain Management

The Agency for Health Care Research and Quality (AHRQ) (www.ahrq.gov or 800-358-9295) offers resources, research, and information on pain and pain guidelines.

The American Pain Foundation (www.painfoundation.org or 888-615-PAIN[7246]) has information for clinicians and patients on causes and management of pain.

The American Pain Society (www.ampainsoc.org) offers extensive educational materials such as "Pain: Current Understanding of Assessment, Management, and Treatments," which is part of a continuing education program, and pain patient guides that are available for purchase.

The Hospice and Palliative Nurses Association (www.hpna.org or 412-787-9301) offers pain resources for patients and caregivers.

The International Association for the Study of Pain (www.iasp-pain.org or 206-547-6409) offers information for consumers and clinicians regarding pain and pain research.

Pain Treatment Topics (www.pain-topics.org or 847-724-0862) provides evidence-based information and research on clinical treatment and better management of pain conditions for consumers and professionals.

www.palliativedrugs.com provides comprehensive and independent information for health professionals about the use of drugs in palliative care.

Palliative Care (see Hospice)

Pulmonary (see Respiratory)

Quality

The Centers for Medicare and Medicaid Services Home Health Quality Initiative (www.cms.hhs.gov/HomeHealthQualityInits) is explained on the website and related links are provided.

The Medicare Quality Improvement Community (www.medqic.org) supports quality improvement organizations and providers in finding, using, and sharing quality improvement resources.

The National Committee for Quality Assurance (www.ncqa.org) seeks to improve healthcare quality by accrediting health programs that pass a rigorous, comprehensive review and report annually on their performance.

The Outcome-Based Quality Improvement (OBQI) Clearinghouse (www.obqi.org) contains a collection of articles, frequently-asked questions, practices, discussion groups, and other resources to help home health agencies successfully apply OBQI strategies.

Regulatory (also see Medicare)

The Office of the Inspector General (OIG) (www.oig.hhs.gov) website provides information on reports issues, guidance, and related information on fraud, waste, and abuse issues in healthcare organizations.

Respiratory (also see Infection Control)

The Agency for Healthcare Research and Quality (AHRQ) (www.ahrq.gov or 800-358-9295) offers resources and clinical guidelines on respiratory and pulmonary problems. In conjunction with the AHRQ, the National Quit Line (www.smokefree.gov or 800-QUIT-NOW [800-784-8669]) offers help and support for smokers who want to quit.

The American Association for Respiratory Care (AARC) (www.aarc.org or 972-243-2272) offers conferences, clinical practice guidelines, and numerous resources including "Breath of Life" and "Empowering COPD Patients to Improve Their Quality of Life".

The American Lung Association (www.lungusa.org or 800-232-5864) has information on treatment and support for patients and healthcare professionals.

The Centers for Disease Control and Prevention (CDC) (www.cdc.gov) has a tuberculosis site with up-to-date information and research resources for patients and healthcare professionals.

The Francis J. Curry National Tuberculosis Center (www.nationaltbcenter.edu) offers information, an e-newsletter through on-line enrollment, web-based workshops, and resources on tuberculosis.

The National Heart Lung and Blood Institute (www.learnaboutcopd.org or 301-592-8573) offers information, research, and news about chronic obstructive pulmonary disease.

The World Health Organization (www.who.org) offers tuberculosis (TB) fact sheets, handouts, and other information. TB-related topics, information, and presentations are available in the "products" area of the website.

RHHI (see Medicare)

Safety (see also Falls and Medications)

The Agency for Healthcare Research and Quality (AHRQ) Patient Safety Tools and Resources (www.ahrq.gov/qual/pstools.htm) summarizes AHRQ patient safety tools and resources designed for health systems, providers, and consumers, and range from system-wide event reporting methods to specific measures to minimize medical errors.

Elder Care Online (www.ec-online.net) is an internet community of caregivers for older adults that includes safety information and support for caregivers.

The John A. Hartford Foundation Institute for Geriatric Nursing (www.hartfordign.org) has a series of assessment tools available called the "Try This: Best Practices in Care for Older Adults" that include a comprehensive "Fall Risk Assessment."

The Joint Commission International Center for Patient Safety (www.jcipatientsafety.org) was established to continuously improve patient safety in all healthcare settings, and includes sections on Patient Safety Practices, Patient Safety Solutions, and Patient Safety Goals.

The National Safety Council (www.nsc.org) was established to educate and influence people to prevent accidental injury and death and offers information and resources related to these safety issues.

The Occupational Health and Safety Administration (www.osha.gov) provides safety regulations and guidelines for workers.

The Safe Lifting Portal (www.safeliftingportal.com) is designed to support safe lifting and caregiver injury prevention programs and offers continuing education units, a "Starter Kit" for injury prevention programs, and a poster of "The Seven Deadly Sins of Unsafe Lifting."

Telehealth/Telemedicine

The American Telemedicine Association (www.americantelemed.org) promotes access to medical care for consumers and health professionals via telecommunications technology.

The Association of Telehealth Service Providers (www.atsp.org) provides educational programs and business support services to healthcare agencies utilizing telehealth technologies.

The Health Resources and Services Administration Telehealth Division (HRSA) (www.hrsa.gov/telehealth)

works to increase and improve the use of telehealth to meet the needs of underserved people.

The National Library of Medicine National Telemedicine Initiative website (www.nlm.nih.gov/research/telemedinit.html) provides information and links on telemedicine initiatives and research.

The Telemedicine Information Exchange (TIE) (http://tie.telemed.org) provides an online platform for information on telemedicine and telehealth aimed at health professionals.

Therapy

The American Speech-Language-Hearing Association (ASHA) (http://www.asha.org or 1-800-498-2071) is the professional, scientific, and credentialing association for audiologists, speech-language pathologists, and speech, language, and hearing scientists. Professional journal: The *Journal of Speech, Language, and Hearing Research* (http://jslhr.asha.org/).

The American Physical Therapy Association (APTA) (http://www.apta.org/ or 1-800-999-2782) is a national professional organization which fosters advancements in physical therapy practice, research, and education. Professional journal: *Physical Therapy* (http://www.ptjournal.org/).

The American Occupational Therapy Association (AOTA) (http://www.aota.org/or 1-800-377-8555 is the national professional association that represents the interests and concerns of occupational therapy practitioners and students of occupational therapy and to improve the quality of occupational therapy services. Professional journal: *The American Journal of Occupational Therapy* (www.aota.org/ajot/index.asp).

Urinary Incontinence (see Genitourinary)

Wellness (see Health Promotion/ Disease Prevention/Wellness)

Wounds

The Agency for Healthcare Research and Quality (AHRQ) (www.ahrq.gov or 1-800-358-9295) offers resources that include "Clinical Practice Guideline Number 3: Preventing Pressure Ulcers: Patient Guide" and "Pressure Ulcers in Adults: Prediction and Prevention." Consumer versions are available in English and Spanish.

The Mayo Clinic website (www.mayoclinic.com) offers information about the causes, risk factors, symptoms, and complications of pressure ulcers. To demonstrate the effects of a pressure ulcer, there is an "Anatomy of Your Skin" diagram showing the layers of skin.

The National Pressure Ulcer Advisory Panel (NPUAP) (www.npuap.org or 202-521-6789) displays examples of extensive pressure ulcers. It offers a frequently asked questions page, an archive of past newsletters, and a site to sign up for the newsletter.

The Paralyzed Veterans of America (PVA) at (www.pva.org or 800-424-8200) offers publications that include "Pressure Ulcer Prevention and Treatment Following Spinal Cord Injury" and "Pressure Ulcers: What You Should Know" available in English and Spanish.

The United Ostomy Associations of America (www.uoaa.org or 800-826-0826) offers information on ostomy care, frequently asked questions, and adjusting to an ostomy.

The Wound, Ostomy and Continence Nurses Society (www.wocn.org or 888-224-9626) offers educational resources and programs that include the WOCN "Guidance on OASIS Skin and Wound Status MO Items" (revised July 2006).

Book Resources:

Baranoski S, Ayello E: *Wound care essentials: practice principles,* ed 2, Philadelphia, 2007, Lippincott Williams & Wilkins.

Hess CT: *Clinical guide: wound care*, ed 5, Philadelphia, 2004, Lippincott Williams & Wilkins.

Sussman C, Bates-Jensen B: *Wound care: a collaboration manual for physical therapists and nurses*, ed 3, Philadelphia, 2007, Lippincott Williams & Wilkins.

HOME CARE CLINICAL JOURNALS AND NEWSLETTERS

Journals

The American Journal of Hospice and Palliative Medicine (www.ajh.sagepub.com)
Caring Magazine (www.nahc.org)
Home Health Aide Digest (www.hhadigest.com)
Home Health Care Management & Practice (http://hhc.sagepub.com)
Home Healthcare Nurse (www.homehealthcarenurseonline.com)
Journal of Hospice and Palliative Nursing (www.jhpn.com)
Journal of Community Health Nursing (http://www.informaworld.com/smpp/title~content=t775648098)

Newsletters

Home Care Week (www.elihealthcare.com)
Home Health ICD-9 Alert (www.elihealthcare.com)
Home Health Line (www.decisionhealth.com)
Medicare Compliance Week (www.elihealthcare.com)
Medline Plus (www.nlm.nih.gov/cgi/medlineplus/listserv.pl?lang=EN)—you can sign up for listserv and e-mail updates on health topics such as diabetes, nutrition, senior health, women's health, men's health
OASIS Alert (www.elihealthcare.com)
Telemedicine Today—The Health News Magazine (www.telemed.com)

APPENDIX A

HOME CARE ORIENTATION

Important Foundation for Success

A

All home care team members need an orientation period, the length of which should be appropriate to the position's responsibilities and requirements. A quality orientation is important to being successful in home care and to functioning safely and competently in the role. Although the term *nurse* may be used, all therapists, speech-language pathologists, social workers, dietitians, home health aides—anyone who makes home visits—need an orientation. Regardless how understaffed a home care program may be, clinicians must try to define or address the orientation each home care team member will receive, including the time span and content, before accepting a new position. The following list addresses some of the information an effective orientation should include. Obviously, if the clinician has been in home care for some time, reviewing all of this information may not be appropriate or necessary; however, all team members need to have an understanding of these "hallmarks" of home care:

1. The organization's orientation manuals.
2. The Medicare Conditions of Participation, the Centers for Medicare and Medicaid Services Outcome and ASsessment Information Set (OASIS) Implementation Manual, the Medicare manual section that specifies the coverage of services, and the specific state rules and regulations governing the particular agency or organization.
3. The schedules of home care team meetings and care coordination and/or case conferences.
4. The role of all home team members—nurse, therapist, aide, social worker, etc. This information, which includes a position description, provides an overview of the role. Often this information is prepared by the specialty service (e.g., occupational therapist about occupational therapy cases, physical therapist about therapy cases). Case management will be addressed as a part of the role description, as well as the model of care at the new organization. Regulatory components, such as accreditation and licensing responsibilities, related to the role also should be addressed.

5. The organization's clinical and administrative policy and procedure manuals.
6. An overview of the organization's clinical records, comprehensive assessment information with the OASIS data elements (if required), documentation system, required forms, clinical paths, and paper flow and timelines for completion and submission.
7. Guidelines for home visits, including verbal orders, the referral process, and scheduling. Personal and community safety "in the field" should also be a part of these guidelines.
8. The opportunity to "buddy" with an experienced nurse or therapist (peer, if possible) from the home care organization.
9. An orientation to the organization's required forms (e.g., daily schedule, mileage tracking form).
10. Medicare and other coverage and documentation requirements, including confidentiality, the Health Insurance Portability and Accountability Act (HIPAA), patient rights and responsibilities, and timeliness of physician orders.
11. Administrative details and processes, such as those involved in payroll and on-call schedules.
12. Acquisition and overview of equipment and supplies, such as lab forms, locations of supplies and related documentation, and drop-off lab locations.
13. Orientation to automated clinical documentation and/or other clinical related systems (if applicable).
14. Quality improvement processes, Outcome-Based Quality Monitoring (OBQM), and Outcome-Based Quality Improvement (OBQI), and the clinician's role in identifying and reporting information. This may include infections, falls, missed visits, drug reactions, variances identified in clinical paths, OASIS data or indicators, information from the OBQM, OBQI, and Home Health Compare reports, and other information required by the organization to establish and maintain quality and other standards.

15. The employee handbook, which may contain information unique to the program, such as mileage, on-call process, pay, lab pickup schedules, and other miscellaneous information unique to the program and community.
16. Occupational Safety and Health Administration (OSHA) requirements, including hepatitis B vaccination, home health agency-related policies and supplies for blood-borne pathogens, tuberculosis surveillance, standard precautions, supplies, and related disposal of supplies, and associated record-keeping activities.
17. Completion of a skills checklist, proficiency test, or validation of competency/credentials (annually), and an on-going schedule for in-service training and continuing education opportunities.
18. Information related to compliance with laws and regulations (e.g., home health aide training and competency testing, the organization's compliance program and each member's role in compliance).
19. An orientation to the specific technology and related protocols for telehealth used by the organization for specific patient populations.
20. An understanding of the clinician's role in the prospective payment system (PPS). Because PPS is driven by clinical data and related practice, financial viability of the organization is based on clinical assessment, interventions, and close management of care and services (i.e., resources)—and ultimately the achievement of patient outcomes.
21. Emergency management program of the organization and each clinician's specific role in the event of a disaster, such as a hurricane, ice storm, earthquake, flood, or other event.
22. Community linkage and clinical resources available to staff and their locations within the agency (e.g., how to access).
23. Overview of Medicare home health benefit, including:
    1. Criteria for home care;
    2. Documenting to meet Medicare standards; and

3. OASIS documentation (using the tool appropriately and correctly).

24. Case management.
25. Assessment and care of wounds.
26. Physical assessment.
27. Other information, depending on the organization's unique mission and particular populations.

APPENDIX B

SAMPLE CASE-MIX GROUPER WORKSHEET

B

Clinical Dimension

M0 Item Response	Points Earned			
Episode #	1 or 2	1 or 2	3+	3+
Therapy Visits	0–13	14+	0–13	14+
1st or 2nd = Blindness/Low Vision	3	3	3	3
1st or 2nd = Blood Disorders	2	5		
1st or 2nd = CA, Selected Benign Neoplasms	4	7	3	10
Primary = Diabetes	5	12	1	8
2nd = Diabetes	2	4	1	4
1st or 2nd = Dysphagia **AND** Neuro 3—Stroke	2	6		6
1st or 2nd = Dysphagia **AND** M0250 (therapy at home) = 3 (Enteral)		6		
1st or 2nd = Gastrointestinal Disorders	2	6	1	4
1st or 2nd = Gastrointestinal Disorders **AND** M0550 (Ostomy) = 1 or 2	3			
1st or 2nd = Gastrointestinal Disorders **AND** 1st or 2nd Neuro 1, 2, 3, or 4			2	
1st or 2nd = Heart Disease OR Hypertension	3	7	1	8
Primary = Neuro 1—Brain Disorders and Paralysis	3	8	5	8
1st or 2nd = Neuro 1—Brain Disorders and Paralysis **AND** M0680 (toileting) = 2 or more	3	10	3	10
1st or 2nd = Neuro 1—Brain Disorders and Paralysis OR Neuro 2—Peripheral neurological disorders **AND** M0650 or M0660 (Dressing ↑ and ↓ body) = 1, 2, or 3	2	4	2	2
1st or 2nd = Neuro 3—Stroke		1		
1st or 2nd = Neuro 3—Stroke **AND** M0650 or M0660 (Dressing ↑ and ↓ body) = 1, 2, or 3	1	3	2	8
1st or 2nd = Neuro 3—Stroke **AND** M0700 (Ambulation) = 3 or more	1	5		
1st or 2nd = Neuro 4—MS **AND** at least 1 of the following: M0670 (bathing) = 2 or more or M0680 (toileting) = 2 or more or M0690 (transfer) = 2 or more or M0700 (ambulation) = 3 or more	3	3	12	18
1st or 2nd = Ortho 1—Leg or Gait Disorders **AND** M0460 (problem PU) = 1, 2, 3, or 4	2			
1st or 2nd = Ortho 1—Leg or Gait Disorders OR Ortho 2—Other orthopedic disorders **AND** M0250 (Therapy at home) = 1 (IV/Infusion) or 2 (Parenteral)	5	5		

M0 Item Response	Points Earned			
Episode #	1 or 2	1 or 2	3+	3+
Therapy Visits	0–13	14+	0–13	14+
1st or 2nd = Psych 1—Affective and other psychoses, depression	3	5	2	5
1st or 2nd = Psych 2—Degenerative and organic psychiatric disorders	1	2		2
1st or 2nd = Pulmonary disorders	1	5	1	5
1st or 2nd = Pulmonary disorders **AND** M0700 (Ambulation) = 1 or more	1			
Primary = Skin 1—Traumatic wounds, burns, & post-op complications	10	20	8	20
2nd = Skin 1—Traumatic wounds, burns, & post-op complications	6	6	4	4
2nd = Skin 1—Traumatic wounds, burns, & post-op OR Skin 2—Ulcers and other skin conditions **AND** M0250 (therapy at home) = 1 (IV/Infusion) or 2 (Parenteral)	2		2	
1st or 2nd = Skin 2—Ulcers and other skin conditions	6	12	5	12
1st or 2nd = Tracheostomy	4	4	4	
1st or 2nd = Urostomy/Cystostomy	6	23	4	23
M0250 (Therapy at home) = 1 (IV/Infusion) or 2 (Parenteral)	8	15	5	12
M0250 (Therapy at home) = 3 (Enteral)	4	12		12
M0390 (Vision) = 1 or more	1			1
M0420 (Pain) = 2 or 3	1			
M0450 = 2 or more pressure ulcers at Stage 3 or 4	3	3	5	5
M0460 (Most problematic pressure ulcer) = 1 or 2	5	11	5	11
M0460 (Most problematic pressure ulcer) = 3 or 4	16	26	12	23
M0476 (Stasis ulcer) = 2	8	8	8	8
M0476 (Stasis ulcer) = 3	11	11	11	11
M0488 (Surgical wound status) = 2		2	3	
M0488 (Surgical wound status) = 3	4	4	4	4
M0490 (Dyspnea) = 2, 3 or 4	2	2		
M0540 (Bowel incontinence) = 2, 3, 4, or 5	1	2	1	
M0550 (Ostomy) = 1 or 2	5	9	3	9
M0800 (Injectable drugs) = 0, 1, or 2	1	1	2	4
TOTAL FOR CLINICAL DIMENSION				

Functional Dimension

M0 Item	Response	Points Earned			
	Episode #	1 or 2	1 or 2	3+	3+
	Therapy Visits	0–13	14+	0–13	14+
M0650 or M0660 (Dressing UB and LB) = 1, 2, or 3		2	4	2	2
M0670 (Bathing) = 2 or more		3	3	6	6
M0680 (Toileting) = 2 or more		2	3	2	
M0690 (Transferring) = 2 or more			2		
M0700 (Ambulation) = 1 or 2		1		1	
M0700 (Ambulation) = 3 or more		3	4	4	5
TOTAL FOR FUNCTIONAL DIMENSION					

Number of Therapy Visits:

CFS Scoring			1st and 2nd Episodes		3rd+ Episodes		All Episodes
	Severity	HIPPS	THERAPY VISITS MADE FOR EPISODE				
Dimension	Levels	Value	0–13	14–19	0–13	14–19	20+
Clinical	C1	A	0–4	0–6	0–2	0–8	0–7
	C2	B	5–8	7–14	3–5	9–16	8–14
	C3	C	9+	15+	6+	17+	15+
Functional	F1	F	0–5	0–6	0–8	0–7	0–6
	F2	G	6	7	9	8	7
	F3	H	7+	8+	10+	9+	8+
Service	S1	K	0–5	14–15	0–5	14–15	20+
	S2	L	6	16–17	6	16–17	
	S3	M	7–9	18–19	7–9	18–19	
	S4	N	10		10		
	S5	P	11–13		11–13		

B

Non-Routine Supply

Severity level	Points	HIPPS value w/NRS	HIPPS value w/o NRS	Payments
1	0	S	1	14.12
2	1–14	T	2	51.00
3	15–27	U	3	139.84
4	28–48	V	4	207.76
5	49–98	W	5	320.76
6	99+	X	6	551.00

Final Scoring

Scoring	Dimension	Value	HIPPS Value	Dollar Amt
	Clinical			
	Functional			
	Service			
	NRS			

APPENDIX C

NON-ROUTINE SUPPLIES (NRS) CASE-MIX ADJUSTMENT VARIABLES AND SCORES

C

TABLE 10A

NRS CASE-MIX ADJUSTMENT VARIABLES AND SCORES

Item	Description	Score
	SELECTED SKIN CONDITIONS:	
1	Primary diagnosis = Anal fissure, fistula and abscess	15
2	Other diagnosis = Anal fissure, fistula and abscess	13
3	Primary diagnosis = Cellulitis and abscess	14
4	Other diagnosis = Cellulitis and abscess	8
5	Primary diagnosis = Diabetic ulcers	20
6	Primary diagnosis = Gangrene	11
7	Other diagnosis = Gangrene	8
8	Primary diagnosis = Malignant neoplasms of skin	15
9	Other diagnosis = Malignant neoplasms of skin	4
10	Primary or Other diagnosis = Non-pressure and non-stasis ulcers	13
11	Primary diagnosis = Other infections of skin and subcutaneous tissue	16
12	Other diagnosis = Other infections of skin and subcutaneous tissue	7
13	Primary diagnosis = Post-operative Complications	23
14	Other diagnosis = Post-operative Complications	15
15	Primary diagnosis = Traumatic Wounds and Burns	19
16	Other diagnosis = Traumatic Wounds and Burns	8
17	Primary or Other diagnosis = V code, Cystostomy care	16
18	Primary or Other diagnosis = V code, Tracheostomy care	23
19	Primary or Other diagnosis = V code, Urostomy care	24
20	OASIS M0450 = 1 or 2 pressure ulcers, stage 1	4
21	OASIS M0450 = 3+ pressure ulcers, stage 1	6
22	OASIS M0450 = 1 pressure ulcer, stage 2	14
23	OASIS M0450 = 2 pressure ulcers, stage 2	22
24	OASIS M0450 = 3 pressure ulcers, stage 2	29
25	OASIS M0450 = 4+ pressure ulcers, stage 2	35
26	OASIS M0450 = 1 pressure ulcer, stage 3	29
27	OASIS M0450 = 2 pressure ulcers, stage 3	41
28	OASIS M0450 = 3 pressure ulcers, stage 3	46
29	OASIS M0450 = 4+ pressure ulcers, stage 3	58
30	OASIS M0450 = 1 pressure ulcer, stage 4	48

Continued

C

TABLE 10A—CONT'D

Item	Description	Score
	SELECTED SKIN CONDITIONS:	
31	OASIS M0450 = 2 pressure ulcers, stage 4	67
32	OASIS M0450 = 3+ pressure ulcers, stage 4	75
33	OASIS M0450e = 1 (unobserved pressure ulcer(s))	17
34	OASIS M0470 = 2 (2 stasis ulcers)	6
35	OASIS M0470 = 3 (3 stasis ulcers)	12
36	OASIS M0470 = 4 (4+ stasis ulcers)	21
37	OASIS M0474 = 1 (unobservable stasis ulcers)	9
38	OASIS M0476 = 1 (status of most problematic stasis ulcer: fully granulating)	6
39	OASIS M0476 = 2 (status of most problematic stasis ulcer: early/partial granulation)	25
40	OASIS M0476 = 3 (status of most problematic stasis ulcer: not healing)	36
41	OASIS M0488 = 2 (status of most problematic surgical wound: early/partial granulation)	4
42	OASIS M0488 = 3 (status of most problematic surgical wound: not healing)	14
	OTHER CLINICAL FACTORS:	
43	OASIS M0550 = 1(ostomy not related to inpt stay/no regimen change)	27
44	OASIS M0550 = 2 (ostomy related to inpt stay/ regimen change)	45
45	Any `Selected Skin Conditions` (rows 1-42 above) AND M0550=1(ostomy not related to inpt stay/no regimen change)	14
46	Any `Selected Skin Conditions` (rows 1-42 above) AND M0550=2(ostomy related to inpt stay/ regimen change)	11
47	OASIS M0250 (Therapy at home) =1 (IV/Infusion)	5
48	OASIS M0520 = 2 (patient requires urinary catheter)	9
49	OASIS M0540 = 4 or 5 (bowel incontinence, daily or >daily)	10

Note: Points are additive, however, points may not be given for the same line item in the table more than once. Points are not assigned for a secondary diagnosis if points are already assigned for a primary diagnosis from the same diagnosis/condition group. See Table 10B (in Appendix D) for definitions of diagnosis/condition groups

Please see Medicare Home Health Diagnosis Coding guidance at http://www.cms.hhs.gov/HomeHealthPPS/03_coding&billing.asp for definitions of primary and secondary diagnoses.

APPENDIX D

HOME HEALTH PROSPECTIVE PAYMENT SYSTEM FINAL RULE

(from the Federal Register 2007)

D

TABLE 2A

CASE-MIX ADJUSTMENT VARIABLES AND SCORES

	Episode number within sequence of adjacent episodes	1 or 2	1 or 2	3+	3+
	Therapy visits	0–13	14+	0–13	14+
	EQUATION:	1	2	3	4
	Clinical Dimension				
1	Primary or Other Diagnosis = Blindness/Low Vision	3	3	3	3
2	Primary or Other Diagnosis = Blood Disorders	2	5		
3	Primary or Other Diagnosis = Cancer, Selected Benign Neoplasms	4	7	3	10
4	Primary Diagnosis = Diabetes	5	12	1	8
5	Other Diagnosis = Diabetes	2	4	1	4
6	Primary or Other Diagnosis = Dysphagia *AND* Primary or Other Diagnosis = Neuro 3—Stroke	2	6		6
7	Primary or Other Diagnosis = Dysphagia *AND* M0250 (Therapy at Home) = 3 (Enteral)		6		
8	Primary or Other Diagnosis = Gastrointestinal Disorders	2	6	1	4
9	Primary or Other Diagnosis = Gastrointestinal disorders *AND* M0550 (Ostomy) = 1 or 2	3			

10	Primary or Other Diagnosis = Gastrointestinal Disorders *AND* Primary or Other Diagnosis = Neuro 1—Brain Disorders and Paralysis, OR Neuro 2—Peripheral Neurological Disorders, OR Neuro 3—Stroke, OR Neuro 4—Multiple Sclerosis			2	
11	Primary or Other Diagnosis = Heart Disease OR Hypertension	3	7	1	8
12	Primary Diagnosis = Neuro 1—Brain Disorders and Paralysis	3	8	5	8
13	Primary or Other Diagnosis = Neuro 1—Brain Disorders and Paralysis *AND* M0680 (Toileting) = 2 or more	3	10	3	10
14	Primary or Other Diagnosis = Neuro 1—Brain Disorders and Paralysis, OR Neuro 2—Peripheral Neurological Disorders *AND* M0650 or M0660 (Dressing Upper or Lower Body) = 1, 2, or 3	2	4	2	2
15	Primary or Other Diagnosis = Neuro 3—Stroke		1		
16	Primary or Other Diagnosis = Neuro 3—Stroke *AND* M0650 or M0660 (Dressing Upper or Lower Body) = 1, 2, or 3	1	3	2	8
17	Primary or Other Diagnosis = Neuro 3—Stroke *AND* M0700 (Ambulation) = 3 or more	1	5		

Continued

D

TABLE 2A—CONT'D

18	Primary or Other Diagnosis = Neuro 4—Multiple Sclerosis *AND AT LEAST ONE OF THE FOLLOWING:* M0670 (Bathing) = 2 or more *OR* M0680 (Toileting) = 2 or more *OR* M0690 (Transferring) = 2 or more *OR* M0700 (Ambulation) = 3 or more	3	3	12	18
19	Primary or Other Diagnosis = Ortho 1—Leg Disorders or Gait Disorders *AND* M0460 (Most Problematic Pressure Ulcer Stage) = 1, 2, 3, or 4	2			
20	Primary or Other Diagnosis = Ortho 1—Leg, OR Ortho 2—Other Orthopedic Disorders *AND* M0250 (Therapy at Home) = 1 (IV/Infusion) or 2 (Parentera)	5	5		
21	Primary or Other Diagnosis = Psych 1—Affective and Other Psychoses, Depression	3	5	2	5
22	Primary or Other Diagnosis = Psych 2 —Degenerative and Other Organic Psychiatric Disorders	1	2		2
23	Primary or Other Diagnosis = Pulmonary Disorders	1	5	1	5
24	Primary or Other Diagnosis = Pulmonary Disorders *AND* M0700 (Ambulation) = 1 or more	1			
25	Primary Diagnosis = Skin 1—Traumatic Wounds, Burns, and Post-operative Complications	10	20	8	20

26	Other Diagnosis = Skin 1—Traumatic Wounds, Burns, Post-operative Complications	6	6	4	4
27	Primary or Other Diagnosis = Skin 1—Traumatic Wounds, Burns, and Post-operative Complications, OR Skin 2—Ulcers and Other Skin Conditions *AND* M0250 (Therapy at Home) = 1 (IV/Infusion) or 2 (Parenteral)	2		2	
28	Primary or Other Diagnosis = Skin 2—Ulcers and Other Skin Conditions	6	12	5	12
29	Primary or Other Diagnosis = Tracheostomy	4	4	4	
30	Primary or Other Diagnosis = Urostomy/Cystostomy	6	23	4	23
31	M0250 (Therapy at Home) = 1 (IV/Infusion) or 2 (Parenteral)	8	15	5	12
32	M0250 (Therapy at Home) = 3 (Enteral)	4	12		12
33	M0390 (Vision) = 1 or more	1			1
34	M0420 (Pain) = 2 or 3	1			
35	M0450 = 2 or More Pressure Ulcers At Stage 3 or 4	3	3	5	5
36	M0460 (Most Problematic Pressure Ulcer Stage) = 1 or 2	5	11	5	11
37	M0460 (Most Problematic Pressure Ulcer Stage) = 3 or 4	16	26	12	23
38	M0476 (Stasis Ulcer Status) = 2	8	8	8	8
39	M0476 (Stasis Ulcer Status) = 3	11	11	11	11
40	M0488 (Surgical Wound Status) = 2		2	3	
41	M0488 (Surgical Wound Status) = 3	4	4	4	4
42	M0490 (Dyspnea) = 2, 3, or 4	2	2		
43	M0540 (Bowel Incontinence) = 2 to 5	1	2	1	
44	M0550 (Ostomy) = 1 or 2	5	9	3	9
45	M0800 (Injectable Drug Use) = 0, 1, or 2	1	1	2	4

Continued

TABLE 2A—CONT'D					
Functional Dimension					
46	M0650 or M0660 (Dressing Upper or Lower Body) = 1, 2, or 3	2	4	2	2
47	M0670 (Bathing) = 2 or more	3	3	6	6
48	M0680 (Toileting) = 2 or more	2	3	2	
49	M0690 (Transferring) = 2 or more		2		
50	M0700 (Ambulation) = 1 or 2	1		1	
51	M0700 (Ambulation) = 3 or more	3	4	4	5

Notes: The data for the regression equations come from a 20% random sample of episodes from CY 2005. The sample excludes LUPA episodes, outlier episodes, and episodes with SCIC or PEP adjustments.

Points are additive, however, points may not be given for the same line item in the table more than once.

Please see Medicare Home Health Diagnosis Coding guidance at http://www.cms.hhs.gov/HomeHealthPPS/03_coding&billing.asp for definitions of primary and secondary diagnoses.

TABLE 2B

DIAGNOSIS CODES, "SECONDARY-ONLY" DIAGNOSIS CODES, DIAGNOSIS GROUPS, AND DIAGNOSIS GROUP VARIABLE NAMES

Diagnostic Category	ICD-9-CM Code	Manifestation Codes	Short Description of ICD-9-CM Code
Blindness and Low Vision	369.01		BETTER EYE: TOTAL IMPAIRMENT; LESSER EYE: TOTAL IMPAIRMENT
	369.02		BETTER EYE: NEAR TOTAL IMPAIRMENT; LESSER EYE: NOT FURTHER SPECIFIED
	369.03		BETTER EYE: NEAR TOTAL IMPAIRMENT; LESSER EYE: TOTAL IMPAIRMENT
	369.04		BETTER EYE: NEAR TOTAL IMPAIRMENT; LESSER EYE: NEAR TOTAL IMPAIRMENT
	369.05		BETTER EYE: PROFOUND IMPAIRMENT; LESSER EYE: NOT FURTHER SPECIFIED
	369.06		BETTER EYE: PROFOUND IMPAIRMENT; LESSER EYE: TOTAL IMPAIRMENT
	369.07		BETTER EYE: PROFOUND IMPAIRMENT; LESSER EYE: NEAR TOTAL IMPAIRMENT

Continued

TABLE 2B—CONT'D			
	369.08		BETTER EYE: PROFOUND IMPAIRMENT; LESSER EYE: PROFOUND IMPAIRMENT
	369.10		IMPAIRMENT LEVEL NOT FURTHER SPECIFIED, BLINDNESS, ONE EYE, LOW VISION OTHER EYE
	369.11		BETTER EYE: SEVERE IMPAIRMENT; LESSER EYE: BLIND, NOT FURTHER SPECIFIED
	369.12		BETTER EYE: SEVERE IMPAIRMENT; LESSER EYE: TOTAL IMPAIRMENT
	369.13		BETTER EYE: SEVERE IMPAIRMENT; LESSER EYE: NEAR TOTAL IMPAIRMENT
	369.14		BETTER EYE: SEVERE IMPAIRMENT; LESSER EYE: PROFOUND IMPAIRMENT
	369.15		BETTER EYE: MODERATE IMPAIRMENT; LESSER EYE: BLIND, NOT FURTHER SPECIFIED
	369.16		BETTER EYE: MODERATE IMPAIRMENT; LESSER EYE: TOTAL IMPAIRMENT
	369.17		BETTER EYE: MODERATE IMPAIRMENT; LESSER EYE: NEAR TOTAL IMPAIRMENT

	369.18		BETTER EYE: MODERATE IMPAIRMENT; LESSER EYE: PROFOUND IMPAIRMENT
	369.20		IMPAIRMENT LEVEL NOT FURTHER SPECIFIED, LOW VISION, BOTH EYES NOS
	369.21		BETTER EYE: SEVERE IMPAIRMENT; LESSER EYE: NOT FURTHER SPECIFIED
	369.22		BETTER EYE: SEVERE IMPAIRMENT; LESSER EYE: SEVERE IMPAIRMENT
	369.23		BETTER EYE: MODERATE IMPAIRMENT; LESSER EYE: NOT FURTHER SPECIFIED
	369.24		BETTER EYE: MODERATE IMPAIRMENT; LESSER EYE: SEVERE IMPAIRMENT
	369.25		BETTER EYE: MODERATE IMPAIRMENT; LESSER EYE: MODERATE IMPAIR
	369.3		BLINDNESS NOS, BOTH EYES
	369.4		LEGAL BLINDNESS—USA DEF
	950		INJURY TO OPTIC NERVE AND PATHWAYS
Blood Disorders	281		OTHER DEFICIENCY ANEMIAS

Continued

TABLE 2B—CONT'D

	282		HEREDITARY HEMOLYTIC ANEMIAS
	283		ACQUIRED HEMOLYTIC ANEMIAS
	284		APLASTIC ANEMIA
	285		OTHER AND UNSPECIFIED ANEMIAS
	287		PURPURA & OTHER HEMORRHAGIC CONDS
	288		DISEASES OF WHITE BLOOD CELLS
	289		OTH DISEASES BLD & BLD-FORMING ORGANS
Cancer and Selected Benign Neoplasms	140		MALIGNANT NEOPLASM OF LIP
	141		MALIGNANT NEOPLASM OF TONGUE
	142		MALIG NEOPLASM MAJOR SALIV GLANDS
	143		MALIGNANT NEOPLASM OF GUM
	144		MALIGNANT NEOPLASM FLOOR MOUTH
	145		MALIG NEOPLSM OTH & UNSPEC PART MOUTH
	146		MALIGNANT NEOPLASM OF OROPHARYNX
	147		MALIGNANT NEOPLASM OF NASOPHARYNX
	148		MALIGNANT NEOPLASM OF HYPOPHARYNX

D

	149		OTH MALIG NEO LIP-MOUTH-PHARYNX
	150		MALIGNANT NEOPLASM OF ESOPHAGUS
	151		MALIGNANT NEOPLASM OF STOMACH
	152		MALIG NEOPLSM SM INTEST INCL DUODUM
	153		MALIGNANT NEOPLASM OF COLON
	154		MAL NEO RECT RECTOSIGMOID JUNC & ANUS
	155		MALIG NEOPLASM LIVER & INTRAHEP BDS
	156		MALIG NEOPLSM GALLBLADD & XTRAHEP BDS
	157		MALIGNANT NEOPLASM OF PANCREAS
	158		MALIG NEOPLASM RETROPERITON & PERITON
	159		MAL NEO DIGES ORGANS & PANCREAS OTH
	160		MAL NEO NASL CAV/ MID EAR & ACSS SINUS
	161		MALIGNANT NEO LARYNX
	162		MALIGNANT NEO TRACHEA/LUNG
	163		MALIGNANT NEOPL PLEURA
	164		MAL NEO THYMUS/ MEDIASTIN

Continued

TABLE 2B—CONT'D

	165		OTH/ILL—DEF MAL NEO RESP
	170		MALIG NEOPLASM BONE & ARTICLR CART
	171		MALIG NEOPLSM CNCTV & OTH SOFT TISSUE
	172		MALIGNANT MELANOMA OF SKIN
	173		OTHER MALIGNANT NEOPLASM OF SKIN
	174		MALIGNANT NEOPLASM OF FEMALE BREAST
	175		MALIGNANT NEOPLASM OF MALE BREAST
	176		KAPOSIS SARCOMA
	179		MALIG NEOPLASM UTERUS PART UNSPEC
	180		MALIGNANT NEOPLASM OF CERVIX UTERI
	181		MALIGNANT NEOPLASM OF PLACENTA
	182		MALIGNANT NEOPLASM BODY UTERUS
	183		MALIG NEOPLSM OVRY & OTH UTERN ADNEXA
	184		MALIG NEOPLSM OTH & UNS FE GENIT ORGN
	185		MALIGNANT NEOPLASM OF PROSTATE
	186		MALIGNANT NEOPLASM OF TESTIS

	187		MAL NEOPLSM PENIS & OTH MALE GNT ORGN
	188		MALIGNANT NEOPLASM OF BLADDER
	189		MAL NEO KIDNEY & OTH & UNS URIN ORGN
	190		MALIGNANT NEOPLASM OF EYE
	192.0		MALIGNANT NEOPLASM, CRANIAL NERVES
	192.8		MALIGNANT NEOPLASM OTHER NERV SYS
	192.9		MALIGNANT NEOPLASM, UNS PART NERV SYS
	193		MALIGNANT NEOPLASM OF THYROID GLAND
	194		MAL NEO OTH ENDOCRN GLND & REL STRCT
	195		MALIG NEOPLASM OTH & ILL-DEFIND SITES
	196		SEC & UNSPEC MALIG NEOPLASM NODES
	197		SEC MALIG NEOPLASM RESP & DIGESTV SYS
	198		SEC MALIG NEOPLASM OTHER SPEC SITES
	199		MALIG NEOPLASM WITHOUT SPEC SITE
	200		LYMPHOSARCOMA AND RETICULOSARCOMA
	201		HODGKINS DISEASE
	202		OTH MAL NEO LYMPHOID & HISTCYT TISS
	203		MX MYELOMA & IMMUNOPROLIFERAT NEOPLSM

Continued

D

TABLE 2B—CONT'D			
	204		LYMPHOID LEUKEMIA
	205		MYELOID LEUKEMIA
	206		MONOCYTIC LEUKEMIA
	207		OTHER SPECIFIED LEUKEMIA
	208		LEUKEMIA OF UNSPECIFIED CELL TYPE
	213 except 213.9		BENIGN NEOPLASM OF BONE AND ARTICULAR CARTILAGE
	225.1		BEN NEOPLSM CRANIAL NERVES
	225.8		BEN NEOPLSM OTH SPEC SITES
	230 except 230.9		CARCINOMA IN SITU OF DIGESTIVE ORGANS
	231 except 231.9		CARCINOMA IN SITU OF RESPIRATORY SYSTEM
	232 except 232.9		CARCINOMA IN SITU OF SKIN
	233 except 233.9		CARCINOMA IN SITU OF BREAST AND GENITOURINARY SYSTEM
	234 except 234.9		CARCINOMA IN SITU OF OTHER AND UNSPECIFIED SITES
Diabetes	250		DIABETES MELLITUS
	357.2	M	POLYNEUROPATHY IN DIABETES
	362.01	M	BACKGROUND DIABETIC RETINOPATHY
	362.02	M	PROLIFERATIVE DIABETIC RETINOPATHY
	366.41	M	DIABETIC CATARACT

Dysphagia	787.20		DYSPHAGIA, UNSPECIFIED
	787.21		DYSPHAGIA, ORAL PHASE
	787.22		DYSPHAGIA, OROPHARYNGEAL PHASE
	787.23		DYSPHAGIA, PHARYNGEAL PHASE
	787.24		DYSPHAGIA, PHARYNGO-ESOPHAGEAL PHASE
	787.29		OTHER DYSPHAGIA
Gait Abnormality	781.2		ABNORM GAIT
Gastroin-testinal Disorders	002		TYPHOID AND PARATYPHOID FEVERS
	003		OTHER SALMONELLA INFECTIONS
	004		SHIGELLOSIS
	005		OTHER FOOD POISONING
	006		AMEBIASIS
	007		OTHER PROTOZOAL INTESTINAL DISEASES
	008		INTESTINAL INFS DUE OTH ORGANISMS
	009		ILL-DEFINED INTESTINAL INFECTIONS
	530		DISEASES OF ESOPHAGUS
	531		GASTRIC ULCER
	532		DUODENAL ULCER
	533		PEPTIC ULCER, SITE UNSPECIFIED
	534		GASTROJEJUNAL ULCER
	535		GASTRITIS AND DUODENITIS
	536		DISORDERS OF FUNCTION OF STOMACH

Continued

TABLE 2B—CONT'D

	537		OTHER DISORDERS OF STOMACH & DUODENUM
	540		ACUTE APPENDICITIS
	541		APPENDICITIS, UNQUALIFIED
	542		OTHER APPENDICITIS
	543		OTHER DISEASES OF APPENDIX
	555		REGIONAL ENTERITIS
	556		ULCERATIVE COLITIS
	557		VASCULAR INSUFFICIENCY OF INTESTINE
	558		OTH NONINF GASTROENTERITIS & COLITIS
	560		INTEST OBST W/O MENTION HERN
	562		DIVERTICULA OF INTESTINE
	564 except 564.0x, 564.9		FUNCTIONAL DIGESTIVE DISORDERS, NOT ELSEWHERE CLASSIFIED
	567.0	M	PERITONITIS IN INFEC DIS CLASS ELSEWH
	567.1		PNEUMOCOCCAL PERITONITIS
	567.21		PERITONITIS (ACUTE) GENERALIZED
	567.22		PERITONEAL ABSCESS
	567.23		SPONTANEOUS BACTERIAL PERITONITIS
	567.29		OTHER SUPPURATIVE PERITONITIS
	567.31		PSOAS MUSCLE ABSCESS
	567.38		OTHER RETROPERITONEAL ABSCESS

	567.39		OTHER RETROPERITONEAL INFECTIONS
	567.81		CHOLEPERITONITIS
	567.82		SCLEROSING MESENTERITIS
	567.89		OTHER SPECIFIED PERITONITIS
	567.9		UNSPECIFIED PERITONITIS
	568		OTHER DISORDERS OF PERITONEUM
	569 except 569.9		OTHER DISORDERS OF INTESTINE
	570		ACUTE & SUBACUTE NECROSIS OF LIVER
	571		CHRONIC LIVER DISEASE AND CIRRHOSIS
	572		LIVER ABSC & SEQUELAE CHRON LIVR DZ
	573.0		CHRONIC PASSIVE CONGESTION OF LIVER
	573.1	M	HEPATITIS IN VIRAL DISEASES CLASS ELSW
	573.2	M	HEPATITIS IN INFEC DISEASES CLASS ELSW
	573.3		HEPATITIS, UNSPECIFIED
	573.4		HEPATIC INFARCTION
	573.8		OTHER SPECIFIED DISORDERS OF LIVER
	573.9		UNSPECIFIED DISORDER OF LIVER
	574		CHOLELITHIASIS
	575		OTHER DISORDERS OF GALLBLADDER
	576		OTHER DISORDERS OF BILIARY TRACT

Continued

TABLE 2B—CONT'D			
	577		DISEASES OF PANCREAS
	578		GASTROINTESTINAL HEMORRHAGE
	579		INTESTINAL MALABSORPTION
	783.21		ABNORMAL LOSS OF WEIGHT
	783.22		ABNORMAL UNDERWEIGHT
Heart Disease	411		OTH AC & SUBAC FORMS ISCHEMIC HRT DZ
	410.02		AMI ANTERO-LATERAL,SUBSEQ
	410.12		AMI ANTERIOR WALL,SUBSEQ
	410.22		AMI INFERO-LATERAL,SUBSEQ
	410.32		AMI INFEROPOST, SUBSEQ
	410.42		AMI INFERIOR WALL,SUBSEQ
	410.52		AMI LATERAL NEC, SUBSEQ
	410.62		TRUE POST INFARCT,SUBSEQ
	410.72		SUBENDO INFARCT, SUBSEQ
	410.82		AMI NEC, SUBSEQUENT
	410.92		AMI NOS, SUBSEQUENT
	414 except 414.9		OTHER FORMS OF CHRONIC ISCHEMIC HEART DISEASE
	428		HEART FAILURE
Hypertension	401.0		ESSENTIAL HYPERTENSION—MALIGNANT
	401.1		BENIGN HYPERTENSION
	401.9		HYPERTENSION, UNSPECIFIED

	402.00		MAL HYP HT DIS W/O HF
	402.01		MAL HYPERT HRT DIS W HF
	402.10		BENIGN HYPERT HRT DIS W/O HF
	402.11		BENIGN HYP HT DIS W HF
	402.90		UNSPECIFIED HYPERT HRT DIS W/O HF
	402.91		HYP HT DIS NOS W HT FAIL
	403		HYPERTENSIVE RENAL DISEASE
	404		HYPERTENSIVE HEART & RENAL DISEASE
	405		SECONDARY HYPERTENSION
Neuro 1—Brain Disorders and Paralysis	013		TB MENINGES & CNTRL NERV SYS
	046		SLOW VIRUS INFECTION CNTRL NERV SYS
	047		MENINGITIS DUE TO ENTEROVIRUS
	048		OTH ENTEROVIRUS DZ CNTRL NERV SYS
	049		OTH NON-ARTHROPOD BORNE VIRL DX—CNS
	191		MALIGNANT NEOPLASM OF BRAIN
	192.2		MALIG NEOPLSM SPINAL CORD
	192.3		MALIG NEOPLSM SPINAL MENINGES
	225.0		BEN NEOPLSM BRAIN
	225.2		BEN NEOPLSM BRAIN MENINGES
	225.3		BEN NEOPLSM SPINAL CORD

Continued

D

TABLE 2B—CONT'D

	225.4		BEN NEOPLSM SPINAL CORD MENINGES
	320.0		HEMOPHILUS MENINGITIS
	320.1		PNEUMOCOCCAL MENINGITIS
	320.2		STREPTOCOCCAL MENINGITIS
	320.3		STAPHYLOCOCCAL MENINGITIS
	320.7	M	MENINGITIS OTH BACT DZ CLASS ELSW
	320.81		ANAEROBIC MENINGITIS
	320.82		MENINGITIS DUE GM—NEG BACTER NEC
	320.89		MENINGITIS DUE OTHER SPEC BACTERIA
	320.9		MENINGITIS DUE UNSPEC BACTERIUM
	321.0	M	CRYPTOCOCCAL MENINGITIS
	321.1	M	MENINGITIS IN OTHER FUNGAL DISEASES
	321.2	M	MENINGITIS DUE TO VIRUSES NEC
	321.3	M	MENINGITIS DUE TO TRYPANOSOMIASIS
	321.4	M	MENINGITIS IN SARCOIDOSIS
	321.8	M	MENINGITIS—OTH NONBCTRL ORGNISMS CE
	322		MENINGITIS OF UNSPECIFIED CAUSE
	323.01	M	ENCEPHALITIS & ENCEPHALOMYELITIS IN VIRAL DIS CLASS ELSW
	323.02	M	MYELITIS IN VIRAL DISEASES CLASSIFIED ELSEWHERE

	323.1	M	ENCEPHALIT RICKETTS DZ CLASS ELSW
	323.2	M	ENCEPHALIT PROTOZOAL DZ CLASS ELSW
	323.41	M	OTH ENCEPHALITIS AND ENCEPHALOMYELITIS DUE TO INF CLASS ELSW
	323.42	M	OTHER MYELITIS DUE TO INFECTION CLASSIFIED ELSEWHERE
	323.51		ENCEPH/MYEL FOLWG IMMUNE
	323.52		MYELITIS FOLLWG IMMUNE
	323.61	M	INFEC ACUTE DISSEM ENCEPHALOMYELITIS (ADEM)
	323.62	M	OTH POSTINFECTIOUS ENCEPHALITIS & ENCEPHALOMYELITIS
	323.63	M	POSTINFECTIOUS MYELITIS
	323.71	M	TOXIC ENCEPHALITIS AND ENCEPHALOMYELITIS
	323.72	M	TOXIC MYELITIS
	323.81		OTHER CAUSES OF ENCEPHALITIS AND ENCEPHALOMYELITIS
	323.82		OTHER CAUSES OF MYELITIS
	323.9		ENCEPHALITIS NOS
	324		INTRACRANIAL & INTRASPINAL ABSCESS
	325		PHLEBIT & THRMBOPHLB INTRACRAN VENUS
	326		LATE EFF INTRACRAN ABSC/PYOGEN INF

Continued

TABLE 2B—CONT'D

	330.0		LEUKODYSTROPHY
	330.1		CEREBRAL LIPIDOSES
	330.2	M	CEREB DEGEN IN LIPIDOSIS
	330.3	M	CERB DEG CHLD IN OTH DIS
	330.8		CEREB DEGEN IN CHILD NEC
	330.9		CEREB DEGEN IN CHILD NOS
	334.1		HERED SPASTIC PARAPLEGIA
	335		ANTERIOR HORN CELL DISEASE
	336.0		SYRINGOMYELIA AND SYRINGOBULBIA
	336.1		VASCULAR MYELOPATHIES
	336.2	M	SUBACUTE COMB DEGEN SPINL CRD DZ CE
	336.3	M	MYELOPATHY OTH DISEASES CLASS ELSW
	336.8		OTHER MYELOPATHY
	337.3		AUTONOMIC DYSREFLEXIA
	344.00		QUADRIPLEGIA, UNSPECIFIED
	344.01		QUADRIPLEGIA, C1–C4, COMPLETE
	344.02		QUADRIPLEGIA, C1–C4, INCOMPLETE
	344.03		QUADRIPLEGIA, C5–C7, COMPLETE
	344.04		QUADRIPLEGIA, C5–C7, INCOMPLETE
	344.09		QUADRIPLEGIA, OTHER
	344.1		PARAPLEGIA
	344.81		OTHER SPECIFIED PARALYTIC SYNDROMES—LOCKED-IN STATE

	344.89		OTHER SPECIFIED PARALYTIC SYNDROMES—OTHER SPECIFIED PARALYTIC SYNDROME
	348		OTHER CONDITIONS OF BRAIN
	349.82		TOXIC ENCEPHALOPATHY
	741		SPINA BIFIDA
	780.01		COMA
	780.03		PERSISTENT VEGETATIVE STATE
	806		FX VERT COLUMN W/ SPINAL CORD INJURY
	851		CEREBRAL LACERATION AND CONTUSION
	852		SUBARACH SUB & XTRADURL HEMOR FLW INJ
	853		OTH & UNS INTRACRAN HEMOR FLW INJURY
	854		INTRACRAN INJURY OTH & UNSPEC NATURE
	907		LATE EFFECTS INJURIES NERVOUS SYS
	952		SP CRD INJR W/O EVIDENCE SP BN INJR
Neuro 2—Peripheral Neurological Disorders	138		LATE EFFECT ACUTE POLIO
	332		PARKINSONS DISEASE
	333		OTH XTRAPYRAMIDAL DZ & ABN MOVMNT D/O
	334.0		FRIEDREICH'S ATAXIA
	334.2		PRIMARY CEREBELLAR DEGEN

Continued

TABLE 2B—CONT'D

	334.3		CEREBELLAR ATAXIA NEC
	334.4	M	CEREBEL ATAX IN OTH DIS
	334.8		SPINOCEREBELLAR DIS NEC
	337.0		IDIOPATH PERIPH AUTONOM NEUROPATHY
	337.1	M	PRIPHERL AUTONOMIC NEUROPTHY D/O CE
	337.20		UNSPEC REFLEX SYMPATHETIC DYSTROPHY
	337.21		REFLX SYMPATHET DYSTROPHY UP LIMB
	337.22		REFLX SYMPATHET DYSTROPHY LOW LIMB
	337.29		REFLX SYMPATHET DYSTROPHY OTH SITE
	337.9		UNSPEC DISORDER AUTONOM NERV SYSTEM
	343		INFANTILE CEREBRAL PALSY
	344.2		DIPLEGIA OF BOTH UPPER LIMBS
	352		DISORDERS OF OTHER CRANIAL NERVES
	353.0		BRACHIAL PLEXUS LESION
	353.1		LUMBOSACRAL PLEXUS LESION
	353.5		NEURALGIC AMYLOTROPHY
	354.5		MONONEURITIS MULTIPLEX
	355.2		OTHER LESION OF FEMORAL NERVE
	355.9		LESION OF SCIATIC NERVE

	356		HEREDIT & IDIOPATH PERIPH NEUROPATHY
	357.0		ACUTE INFECTIVE POLYNEURITIS
	357.1	M	POLYNEUROPATHY COLL VASC DISEASE
	357.3	M	POLYNEUROPATHY IN MALIGNANT DISEASE
	357.4	M	POLYNEUROPATHY OTH DZ CLASS ELSW
	357.5		ALCOHOLIC POLYNEUROPATHY
	357.6		POLYNEUROPATHY DUE TO DRUGS
	357.7		POLYNEUROPATHY DUE OTH TOXIC AGENTS
	357.81		CHRONIC INFLAMMATORY DEMYELINATING POLYNEURITIS
	357.82		CRIT ILLNESS NEUROPATHY
	357.89		INFLAM/TOX NEUROPATHY
	358.00		MYASTHENIA GRAVIS W/O ACUTE
	358.01		MYASTHENIA GRAVIS W/ACUTE
	358.1	M	MYASTHENIC SYNDROMES DZ CLASS ELSW
	358.2		TOXIC MYONEURAL DISORDERS
	359.0		CONGEN HEREDIT MUSCULAR DYSTROPHY
	359.1		HEREDITARY PROGRESSIVE MUSC DYSTROPH
	359.3		PERIODIC PARALYSIS
	359.4		TOXIC MYOPATHY
	359.5	M	MYOPATHY ENDOCRINE DZ CLASS ELSW

Continued

TABLE 2B—CONT'D			
	359.6	M	SX INFLAM MYOPATHY DZ CLASS ELSW
	359.81		CRITICAL ILLNESS MYOPATHY
	359.89		OTHER MYOPATHIES
	386.00		MÉNIÉRE'S DISEASE, UNSPECIFIED, MÉNIÉRE'S DISEASE (ACTIVE)
	386.01		ACTIVE MÉNIÉRE'S DISEASE, COCHLEOVES-TIBULAR
	386.02		ACTIVE MÉNIÉRE'S DISEASE, COCHLEAR
	386.03		ACTIVE MÉNIÉRE'S DISEASE, VESTIBULAR
	386.2		VERTIGO OF CENTRAL ORIGIN
	386.30		LABYRINTHITIS, UNSPECIFIED
	386.31		SEROUS LABYRINTHITIS, DIFFUSE LABYRINTHITIS
	386.32		CIRCUMSCRIBED LABYRINTHITIS, FOCAL LABYRINTHITIS
	386.33		SUPPURATIVE LABYRINTHITIS, PURULENT LABYRINTHITIS
	386.34		TOXIC LABYRINTHITIS
	386.35		VIRAL LABYRINTHITIS
	392		RHEUMATIC CHOREA
	953		INJURY TO NERVE ROOTS & SPINAL PLEXUS
	954		INJR OTH NRV TRNK NO SHLDR & PLV GIRD
	955.8		INJR PERIPH NRV SHLDR GIRDL & UP LIMB

D

	956.0		INJR TO SCIATIC NERVE
	956.1		INJ TO FEMORAL NERVE
	956.8		INJR TO MULTIPLE PELVIC AND LE NERVES
Neuro 3—Stroke	342		HEMIPLEGIA AND HEMIPARESIS
	344.30		MONOPLEGIA OF LOWER LIMB, AFFECTING UNSPECIFIED SIDE
	344.31		MONOPLEGIA OF LOWER LIMB, AFFECTING DOMINANT SIDE
	344.32		MONOPLEGIA OF LOWER LIMB, AFFECTING NONDOMINANT SIDE
	344.40		MONOPLEGIA OF UPPER LIMB, AFFECTING UNSPECIFIED SIDE
	344.41		MONOPLEGIA OF UPPER LIMB, AFFECTING DOMINANT SIDE
	344.42		MONOPLEGIA OF UPPER LIMB, AFFECTING NONDOMINANT SIDE
	344.60		CAUDA EQUINA SYNDROME, WITHOUT MENTION OF NEUROGENIC BLADDER
	344.61		CAUDA EQUINA SYNDROME, WITH NEUROGENIC BLADDER
	438		LATE EFF CEREBROVASCULAR DZ

Continued

TABLE 2B—CONT'D			
	781.8		NEURO NEGLECT SYNDROME
Neuro 4—Multiple Sclerosis	340		MULTIPLE SCLEROSIS
	341.0		NEUROMYELITIS OPTICA
	341.1		SCHILDER'S DISEASE
	341.20		ACUTE (TRANSVERSE) MYELITIS NOS
	341.21	M	ACUTE (TRANSVERSE) MYELITIS IN CONDITIONS CLASSIFIED ELSEWHERE
	341.22		IDIOPATHIC TRANSVERSE MYELITIS
	341.8		OTHER DEMYELINATING DISEASES OF CENTRAL NERVOUS SYSTEM
	341.9		DEMYELINATING DISEASE OF CENTRAL NERVOUS SYSTEM, UNSPECIFIED
Ortho 1—Leg Disorders	711.05		PYOGEN ARTHRITIS—PELVIS
	711.06		PYOGEN ARTHRITIS—L/LEG
	711.07		PYOGEN ARTHRITIS—ANKLE
	711.15	M	REITER ARTHRITIS—PELVIS
	711.16	M	REITER ARTHRITIS—L/LEG
	711.17	M	REITER ARTHRITIS—ANKLE
	711.25	M	BEHCET ARTHRITIS—PELVIS
	711.26	M	BEHCET ARTHRITIS—L/LEG

	711.27	M	BEHCET ARTHRITIS—ANKLE
	711.35	M	DYSENTER ARTHRIT—PELVIS
	711.36	M	DYSENTER ARTHRIT—L/LEG
	711.37	M	DYSENTER ARTHRIT—ANKLE
	711.45	M	BACT ARTHRITIS—PELVIS
	711.46	M	BACT ARTHRITIS—L/LEG
	711.47	M	BACT ARTHRITIS—ANKLE
	711.55	M	VIRAL ARTHRITIS—PELVIS
	711.56	M	VIRAL ARTHRITIS—L/LEG
	711.57	M	VIRAL ARTHRITIS—ANKLE
	711.65	M	MYCOTIC ARTHRITIS—PELVI
	711.66	M	MYCOTIC ARTHRITIS—L/LEG
	711.67	M	MYCOTIC ARTHRITIS—ANKLE
	711.75	M	HELMINTH ARTHRIT—PELVIS
	711.76	M	HELMINTH ARTHRIT—L/LEG
	711.77	M	HELMINTH ARTHRIT—ANKLE
	711.85	M	INF ARTHRITIS NEC—PELVI
	711.86	M	INF ARTHRITIS NEC—L/LEG
	711.87	M	INF ARTHRITIS NEC—ANKLE
	711.95		INF ARTHRIT NOS—PELVIS
	711.96		INF ARTHRIT NOS—L/LEG

Continued

TABLE 2B—CONT'D			
	711.97		INF ARTHRIT NOS—ANKLE
	712.15	M	DICALC PHOS CRYST—PELVI
	712.16	M	DICALC PHOS CRYST—L/LEG
	712.17	M	DICALC PHOS CRYST—ANKLE
	712.25	M	PYROPHOSPH CRYST—PELVIS
	712.26	M	PYROPHOSPH CRYST—L/LEG
	712.27	M	PYROPHOSPH CRYST—ANKLE
	712.35	M	CHONDROCALCIN NOS—PELVI
	712.36	M	CHONDROCALCIN NOS—L/LEG
	712.37	M	CHONDROCALCIN NOS—ANKLE
	712.85		CRYST ARTHROP NEC—PELVI
	712.86		CRYST ARTHROP NEC—L/LEG
	712.87		CRYST ARTHROP NEC—ANKLE
	716.05		KASCHIN-BECK DIS—PELVIS
	716.06		KASCHIN-BECK DIS—L/LEG
	716.07		KASCHIN-BECK DIS—ANKLE
	716.15		TRAUM ARTHROPATHY—PELVIS
	716.16		TRAUM ARTHROPATHY—L/LEG
	716.17		TRAUM ARTHROPATHY—ANKLE
	716.25		ALLERG ARTHRITIS—PELVIS

	716.26		ALLERG ARTHRITIS—L/LEG
	716.27		ALLERG ARTHRITIS—ANKLE
	716.35		CLIMACT ARTHRITIS—PELVIS
	716.36		CLIMACT ARTHRITIS—L/LEG
	716.37		CLIMACT ARTHRITIS—ANKLE
	716.45		TRANS ARTHROPATHY—PELVIS
	716.46		TRANS ARTHROPATHY—L/LEG
	716.47		TRANS ARTHROPATHY—ANKLE
	716.85		ARTHROPATHY NEC—PELVIS
	716.86		ARTHROPATHY NEC—L/LEG
	716.87		ARTHROPATHY NEC—ANKLE
	717		INTERNAL DERANGEMENT OF KNEE
	718.05		ART CARTIL DISORDER PELVIS AND THIGH
	718.07		ART CARTIL DIS ANKLE FOOT
	718.15		LOOSE BODY—PELVIS
	718.17		LOOSE BODY—ANKLE
	718.25		PATHOLOGIC DISLOCATION PELVIS AND THIGH
	718.26		PATHOLOGIC DISLOCATION LOWER LEG
	718.27		PATHOLOGIC DISLOCATION ANKLE FOOT

Continued

TABLE 2B—CONT'D			
	718.35		RECURRENT DISLOCATION PELVIS AND THIGH
	718.36		RECURRENT DISLOCATION LOW LEG
	718.37		RECURRENT DISLOCATION ANKLE FOOT
	718.45		CONTRACTURE PELVIS AND THIGH
	718.46		CONTRACTURE LOWER LEG
	718.47		CONTRACTURE OF JOINT ANKLE FOOT
	718.55		ANKYLOSIS OF PELVIS AND THIGH
	718.56		ANKYLOSIS OF LOWER LEG
	718.57		ANKYLOSIS OF JOINT ANKLE FOOT
	718.75		DEVELOPMENTAL DISLOCATION OF JOINT -PELVIC REGION AND THIGH
	718.76		DEVELOPMENTAL DISLOCATION OF JOINT—LOWER LEG
	718.77		DEVELOPMENTAL DISLOCATION OF JOINT—ANKLE AND FOOT
	719.15		HEMARTHROSIS PELVIS AND THIGH
	719.16		HEMARTHROSIS LOWER LEG
	719.17		HEMARTHROSIS ANKLE AND FOOT
	719.25		VILLONODULAR SYNOVITIS PELVIS AND THIGH

	719.26		VILLONODULAR SYNOVITIS LOWER LEG
	719.27		VILLONODULAR SYNOVITIS ANKLE AND FOOT
	719.35		PALANDROMIC RHEUMATISM PELVIS AND THIGH
	719.36		PALANDROMIC RHEUMATISM LOWER LEG
	719.37		PALANDROMIC RHEUMATISM ANKLE AND FOOT
	727.65		RUPTURE OF TENDON QUADRACEPS
	727.66		RUPTURE OF TENDON PATELLAR
	727.67		RUPTURE OF TENDON ACHILLES
	727.68		RUPTURE OTHER TENDONS FOOT AND ANKLE
	730.05		AC OSTEOMYELITIS—PELVIS
	730.06		AC OSTEOMYELITIS—L/LEG
	730.07		AC OSTEOMYELITIS—ANKLE
	730.15		CHR OSTEOMYELIT—PELVIS
	730.16		CHR OSTEOMYELIT—L/LEG
	730.17		CHR OSTEOMYELIT—ANKLE
	730.25		OSTEOMYELITIS NOS—PELVI
	730.26		OSTEOMYELITIS NOS—L/LEG
	730.27		OSTEOMYELITIS NOS—ANKLE
	730.35		PERIOSTITIS—PELVIS

Continued

TABLE 2B—CONT'D			
	730.36		PERIOSTITIS—L/LEG
	730.37		PERIOSTITIS—ANKLE
	730.75	M	POLIO OSTEOPATHY—PELVIS
	730.76	M	POLIO OSTEOPATHY—L/LEG
	730.77	M	POLIO OSTEOPATHY—ANKLE
	730.85	M	BONE INFECT NEC—PELVIS
	730.86	M	BONE INFECT NEC—L/LEG
	730.87	M	BONE INFECT NEC—ANKLE
	730.95		BONE INFECT NOS—PELVIS
	730.96		BONE INFECT NOS—L/LEG
	730.97		BONE INFECT NOS—ANKLE
	733.14		PATHOLOGIC FRACTURE OF NECK OF FEMUR
	733.15		PATHOLOGIC FRACTURE OF FEMUR
	733.16		PATHOLOGIC FRACTURE OF TIBIA OR FIBULA
	733.42		ASEPTIC NECROSIS OF HEAD AND NECK OF FEMUR
	733.43		ASEPTIC NECROSIS OF MEDIAL FEMORAL CONDYLE
	808		FRACTURE OF PELVIS
	820		FRACTURE OF NECK OF FEMUR
	821		FRACTURE OTHER & UNSPEC PARTS FEMUR
	822		FRACTURE OF PATELLA

D

	823		FRACTURE OF TIBIA AND FIBULA
	824		FRACTURE OF ANKLE
	825		FRACTURE 1/MORE TARSAL & MT BNS
	827		OTH MX & ILL-DEFINED FX LOWER LIMB
	828		MX FX LEGS—LEG W/ ARM—LEGS W/RIBS
	835		DISLOCATION OF HIP
	836		DISLOCATION OF KNEE
	897		TRAUMATIC AMPUTATION OF LEG
	928		CRUSHING INJURY OF LOWER LIMB
Ortho 2—Other Orthopedic Disorders	711.01		PYOGEN ARTHRITIS—SHLDER
	711.02		PYOGEN ARTHRITIS—UP/ARM
	711.03		PYOGEN ARTHRITIS—FOREAR
	711.04		PYOGEN ARTHRITIS—HAND
	711.08		PYOGEN ARTHRITIS NEC
	711.09		PYOGEN ARTHRITIS—MULT
	711.10	M	REITER ARTHRITIS—UNSPEC
	711.11	M	REITER ARTHRITIS—SHLDER
	711.12	M	REITER ARTHRITIS—UP/ARM
	711.13	M	REITER ARTHRITIS—FOREAR
	711.14	M	REITER ARTHRITIS—HAND
	711.18	M	REITER ARTHRITIS NEC
	711.19	M	REITER ARTHRITIS—MULT

Continued

D

TABLE 2B—CONT'D			
	711.20	M	BEHCET ARTHRITIS—UNSPEC
	711.21	M	BEHCET ARTHRITIS—SHLDER
	711.22	M	BEHCET ARTHRITIS—UP/ARM
	711.23	M	BEHCET ARTHRITIS—FOREAR
	711.24	M	BEHCET ARTHRITIS—HAND
	711.28	M	BEHCET ARTHRITIS NEC
	711.29	M	BEHCET ARTHRITIS—MULT
	711.30	M	DYSENTER ARTHRIT—UNSPEC
	711.31	M	DYSENTER ARTHRIT—SHLDER
	711.32	M	DYSENTER ARTHRIT—UP/ARM
	711.33	M	DYSENTER ARTHRIT—FOREAR
	711.34	M	DYSENTER ARTHRIT—HAND
	711.38	M	DYSENTER ARTHRIT NEC
	711.39	M	DYSENTER ARTHRIT—MULT
	711.40	M	BACT ARTHRITIS—UNSPEC
	711.41	M	BACT ARTHRITIS—SHLDER
	711.42	M	BACT ARTHRITIS—UP/ARM
	711.43	M	BACT ARTHRITIS—FOREARM
	711.44	M	BACT ARTHRITIS—HAND
	711.48	M	BACT ARTHRITIS NEC
	711.49	M	BACT ARTHRITIS—MULT

	711.50	M	VIRAL ARTHRITIS—UNSPEC
	711.51	M	VIRAL ARTHRITIS—SHLDER
	711.52	M	VIRAL ARTHRITIS—UP/ARM
	711.53	M	VIRAL ARTHRITIS—FOREARM
	711.54	M	VIRAL ARTHRITIS—HAND
	711.58	M	VIRAL ARTHRITIS NEC
	711.59	M	VIRAL ARTHRITIS—MULT
	711.60	M	MYCOTIC ARTHRITIS—UNSPE
	711.61	M	MYCOTIC ARTHRITIS—SHLDE
	711.62	M	MYCOTIC ARTHRITIS—UP/AR
	711.63	M	MYCOTIC ARTHRIT—FOREARM
	711.64	M	MYCOTIC ARTHRITIS—HAND
	711.68	M	MYCOTIC ARTHRITIS NEC
	711.69	M	MYCOTIC ARTHRITIS—MULT
	711.70	M	HELMINTH ARTHRIT—UNSPEC
	711.71	M	HELMINTH ARTHRIT—SHLDER
	711.72	M	HELMINTH ARTHRIT—UP/ARM
	711.73	M	HELMINTH ARTHRIT—FOREAR
	711.74	M	HELMINTH ARTHRIT—HAND
	711.78	M	HELMINTH ARTHRIT NEC
	711.79	M	HELMINTH ARTHRIT—MULT
	711.80	M	INF ARTHRITIS NEC—UNSPE

Continued

TABLE 2B—CONT'D			
	711.81	M	INF ARTHRITIS NEC—SHLDE
	711.82	M	INF ARTHRITIS NEC—UP/AR
	711.83	M	INF ARTHRIT NEC—FOREARM
	711.84	M	INF ARTHRITIS NEC—HAND
	711.88	M	INF ARTHRIT NEC—OTH SIT
	711.89	M	INF ARTHRITIS NEC—MULT
	711.90		INF ARTHRITIS NOS—UNSPE
	711.91		INF ARTHRITIS NOS—SHLDE
	711.92		INF ARTHRITIS NOS—UP/AR
	711.93		INF ARTHRIT NOS—FOREARM
	711.94		INF ARTHRIT NOS—HAND
	711.98		INF ARTHRIT NOS—OTH SIT
	711.99		INF ARTHRITIS NOS—MULT
	712.10	M	DICALC PHOS CRYST—UNSPE
	712.11	M	DICALC PHOS CRYST—SHLDE
	712.12	M	DICALC PHOS CRYST—UP/AR
	712.13	M	DICALC PHOS CRYS—FOREAR
	712.14	M	DICALC PHOS CRYST—HAND
	712.18	M	DICALC PHOS CRY—SITE NE
	712.19	M	DICALC PHOS CRYST—MULT
	712.20	M	PYROPHOSPH CRYST—UNSPEC

	712.21	M	PYROPHOSPH CRYST—SHLDER
	712.22	M	PYROPHOSPH CRYST—UP/ARM
	712.23	M	PYROPHOSPH CRYST—FOREAR
	712.24	M	PYROPHOSPH CRYST—HAND
	712.28	M	PYROPHOS CRYST—SITE NEC
	712.29	M	PYROPHOS CRYST—MULT
	712.30	M	CHONDROCALCIN NOS—UNSPE
	712.31	M	CHONDROCALCIN NOS—SHLDE
	712.32	M	CHONDROCALCIN NOS—UP/AR
	712.33	M	CHONDROCALC NOS—FOREARM
	712.34	M	CHONDROCALCIN NOS—HAND
	712.38	M	CHONDROCALC NOS—OTH SIT
	712.39	M	CHONDROCALCIN NOS—MULT
	712.80		CRYST ARTHROP NEC—UNSPE
	712.81		CRYST ARTHROP NEC—SHLDE
	712.82		CRYST ARTHROP NEC—UP/AR
	712.83		CRYS ARTHROP NEC—FOREAR
	712.84		CRYST ARTHROP NEC—HAND
	712.88		CRY ARTHROP NEC—OTH SIT
	712.89		CRYST ARTHROP NEC—MULT
	713.0	M	ARTHROP W ENDOCR/MET DI

Continued

TABLE 2B—CONT'D			
	713.1	M	ARTHROP W NONINF GI DIS
	713.2	M	ARTHROPATH W HEMATOL DI
	713.3	M	ARTHROPATHY W SKIN DIS
	713.4	M	ARTHROPATHY W RESP DIS
	713.5	M	ARTHROPATHY W NERVE DIS
	713.6	M	ARTHROP W HYPERSEN REAC
	713.7	M	ARTHROP W SYSTEM DIS NE
	713.8	M	ARTHROP W OTH DIS NEC
	714		RA & OTH INFLAM POLYARTHROPATHIES
	715.15		OSTEOARTHROSIS, LOCALIZED, PRIMARY, PELVIS AND THIGH
	715.16		OSTEOARTHROSIS, LOCALIZED, PRIMARY, LOWER LEG
	715.25		OSTEOARTHROSIS, LOCALIZED, SECONDARY, PELVIS AND THIGH
	715.26		OSTEOARTHROSIS, LOCALIZED, SECONDARY, LOWER LEG
	715.35		OSTEOARTHROSIS, LOCALIZED, NOT SPEC PRIMARY OR SECONDARY, PELVIS AND THIGH
	715.36		OSTEOARTHROSIS, LOCALIZED, NOT SPEC PRIMARY OR SECONDARY, LOWER LEG

	715.95		OSTEOARTHROSIS, UNSPECIFIED, PELVIS AND THIGH
	715.96		OSTEOARTHROSIS, UNSPECIFIED, LOWER LEG
	716.00		KASCHIN-BECK DIS—UNSPEC
	716.01		KASCHIN-BECK DIS—SHLDER
	716.02		KASCHIN-BECK DIS—UP/ARM
	716.03		KASCHIN-BECK DIS—FOREARM
	716.04		KASCHIN-BECK DIS—HAND
	716.08		KASCHIN-BECK DIS NEC
	716.09		KASCHIN-BECK DIS—MULT
	716.10		TRAUM ARTHROPATHY—UNSPEC
	716.11		TRAUM ARTHROPATHY—SHLDER
	716.12		TRAUM ARTHROPATHY—UP/ARM
	716.13		TRAUM ARTHROPATH—FOREARM
	716.14		TRAUM ARTHROPATHY—HAND
	716.18		TRAUM ARTHROPATHY NEC
	716.19		TRAUM ARTHROPATHY—MULT
	716.20		ALLERG ARTHRITIS—UNSPEC
	716.21		ALLERG ARTHRITIS—SHLDER

Continued

D

TABLE 2B—CONT'D			
	716.22		ALLERG ARTHRITIS—UP/ARM
	716.23		ALLERG ARTHRITIS—FOREARM
	716.24		ALLERG ARTHRITIS—HAND
	716.28		ALLERG ARTHRITIS NEC
	716.29		ALLERG ARTHRITIS—MULT
	716.30		CLIMACT ARTHRITIS—UNSPEC
	716.31		CLIMACT ARTHRITIS—SHLDER
	716.32		CLIMACT ARTHRITIS—UP/ARM
	716.33		CLIMACT ARTHRIT—FOREARM
	716.34		CLIMACT ARTHRITIS—HAND
	716.38		CLIMACT ARTHRITIS NEC
	716.39		CLIMACT ARTHRITIS—MULT
	716.40		TRANS ARTHROPATHY—UNSPEC
	716.41		TRANS ARTHROPATHY—SHLDER
	716.42		TRANS ARTHROPATHY—UP/ARM
	716.43		TRANS ARTHROPATH—FOREARM
	716.44		TRANS ARTHROPATHY—HAND
	716.48		TRANS ARTHROPATHY NEC
	716.49		TRANS ARTHROPATHY—MULT

	716.80		ARTHROPATHY NEC—UNSPEC
	716.81		ARTHROPATHY NEC—SHLDER
	716.82		ARTHROPATHY NEC—UP/ARM
	716.83		ARTHROPATHY NEC—FOREARM
	716.84		ARTHROPATHY NEC—HAND
	716.88		ARTHROPATHY NEC—OTH SITE
	716.89		ARTHROPATHY NEC—MULT
	718.01		ART CARTIL DISORDER SHOULDER
	718.02		ART CARTIL DIS UPPER ARM
	718.03		ART CARTIL DIS FOREARM
	718.04		ART CARTIL DIS HAND
	718.08		ART CART DIS OTH SITES
	718.09		ART CART DIS MULT
	718.10		LOOSE BODY—UNSPEC
	718.11		LOOSE BODY—SHLDER
	718.12		LOOSE BODY—UP/ARM
	718.13		LOOSE BODY—FOREARM
	718.14		LOOSE BODY—HAND
	718.18		LOOSE BODY—JOINT NEC
	718.19		LOOSE BODY—MULT JOINTS
	718.20		PATHOLOGIC DISLOCATION UNSPEC SITE
	718.21		PATHOLOGIC DISLOCATION SHOULDER
	718.22		PATHOLOGIC DISLOCATION UPPER ARM

Continued

TABLE 2B—CONT'D			
	718.23		PATHOLOGIC DISLOCATION FOREARM
	718.24		PATHOLOGIC DISLOCATION HAND
	718.28		PATHOLOGIC DISLOCATION OTH LOC
	718.29		PATHOLOGIC DISLOCATION MULT LOC
	718.30		RECURRENT DISLOCATION UNSPEC SITE
	718.31		RECURRENT DISLOCATION SHOULDER
	718.32		RECURRENT DISLOCATION UPPER ARM
	718.33		RECURRENT DISLOCATION FOREARM
	718.34		RECURRENT DISLOCATION HAND
	718.38		RECURRENT DISLOCATION OTH LOC
	718.39		RECURRENT DISLOCATION MULT LOC
	718.40		CONTRACTURE OF JOINT UNSPEC SITE
	718.41		CONTRACTURE SHOULDER
	718.42		CONTRACTURE OF JOINT UPPER ARM
	718.43		CONTRACTURE OF JOINT FOREARM
	718.44		CONTRACTURE OF JOINT HAND

	718.48		CONTRACTURE OF JOINT OTH LOC
	718.49		CONTRACTURE OF JOINT MULT LOC
	718.50		ANKYLOSIS OF JOINT UNSPEC SITE
	718.51		ANKYLOSIS OF SHOULDER
	718.52		ANKYLOSIS OF JOINT UPPER ARM
	718.53		ANKYLOSIS OF JOINT FOREARM
	718.54		ANKYLOSIS OF JOINT HAND
	718.58		ANKYLOSIS OF JOINT OTH LOC
	718.59		ANKYLOSIS OF JOINT MULT LOC
	718.60		UNSPEC INTRAPELVIC PROTRUSION ACETAB
	718.70		DEVELOPMENTAL DISLOCATION OF JOINT—SITE UNSPECIFIED
	718.71		DEVELOPMENTAL DISLOCATION OF JOINT—SHOULDER REGION
	718.72		DEVELOPMENTAL DISLOCATION OF JOINT—UPPER ARM
	718.73		DEVELOPMENTAL DISLOCATION OF JOINT—FOREARM
	718.74		DEVELOPMENTAL DISLOCATION OF JOINT—HAND
	718.78		DEVELOPMENTAL DISLOCATION OF JOINT—OTHER SPECIFIED SITES

Continued

TABLE 2B—CONT'D			
	718.79		DEVELOPMENTAL DISLOCATION OF JOINT—MULTIPLE SITES
	719.10		HEMARTHROSIS UNSPECIFIED SITE
	719.11		HEMARTHROSIS SHOULDER
	719.12		HEMARTHROSIS UPPER ARM
	719.13		HEMARTHROSIS FOREARM
	719.14		HEMARTHROSIS HAND
	719.18		HEMARTHROSIS OTHER SPECIFIED
	719.19		HEMARTHROSIS MULTIPLE SITES
	719.20		VILLONODULAR SYNOVITIS UNSPECIFIED SITE
	719.21		VILLONODULAR SYNOVITIS SHOULDER
	719.22		VILLONODULAR SYNOVITIS UPPER ARM
	719.23		VILLONODULAR SYNOVITIS FOREARM
	719.24		VILLONODULAR SYNOVITIS HAND
	719.28		VILLONODULAR SYNOVITIS OTHER SITES
	719.29		VILLONODULAR SYNOVITIS MULTIPLE SITES
	719.30		PALANDROMIC RHEUMATISM UNSPECIFIED SITE
	719.31		PALANDROMIC RHEUMATISM SHOULDER

	719.32		PALANDROMIC RHEUMATISM UPPER ARM
	719.33		PALANDROMIC RHEUMATISM FOREARM
	719.34		PALANDROMIC RHEUMATISM HAND
	719.38		PALANDROMIC RHEUMATISM OTHER SITES
	719.39		PALANDROMIC RHEUMATISM MULTIPLE SITES
	720.0		ANKYLOSING SPONDYLITIS
	720.1		SPINAL ENTHESOPATHY
	720.2		SACROILIITIS NEC
	720.81	M	SPONDYLOPATHY IN OTH DI
	720.89		OTHER INFLAMMATORY SPONDYLOPATHIES
	720.9		UNSPEC INFLAMMATORY SPONDYLOPATHY
	721		SPONDYLOSIS AND ALLIED DISORDERS
	722 except 722.3x		INTERVERTEBRAL DISC DISORDERS
	723.0		SPINAL STENOSIS OF CERVICAL REGION
	723.2		CERVICOCRANIAL SYNDROME
	723.3		CERVICOBRACHIAL SYNDROME
	723.4		BRACHIA NEURITIS OR RADICULITIS
	723.5		TORTICOLLIS, UNSPECIFIED

Continued

TABLE 2B—CONT'D			
	723.7		OSSIFICATION OF POSTERIOR LONGITUDINAL LIGAMENT IN CERVICAL REGION
	724.00		SPINAL STENOSIS NOS
	724.01		SPINAL STENOSIS—THORACIC
	724.02		SPINAL STENOSIS—LUMBAR
	724.09		SPINAL STENOSIS—OTH SITE
	724.3		SCIATICA
	724.4		LUMBOSACRAL NEURITIS NOS
	724.6		DISORDERS OF SACRUM
	725		POLYMYALGIA RHEUMATICA
	726.0		ADHESIVE CAPSULITIS
	726.10		DISORDERS OF BURSAE AND TENDONS
	726.11		CALCIFYING TENDINITIS
	726.12		BICIPITAL TENOSYNOVITIS
	726.19		ROTATOR CUFF SYNDROME OTHER
	727.61		COMPLETE RUPTURE OF ROTATOR CUFF
	728.0		INFECTIVE MYOSITIS
	728.10		CALCIFICATION AND OSSIFICATION, UNSPECIFIED
	728.11		PROGRESSIVE MYOSITIS OSSIFICANS
	728.12		TRAUMATIC MYOSITIS OSSIFICATIONS
	728.13		POST OP HETEROTOPIC CALCIFICATION

	728.19		OTHER MUSCULAR CALCIFICATION AND OSSIFICATION
	728.6		CONTRACTURE OF PALMAR FASCIA
	730.00		AC OSTEOMYELITIS—UNSPEC
	730.01		AC OSTEOMYELITIS—SHLDER
	730.02		AC OSTEOMYELITIS—UP/ARM
	730.03		AC OSTEOMYELITIS—FOREAR
	730.04		AC OSTEOMYELITIS—HAND
	730.08		AC OSTEOMYELITIS NEC
	730.09		AC OSTEOMYELITIS—MULT
	730.10		CHR OSTEOMYELITIS—UNSP
	730.11		CHR OSTEOMYELIT—SHLDER
	730.12		CHR OSTEOMYELIT—UP/ARM
	730.13		CHR OSTEOMYELIT—FOREARM
	730.14		CHR OSTEOMYELIT—HAND
	730.18		CHR OSTEOMYELIT NEC
	730.19		CHR OSTEOMYELIT—MULT
	730.20		OSTEOMYELITIS NOS—UNSPE
	730.21		OSTEOMYELITIS NOS—SHLDE
	730.22		OSTEOMYELITIS NOS—UP/AR
	730.23		OSTEOMYELIT NOS—FOREARM
	730.24		OSTEOMYELITIS NOS—HAND

Continued

TABLE 2B—CONT'D			
	730.28		OSTEOMYELIT NOS—OTH SIT
	730.29		OSTEOMYELITIS NOS—MULT
	730.30		PERIOSTITIS—UNSPEC
	730.31		PERIOSTITIS—SHLDER
	730.32		PERIOSTITIS—UP/ARM
	730.33		PERIOSTITIS—FOREARM
	730.34		PERIOSTITIS—HAND
	730.38		PERIOSTITIS NEC
	730.39		PERIOSTITIS—MULT
	730.70	M	POLIO OSTEOPATHY—UNSPEC
	730.71	M	POLIO OSTEOPATHY—SHLDER
	730.72	M	POLIO OSTEOPATHY—UP/ARM
	730.73	M	POLIO OSTEOPATHY—FOREAR
	730.74	M	POLIO OSTEOPATHY—HAND
	730.78	M	POLIO OSTEOPATHY NEC
	730.79	M	POLIO OSTEOPATHY—MULT
	730.80	M	BONE INFECT NEC—UNSPEC
	730.81	M	BONE INFECT NEC—SHLDER
	730.82	M	BONE INFECT NEC—UP/ARM
	730.83	M	BONE INFECT NEC—FOREARM
	730.84	M	BONE INFECT NEC—HAND
	730.88	M	BONE INFECT NEC—OTH SIT
	730.89	M	BONE INFECT NEC—MULT
	730.90		BONE INFEC NOS—UNSP SIT

	730.91		BONE INFECT NOS—SHLDER
	730.92		BONE INFECT NOS—UP/ARM
	730.93		BONE INFECT NOS—FOREARM
	730.94		BONE INFECT NOS—HAND
	730.98		BONE INFECT NOS—OTH SIT
	730.99		BONE INFECT NOS—MULT
	731.0		OSTEITIS DEFORMANS W/O BN TUMR
	731.1	M	OSTEITIS DEFORMANS DZ CLASS ELSW
	731.2		HYPERTROPH PULM OSTEOARTHROPATHY
	731.8	M	OTH BONE INVOLVEMENT DZ CLASS ELSW
	732		OSTEOCHONDRO-PATHIES
	733.10		PATHOLOGIC FRACTURE UNSPEC
	733.11		PATHOLOGIC FRACTURE HUMERUS
	733.12		PATHOLOGIC FRACTURE DISTAL RADIUS ULNA
	733.13		PATHOLOGIC FRACTURE OF VERTEBRAE
	733.19		PATHOLOGIC FRACTURE OTH SPEC SITE
	800		FRACTURE OF VAULT OF SKULL
	801		FRACTURE OF BASE OF SKULL
	802		FRACTURE OF FACE BONES

Continued

D

TABLE 2B—CONT'D			
	803		OTHER & UNQUALIFIED SKULL FRACTURES
	804		MX FX INVLV SKULL/ FACE W/OTH BNS
	805		FX VERT COLUMN W/O SP CRD INJR
	807		FRACTURE RIB STERNUM LARYNX & TRACHEA
	809		ILL-DEFINED FRACTURES BONES TRUNK
	810		FRACTURE OF CLAVICLE
	811		FRACTURE OF SCAPULA
	812		FRACTURE OF HUMERUS
	813		FRACTURE OF RADIUS AND ULNA
	814		FRACTURE OF CARPAL BONE
	815		FRACTURE OF METACARPAL BONE
	816		FRACTURE ONE OR MORE PHALANGES HAND
	817		MULTIPLE FRACTURES OF HAND BONES
	818		ILL-DEFINED FRACTURES OF UPPER LIMB
	819		MX FX UP LIMBS & LIMBS W/RIB & STERNUM
	831		DISLOCATION OF SHOULDER
	832		DISLOCATION OF ELBOW
	833		DISLOCATION OF WRIST

	837		DISLOCATION OF ANKLE
	838		DISLOCATION OF FOOT
	846		SPRAINS & STRAINS SACROILIAC REGION
	847		SPRAINS & STRAINS OTH & UNS PART BACK
Psych 1—Affective and Other Psychoses, Depression	295		SCHIZOPHRENIA
	296.0x except 296.06		BIPOLAR I DISORDER, SINGLE MANIC EPISODE
	296.1x except 296.16		MANIC DISORDER, RECURRENT EPISODE
	296.2x except 296.26		MAJOR DEPRESSIVE DISORDER, SINGLE EPISODE
	296.3x except 296.36		MAJOR DEPRESSIVE DISORDER RECURRENT EPISODE
	296.4x except 296.46		BIPOLAR I DISORDER, MOST RECENT EPISODE (OR CURRENT) MANIC
	296.5x except 296.56		BIPOLAR I DISORDER, MOST RECENT EPISODE (OR CURRENT) DEPRESSED
	296.6x except 296.66		BIPOLAR I DISORDER, MOST RECENT EPISODE (OR CURRENT) MIXED
	296.7		BIPOLAR I DISORDER, MOST RECENT EPISODE (OR CURRENT) UNSPECIFIED

Continued

TABLE 2B—CONT'D			
	296.80		BIPOLAR DISORDER, UNSPECIFIED
	296.81		ATYPICAL MANIC DISORDER
	296.82		ATYPICAL DEPRESSIVE DISORDER
	296.89		OTHER AND UNSPECIFIED BIPOLAR DISORDERS
	296.90		UNSPECIFIED EPISODIC MOOD DISORDER
	296.99		OTHER SPECIFIED EPISODIC MOOD DISORDER
	297		DELUSIONAL DIS
	298		OTH PSYCHOSES
	311		DEPRESSIVE DISORDER NEC
Psych 2—Degenerative and Other Organic Psychiatric Disorders	290 except 290.8, 290.9		DEMENTIAS
	291.1		ALCOHOL PSYCHOSIS
	291.2		ALCOHOL DEMENTIA
	292.81		DRUG INDUCED DELIRIUM
	292.82		DRUG INDUCED PERSISTING DEMENTIA
	292.83		DRUG INDUCED PERSISTING AMNESTIC DISORDER
	292.84		DRUG INDUCED MOOD DISORDER
	292.85		DRUG INDUCED SLEEP DISORDERS
	292.89		OTHER DEPRESSIVE STATE INDUCED BY DRUGS

	294.0		AMNESTIC DISORD OTH DIS
	294.10	M	DEMENTIA IN COND CLASS ELSW NOS
	294.11	M	DEMENTIA IN COND CLASS ELSW W BEHAV DISTURB
	294.8		MENTAL DISOR NEC OTH DIS
	331.0		ALZHEIMER'S DISEASE
	331.11		PICK'S DISEASE
	331.19		OTH FRONTO-TEMPORAL DEMENTIA
	331.2		SENILE DEGENERAT BRAIN
	331.3		COMMUNICAT HYDROCEPHALUS
	331.4		OBSTRUCTIV HYDROCEPHALUS
	331.5		IDIOPATHIC NORMAL PRESSURE HYDROCEPHALUS (INPH)
	331.7	M	CEREB DEGEN IN OTH DIS
	331.81		REYE'S SYNDROME
	331.82		DEMENTIA WITH LEWY BODIES
	331.89		CEREB DEGENERATION NEC
Pulmonary Disorders	491 except 491.9		CHRONIC BRONCHITIS
	492		EMPHYSEMA
	493.20		CHRONIC OBSTRUCTIVE ASTHMA UNSPECIFIED
	493.21		CHRONIC OBSTRUCTIVE ASTHMA WITH STATUS ASTHMATICUS

Continued

TABLE 2B—CONT'D

	493.22		CHRONIC OBSTRUCTIVE ASTHMA WITH (ACUTE) EXACERBATION
Skin 1—Traumatic Wounds, Burns and Post-operative Complications	870		OPEN WOUND OF OCULAR ADNEXA
	872		OPEN WOUND OF EAR
	873		OTHER OPEN WOUND OF HEAD
	874		OPEN WOUND OF NECK
	875		OPEN WOUND OF CHEST
	876		OPEN WOUND OF BACK
	877		OPEN WOUND OF BUTTOCK
	878		OPEN WND GNT ORGN INCL TRAUMAT AMP
	879		OPEN WOUND OTH & UNSPEC SITE NO LIMBS
	880		OPEN WOUND OF SHOULDER & UPPER ARM
	881		OPEN WOUND OF ELBOW FOREARM & WRIST
	882		OPEN WOUND HAND EXCEPT FINGER ALONE
	883		OPEN WOUND OF FINGER
	884		MX & UNSPEC OPEN WOUND UPPER LIMB

	885		TRAUMATIC AMPUTATION OF THUMB
	886		TRAUMATIC AMPUTATION OTHER FINGER
	887		TRAUMATIC AMPUTATION OF ARM & HAND
	890		OPEN WOUND OF HIP AND THIGH
	891		OPEN WOUND OF KNEE, LEG, AND ANKLE
	892		OPEN WOUND OF FOOT EXCEPT TOE ALONE
	893		OPEN WOUND OF TOE
	894		MX & UNSPEC OPEN WOUND LOWER LIMB
	895		TRAUMATIC AMPUTATION OF TOE
	896		TRAUMATIC AMPUTATION OF FOOT
	927		CRUSHING INJURY OF UPPER LIMB
	941 except 941.0x, 941.1x		BURN OF FACE, HEAD, AND NECK
	942 except 942.0x, 942.1x		BURN OF TRUNK
	943 except 943.0x, 943.1x		BURN OF UPPER LIMB, EXCEPT WRIST AND HAND
	944 except 944.0x, 944.1x		BURN OF WRIST(S) AND HAND(S)

Continued

TABLE 2B—CONT'D			
	945 except 945.0x, 945.1x		BURN OF LOWER LIMB(S)
	946.2		BURNS OF MULTIPLE SPECIFIED SITES, BLISTERS, EPIDERMAL LOSS [SECOND DEGREE]
	946.3		BURNS OF MULTIPLE SPECIFIED SITES, FULL-THICKNESS SKIN LOSS [THIRD DEGREE NOS]
	946.4		BURNS OF MULTIPLE SPECIFIED SITES, DEEP NECROSIS OF UNDERLYING TISSUES [DEEP THIRD DEGREE] WITHOUT MENTION OF LOSS OF A BODY PART
	946.5		BURNS OF MULTIPLE SPECIFIED SITES, DEEP NECROSIS OF UNDERLYING TISSUES [DEEP THIRD DEGREE] WITH LOSS OF A BODY PART
	948		BURNS CLASSIFIED ACCORDING TO THE EXTENT OF BODY SURFACE INVOLVED
	951		INJURY TO OTHER CRANIAL NERVE
	955.0		INJURY TO AXILLARY NERVE
	955.1		INJURY TO MEDIAN NERVE
	955.2		INJURY TO ULNAR NERVE

D

	955.3		INJURY TO RADIAL NERVE
	955.4		INJURY TO MUSCULO-CUTANEOUS NERVE
	955.6		INJURY TO DIGITAL NERVE
	955.7		INJURY TO OTHER SPECIFIED NERVE(S) SHOULDER GIRDLE AND UPPER LIMB
	956.2		INJURY TO POSTERIOR TIBIAL NERVE
	956.3		INJURY TO PERONEAL NERVE
	956.5		INJURY TO OTHER SPECIFIED NERVE(S) OF PELVIC GIRDLE AND LOWER LIMB
	998.11		HEMORRHAGE COMPLICATING A PROCEDURE
	998.12		HEMATOMA COMPLICATING A PROCEDURE
	998.13		SEROMA COMPLICATING A PROCEDURE
	998.2		ACC PUNCT/ LACRATION DURING PROC NEC
	998.31		DISRUPTION OF INTERNAL OPERATION WOUND
	998.32		DISRUPTION OF EXTERNAL OPERATION WOUND
	998.4		FB ACC LEFT DURING PROC NEC
	998.51		INFECTED POSTOPERATIVE SEROMA
	998.59		OTHER POSTOPERATIVE INFECTION

Continued

TABLE 2B—CONT'D			
	998.6		PERSISTENT POSTOPERATIVE FIST NEC
	998.83		NON-HEALING SURGICAL WOUND NEC
Skin 2—Ulcers and Other Skin Conditions	440.23		ATHEROSCLER—ART EXTREM W/ ULCERATION
	440.24		ATHERSCLER—ART EXTREM W/ GANGRENE
	447.2		RUPTURE OF ARTERY
	447.8		ARTERIAL DISEASE NEC
	565		ANAL FISSURE AND FISTULA
	566		ABSCESS OF ANAL AND RECTAL REGIONS
	680		CARBUNCLE AND FURUNCLE
	681.00		FINGER—CELLULITIS AND ABSCESS, UNSPECIFIED
	681.01		FELON
	681.10		TOE—CELLULITIS AND ABSCESS, UNSPECIFIED
	681.9		CELLULITIS AND ABSCESS OF UNSPECIFIED DIGIT
	682		OTHER CELLULITIS AND ABSCESS
	683		ACUTE LYMPHADENITIS
	685		PILONIDAL CYST
	686		OTH LOCAL INF SKIN & SUBCUT TISSUE
	707.10		ULCER OF LOWER LIMB, UNSPECIFIED
	707.11		ULCER OF THIGH
	707.12		ULCER OF CALF

	707.13		ULCER OF ANKLE
	707.14		ULCER OF HEEL AND MIDFOOT
	707.15		ULCER OF OTHER PART OF FOOT
	707.19		ULCER OF OTHER PART OF LOWER LIMB
	707.8		CHRONIC ULCER OTHER SPECIFIED SITE
	707.9		CHRONIC ULCER OF UNSPECIFIED SITE
	785.4	M	GANGRENE
Tracheostomy	V55.0		TRACHEOSTOMY
Urostomy/ Cystostomy	V55.5		CYSTOSTOMY
	V55.6		OTHER ARTIFICIAL OPENING OF URINARY TRACT—NEPHROSTOMY, URETEROSTOMY, URETHROSTOMY

Note: The category codes listed in Table 2b include all the related four- and five-digit codes. "ICD-9-CM Official Guidelines for Coding and Reporting" dictate the following:

A three-digit code is to be used only if it is not further subdivided.

Where fourth-digit subcategories and/or fifth-digit subclassifications are provided, they must be assigned.

A code is invalid if it has not been coded to the full number of digits required for that code.

Codes with three digits are included in ICD-9-CM as the heading of a category of codes that may be further subdivided by the use of fourth and/or fifth digits, which provide greater detail.

Manifestation codes are required when "M" appears in the column. ICD-9-CM guidelines pertaining to multiple coding and sequencing of diagnosis codes apply to OASIS diagnosis items.

For official ICD-9-CM coding guidance, please go to: http://www.cdc.gov/nchs/datawh/ftpserv/ftpicd9/ftpicd9.htm

TABLE 2C

DELETIONS AND ADDITIONS TO TABLE 2B OF THE PROPOSED RULE

ICD-9-CM Codes Deleted	Code Description	Diagnostic Category
286	Coagulation defects	*Blood Disorders*
213.9	Benign neoplasm bone and articular cartilage, site unspecified	*Cancer and Selected Benign Neoplasm*
225.9	Benign nervous system, part unspecified	
230.9	CA IN SITU, other and unspecified digestive organs	
231.9	CA IN SITU, respiratory system, part unspecified	
232.9	CA IN SITU, skin site unspecified	
233.9	CA. IN SITU, other and unspecified urinary organs	
234.9	CA IN SITU site unspecified	
564.00	Constipation unspecified	*Gastrointestinal Disorders*
564.01	Slow transit constipation	
564.02	Dysfunctional constipation	
564.09	Other constipation	
564.9	Unspecified functional disorder of intestine	
569.9	Unspecified disorder of intestine	
410.0x EXCEPT FOR 410.02	Acute myocardial infarction of anterolateral wall, subsequent episode of care	*Heart Disease*
410.1x EXCEPT FOR 410.12	Acute myocardial infarction of other anterior wall, subsequent episode of care.	

410.2x EXCEPT FOR 410.22	Acute myocardial infarction of inferolateral wall, subsequent episode of care	
410.3x EXCEPT FOR 410.32	Acute myocardial infarction of inferoposterior wall, subsequent episode of care	
410.4x EXCEPT FOR 410.42	Acute myocardial infarction of other inferior wall, subsequent episode of care	
410.5x EXCEPT FOR 410.52	Acute myocardial infarction of other lateral wall, subsequent episode of care	
410.6x EXCEPT FOR 410.62	Acute myocardial infarction, true posterior wall infarction, subsequent episode of care	
410.7x EXCEPT FOR 410.72	Acute myocardial infarction, subendocardial infarction, subsequent episode of care	
410.8x EXCEPT FOR 410.82	Acute myocardial infarction, of other specified sites, subsequent episode of care	
410.9x EXCEPT FOR 410.92	Acute myocardial infarction, of unspecified site, subsequent episode of care	
336.9	Unspecified disorder of autonomic nervous system	*Neuro 1—Brain Disorders and Paralysis*
344.9	Paralysis unspecified	
045	Acute poliomyelitis	*Neuro 2—Peripheral Neurological disorders*
334.9	Spinocerebellar disease, unspecified	

Continued

TABLE 2C—CONT'D		
357.9	Unspecified, inflammatory and toxic neuropathy	
358.9	Myoneural disorders, unspecified	
359.9	Myopathy, unspecified	
386.04	Inactive Meniere's disease; Meniere's disease in remission	
430	Subarachnoid hemorrhage	*Neuro—3 Stroke*
431	Intracerebral hemorrhage	
432	Other and unspecified intracranial hemorrhage	
433.01	Occlusion and stenosis, basilar artery, with infarction	
433.11	Occlusion and stenosis, carotid artery, with infarction	
433.21	Occlusion and stenosis, vertebral artery, with infarction	
433.31	Occlusion and stenosis, multiple and bilateral with infarction	
433.81	Occlusion and stenosis, other	
	Specified precerebral artery, with infarction	
434.01	Cerebral thrombosis with infarction	
434.11	Cerebral embolism with infarction	
435	Transient cerebral ischemia	
436	Acute but ill-defined cerebrovascular disease.	
716.5x	Unspecified polyarthropathy or polyarthritis	*Ortho 1—Leg Disorders*
716.6x	Unspecified monoarthritis	
716.9x	Arthropathy, unspecified	
718.8x	Other joint derangement, not elsewhere classified	
718.9x	Unspecified derangement of joint	
712.9x	Unspecified crystal arthropathy	*Ortho 2—Other Orthopedic Disorders*

723.1	Cervicalgia (pain in the neck)	
723.6	Panniculitis specified as affecting neck	
723.8	Other syndromes affecting cervical region	
723.9	Unspecified musculoskeletal disorders and symptoms referable to neck	
724.1	Pain in thoracic spine	
724.2	Lumbago	
724.5	Backache unspecified	
724.7x	Disorders of coccyx	
724.8	Other symptoms referable to back	
724.9	Other unspecified back disorders	
728.2	Muscular wasting and disuse atrophy, not elsewhere classified	
728.3	Other specific muscle disorders	
728.4	Laxity of ligament	
728.5	Hypermobility syndrome	
296.06	Bipolar 1 disorder, single manic episode, in full remission	*Psych. 1—Affective and Other Psychoses, Depression*
296.16	Manic disorder, recurrent episode, in full remission	
296.26	Major depressive disorder, single episode, in full remission	
296.36	Major depressive disorder, recurrent episode, in full remission	
296.46	Bipolar 1 disorder, most recent episode (or current) manic, in full remission	
296.56	Bipolar 1 disorder, most recent episode (or current) depressed, in full remission	

Continued

TABLE 2C—CONT'D		
296.66	Bipolar 1 disorder, most recent episode (or current) unspecified	
294.9	Unspecified persistent mental disorders due to conditions classified elsewhere	*Psych 2—Degenerative and Other Organic Psychiatric Disorders*
331.9	Cerebral degeneration, unspecified	
491.9	Unspecified chronic bronchitis	*Pulmonary Disorders*
496	Chronic airway obstruction, not elsewhere classified	
941.0x	Burn of face, head and neck	*Skin 1—Traumatic Wounds, Burns and Post-operative Complications*
	Unspecified degree	
941.1x	Erythema (first degree)	
942.0x	Burn of trunk, unspecified degree	
942.1x	Burn of trunk, erythema (first degree)	
943.0x	Burn of upper limb, except wrist and hand, unspecified degree	
943.1x	Burn of upper limb, except wrist and hand, erythema (first degree)	
944.0x	Burn of wrist(s) and hand(s)	
	Unspecified degree	
944.1x	Burn of wrist(s) and hand(s)	
	Erythema (first degree)	
945.0x	Burn of lower limb(s), unspecified degree	
945.1x	Burn of lower limb(s), erythema (first degree)	

946.0	Burns of multiple sites, unspecified degree	
946.1	Burns of multiple specified sites, erythema (first degree)	
949	Burn, unspecified	
955.5	Injury to cutaneous sensory nerve, upper limb	
955.9	Injury to unspecified nerve of shoulder girdle and upper limb	
956.4	Injury to cutaneous sensory nerve, lower limb	
956.9	Injury to unspecified nerve of pelvic girdle and lower limb	
681.11	Onychia and paronychia of toe	*Skin 2—Ulcers and Other Skin Conditions*
681.02	Onychia and paronychia of finger	
684	Impetigo	
ICD-9-CM Codes Added	Code Description	*Diagnostic Category*
414.00	Coronary atherosclerosis of unspecified type of vessel, native or graft	*Heart Disease*
414.01	Coronary atherosclerosis, of native coronary artery	
414.02	Coronary atherosclerosis, of autologous vein bypass graft	
414.03	Coronary atherosclerosis, of nonautologous biological bypass graft	
414.04	Coronary atherosclerosis of artery bypass graft	
414.05	Coronary atherosclerosis of unspecified type of bypass graft	
414.06	Coronary atherosclerosis of native coronary artery of transplanted heart	

Continued

TABLE 2C—CONT'D		
414.07	Coronary atherosclerosis of bypass graft (artery) (vein) of transplanted heart	
414.10	Aneurysm of heart (wall)	
414.11	Aneurysm of coronary vessels	
414.12	Dissection of coronary artery	
414.19	Other aneurysm of heart	
414.2	Chronic total occlusion of coronary artery	
414.8	Other specified forms of chronic ischemic heart disease	
138	Late effects of acute poliomyelitis	*Neuro 2—Peripheral Neurological Disorders*
357.81	Chronic inflammatory demyelinating polyneuritis	
447.2	Rupture of an artery	*Skin 2—Ulcers and Other Skin Conditions*
447.8	Other specified disorders of arteries and arterioles	
V55.0	Tracheostomy	*Tracheostomy Care*
V55.5	Cystostomy	*Urostomy/ Cystostomy Care*
V55.6	Other artificial opening of urinary tract—nephrostomy, ureterostomy, urethrostomy	

TABLE 10B

ICD-9-CM DIAGNOSES INCLUDED IN THE DIAGNOSTIC CATEGORIES FOR THE NON-ROUTINE SUPPLIES (NRS) CASE-MIX ADJUSTMENT MODEL

Diagnostic Category	ICD-9-CM Code*	Manifestation	Short Description of ICD-9-CM Code
Anal Fissure, Fistula and Abscess	565		ANAL FISSURE AND FISTULA
	566		ABSCESS OF ANAL AND RECTAL REGIONS
Cellulitis and Abscess	681.00		FINGER—CELLULITIS AND ABSCESS, UNSPECIFIED
	681.01		FELON
	681.10		TOE—CELLULITIS AND ABSCESS, UNSPECIFIED
	681.9		CELLULITIS AND ABSCESS OF UNSPECIFIED DIGIT
	682		OTHER CELLULITIS AND ABSCESS
Diabetic Ulcers	250.8x and 707.10-707.9		(PRIMARY DIAGNOSIS = 250.8X AND OTHER DIAGNOSIS = 707.10-707.9)
Gangrene	440.24		ATHERSCLER-ART EXTREM WITH GANGRENE
	785.4	M	GANGRENE
Malignant Neoplasms of Skin	172		MALIGNANT MELANOMA OF SKIN

Continued

D

TABLE 10B—CONT'D

	173		OTHER MALIGNANT NEOPLASM OF SKIN
Non-pressure and Non-stasis Ulcers (Other than Diabetic)	440.23		ATHEROSCLER-ART EXTREM WITH ULCERATION
	447.2		RUPTURE OF ARTERY
	447.8		OTHER SPECIFIED DISORDERS OF ARTERIES AND ARTERIOLES
	707.10		ULCER OF LOWER LIMB, UNSPECIFIED
	707.11		ULCER OF THIGH
	707.12		ULCER OF CALF
	707.13		ULCER OF ANKLE
	707.14		ULCER OF HEEL AND MIDFOOT
	707.15		ULCER OF OTHER PART OF FOOT
	707.19		ULCER OF OTHER PART OF LOWER LIMB
	707.8		CHRONIC ULCER OTHER SPECIFIED SITE
	707.9		CHRONIC ULCER OF UNSPECIFIED SITE
Other Infections of Skin and Subcutaneous Tissue	680		CARBUNCLE AND FURUNCLE
	683		ACUTE LYMPHADENITIS
	685		PILONIDAL CYST

	686		OTH LOCAL INF SKIN AND SUBCUTANEOUS TISSUE
Post-operative Complications	998.11		HEMORRHAGE COMPLICATING A PROCEDURE
	998.12		HEMATOMA COMPLICATING A PROCEDURE
	998.13		SEROMA COMPLICATING A PROCEDURE
	998.2		ACC PUNCT/ LACERATION DURING PROC NEC
	998.4		FB ACC LEFT DURING PROC NEC
	998.6		PERSISTENT POST-OPERATIVE FIST NEC
	998.83		NON-HEALING SURGICAL WOUND NEC
Traumatic Wounds, Burns, and Post-operative Complications	870		OPEN WOUND OF OCULAR ADNEXA
	872		OPEN WOUND OF EAR
	873		OTHER OPEN WOUND OF HEAD.
	874		OPEN WOUND OF NECK
	875		OPEN WOUND OF CHEST
	876		OPEN WOUND OF BACK
	877		OPEN WOUND OF BUTTOCK

Continued

TABLE 10B—CONT'D			
	878		OPEN WND GNT ORGN INCL TRAUMATIC AMP
	879		OPEN WOUND OTH AND UNSPEC SITE NO LIMBS
	880		OPEN WOUND OF SHOULDER AND UPPER ARM.
	881		OPEN WOUND OF ELBOW, FOREARM, AND WRIST
	882		OPEN WOUND HAND EXCEPT FINGER ALONE
	883		OPEN WOUND OF FINGER
	884		MX AND UNSPEC OPEN WOUND, UPPER LIMB
	885		TRAUMATIC AMPUTATION OF THUMB
	886		TRAUMATIC AMPUTATION OTHER FINGER
	887		TRAUMATIC AMPUTATION OF ARM AND HAND
	890		OPEN WOUND OF HIP AND THIGH
	891		OPEN WOUND OF KNEE, LEG, AND ANKLE
	892		OPEN WOUND OF FOOT EXCEPT TOE ALONE
	893		OPEN WOUND OF TOE
	894		MX AND UNSPEC OPEN WOUND, LOWER LIMB

	895		TRAUMATIC AMPUTATION OF TOE
	896		TRAUMATIC AMPUTATION OF FOOT
	897		TRAUMATIC AMPUTATION OF LEG
	941 except 941.0x and 941.1x		BURN OF FACE, HEAD, AND NECK
	942 except 942.0x and 942.1x		BURN OF TRUNK
	943 except 943.0x and 943.1x		BURN OF UPPER LIMB, EXCEPT WRIST AND HAND
	944 except 944.0x and 944.1x		BURN OF WRIST(S) AND HAND(S)
	945 except 945.0x and 945.1x		BURN OF LOWER LIMB(S)
	946.2		BURNS OF MULTIPLE SPECIFIED SITES, BLISTERS, EPIDERMAL LOSS (SECOND DEGREE)
	946.3		BURNS OF MULTIPLE SPECIFIED SITES, FULL-THICKNESS SKIN LOSS (THIRD DEGREE NOS)
	946.4		BURNS OF MULTIPLE SPECIFIED SITES, DEEP

Continued

TABLE 10B—CONT'D			
			NECROSIS OF UNDERLYING TISSUES (DEEP THIRD DEGREE) WITHOUT MENTION OF LOSS OF A BODY PART
			BURNS OF MULTIPLE SPECIFIED SITES, DEEP
	946.5		NECROSIS OF UNDERLYING TISSUES (DEEP THIRD DEGREE) WITH LOSS OF A BODY PART
	948		BURN CLASS ACCORD-BODY SURF INVOLVED
	998.31		DISRUPTION OF INTERNAL OPERATION WOUND
	998.32		DISRUPTION OF EXTERNAL OPERATION WOUND
	998.51		INFECTED POST-OPERATIVE SEROMA
	998.59		OTHER POST-OPERATIVE INFECTION
V-Code, Cystostomy	V55.5		CYSTOSTOMY
V-Code, Tracheostomy	V55.0		TRACHEOSTOMY

V-Code, Urostomy	V55.6		OTHER ARTIFICIAL OPENING OF URINARY TRACT—NEPHROSTOMY, URETEROSTOMY, URETHROSTOMY

APPENDIX E

DRAFT OF OASIS C

Home Health Patient Tracking Sheet

(M0010) Agency Medicare Provider Number: __ __ __ __ __ __

(M0014) Branch State: __ __

(M0016) Branch ID Number: __ __ __ __ __ __ __ __ __ __

(M0020) Patient ID Number: __

(M0030) Start of Care Date: __ __/__ __/__ __ __ __
month / day / year

(M0032) Resumption of Care Date: __ __/__ __/__ __ __ __ ☐ NA - Not Applicable
month / day / year

(M0040) Patient Name:

__ __ __ __ __ __ __ __ __ __ __ __ __ __ (First) __ (MI) __ __ __ __ __ __ __ __ __ __ __ __ __ __ __ __ __ __ (Last) __ __ __ (Suffix)

(M0050) Patient State of Residence: __ __

(M0060) Patient Zip Code: __ __ __ __ __ __ __ __ __

(M0063) Medicare Number: __ __ __ __ __ __ __ __ __ __ __ __ (including suffix) ☐ **NA – No Medicare**

(M0064) Social Security Number: __ __ __-__ __-__ __ __ __ ☐ **UK – Unknown or Not Available**

(M0065) Medicaid Number: __ __ __ __ __ __ __ __ __ __ __ __ __ __ ☐ **NA – No Medicaid**

(M0066) Birth Date: __ __/__ __/__ __ __ __
month / day / year

(M0069) Gender:

☐ 1 - Male
☐ 2 - Female

(M0072) Primary Referring Physician ID:

__ __ __ __ __ __ __ __ __ __ ☐ **UK – Unknown or Not Available**

(M0140) Race/Ethnicity (as identified by patient): **(Mark all that apply.)**

☐ 1 - American Indian or Alaska Native
☐ 2 - Asian
☐ 3 - Black or African-American
☐ 4 - Hispanic or Latino
☐ 5 - Native Hawaiian or Pacific Islander
☐ 6 - White
☐ UK - Unknown

(M0150) Current Payment Sources for Home Care: (Mark all that apply.)

☐ 0 - None; no charge for current services
☐ 1 - Medicare (traditional fee-for-service)
☐ 2 - Medicare (HMO/managed care/Advantage plan)
☐ 3 - Medicaid (traditional fee-for-service)
☐ 4 - Medicaid (HMO/managed care)
☐ 5 - Workers' compensation
☐ 6 - Title programs (e.g., Title III, V, or XX)
☐ 7 - Other government (e.g., CHAMPUS, VA, etc.)
☐ 8 - Private insurance
☐ 9 - Private HMO/managed care
☐ 10 - Self-pay
☐ 11 - Other (specify) ______________________
☐ UK - Unknown

According to the Paperwork Reduction Act of 1995, no persons are required to respond to a collection of information unless it displays a valid OMB control number. The valid OMB control numbers for this information are 0938-0760 and 0938-0761. The time required to complete this information collection is estimated to average 0.7 minute per response, including the time to review instructions, search existing data resources, gather the data needed, and complete and review the information collection. If you have comments concerning the accuracy of the time estimate(s) or suggestions for improving this form, please write to: CMS, 7500 Security Boulevard, Attn: PRA Reports

Clearance Officer, Baltimore, Maryland 21244-1850.

Outcome and Assessment Information Set (OASIS-C draft)

Items to be Used at Specific Time Points

Start of Care --- Start of care—further visits planned	Home Health Patient Tracking Sheet, M0080-M0826, M1010, M1020, M1030, M1040, M1050, M1060, M1070, M1072, M1080, M1090, M1102, M1110, M1120, M1130, M1140, M1150, M1160, M1170, M1180
Resumption of Care --- Resumption of care (after inpatient stay)	M0032, M0080-M0826, M1010, M1020, M1030, M1040, M1050, M1060, M1070, M1072, M1080, M1090, M1102, M1110, M1120, M1130, M1140, M1150, M1160, M1170, M1180
Follow-Up --- Recertification (follow-up) assessment Other follow-up assessment	M0080-M0100, M0110, M0230-M0250, M0390, M0420-M0452, M0465-M0490, M0520-M0550, M0652-M0702, M0802, M0826, M1021, M1025, M1031, M1035, M1050, M1060, M1065, M1070, M1073, M1085, M1095, M1105, M1110, M1155, M1160, M1170, M1180
Transfer to an Inpatient Facility --- Transferred to an inpatient facility—patient not discharged from an agency Transferred to an inpatient facility—patient discharged from agency	M0080-M0100, M0831-M0855, M0890-M0906, M1021, M1025, M1031, M1035, M1050, M1060, M1065, M1073, M1085, M1095, M1105, M1110, M1155, M1160, M1170, M1180
Discharge from Agency — Not to an Inpatient Facility	
Death at home ---	M0080-M0100, M0906
Discharge from agency---	M0080-M0100, M0250-M0345, M0406-M0540, M0560-M0712, M0722-M0772, M0782 - M0802, M0810, M0822-M0824, M0831-M0870, M0896, M0900, M0903-M0906, M1021, M1025, M1031, M1035, M1050, M1060, M1065, M1070, M1073, M1085, M1095, M1105, M1110, M1120, M1130, M1140, M1155, M1160, M1170, M1180

CLINICAL RECORD ITEMS

(M0080) Discipline of Person Completing Assessment:

☐ 1-RN ☐ 2-PT ☐ 3-SLP/ST ☐ 4-OT

(M0090) Date Assessment Completed: __ __/__ __/__ __ __ __
month / day / year

(M0100) This Assessment is Currently Being Completed for the Following Reason:

Start/Resumption of Care
- ☐ 1 – Start of care—further visits planned
- ☐ 3 – Resumption of care (after inpatient stay)

Follow-Up
- ☐ 4 – Recertification (follow-up) reassessment **[Go to *M0110*]**
- ☐ 5 – Other follow-up **[Go to *M0110*]**

Transfer to an Inpatient Facility
- ☐ 6 – Transferred to an inpatient facility—patient not discharged from agency **[Go to *M0830*]**
- ☐ 7 – Transferred to an inpatient facility—patient discharged from agency **[Go to *M0830*]**

Discharge from Agency — Not to an Inpatient Facility
- ☐ 8 – Death at home **[Go to *M0906*]**
- ☐ 9 – Discharge from agency **[Go to *M0110*]**

(M0102) Date of Referral: Indicate the date this referral for home health services was made.

__ __/__ __/__ __ __ __
month / day / year

E

(M0104) Date of Physician-ordered Start of Care: If the physician indicated a specific start of care date when the patient was referred for home health services, record the date specified.

__ __/__ __/__ __ __ __
month / day / year

☐ NA – No specific SOC date ordered by physician.

(M0110) Episode Timing: Is the Medicare home health payment episode for which this assessment will define a case mix group an "early" episode or a "later" episode in the patient's current sequence of adjacent Medicare home health payment episodes?

☐ 1 - Early
☐ 2 - Later
☐ UK - Unknown
☐ NA - Not Applicable: No Medicare case mix group to be defined by this assessment.

DEMOGRAPHICS AND PATIENT HISTORY

(M0175) From which of the following **Inpatient Facilities** was the patient discharged during the past 14 days? **(Mark all that apply.)**

☐ 1 - Hospital
☐ 2 - Rehabilitation facility
☐ 3 - Skilled nursing facility
☐ 4 - Other nursing home
☐ 5 - Other (specify) ____________________
☐ NA - Patient was not discharged from an inpatient facility **[If NA go to *M0200*]**

(M0180) Inpatient Discharge Date (most recent):

__ __/__ __/__ __ __ __
month / day / year

☐ UK - Unknown

(M0190) List each **Inpatient Diagnosis** and ICD-9-CM code at the level of highest specificity for only those conditions treated during an inpatient stay within the last 14 days (no surgical, E-codes, or V-codes):

	Inpatient Facility Diagnosis	ICD-9-CM
a.	____________________	(____.__)
b.	____________________	(____.__)

(M0200) Medical or Treatment Regimen Change Within Past 14 Days: Has this patient experienced a change in medical or treatment regimen (e.g., medication, treatment, or service change due to new or additional diagnosis, etc.) within the last 14 days?

☐ 0 - No **[If No, go to *M0220*; if No at Discharge, go to *M0250*]**
☐ 1 - Yes

(M0210) List the patient's **Medical Diagnoses** and ICD-9-CM codes at the level of highest specificity for those conditions requiring changed medical or treatment regimen (no surgical, E-codes, or V-codes):

	Changed Medical Regimen Diagnosis	ICD-9-CM
a.	____________________	(____.__)
b.	____________________	(____.__)
c.	____________________	(____.__)
d.	____________________	(____.__)

(M0220) Conditions Prior to Medical or Treatment Regimen Change or Inpatient Stay Within Past 14 Days: If this patient experienced an inpatient facility discharge or change in medical or treatment regimen within the past 14 days, indicate any conditions which existed prior to the inpatient stay or change in medical or treatment regimen. **(Mark all that apply.)**

☐ 1 - Urinary incontinence
☐ 2 - Indwelling/suprapubic catheter
☐ 3 - Intractable pain
☐ 4 - Impaired decision-making
☐ 5 - Disruptive or socially inappropriate behavior
☐ 6 - Memory loss to the extent that supervision required
☐ 7 - None of the above
☐ NA - No inpatient facility discharge and no change in medical or treatment regimen in past 14 days
☐ UK - Unknown

(M0230/240/246) Diagnoses, Severity Index, and Payment Diagnoses: List each diagnosis for which the patient is receiving home care (Column 1) and enter its ICD-9-CM code at the level of highest specificity (no surgical/procedure codes) (Column 2). Rate each condition (Column 2) using the severity index. (Choose one value that represents the most severe rating appropriate for each diagnosis.) V codes (for M0230 or M0240) or E codes (for M0240 only) may be used. ICD-9-CM sequencing requirements must be followed if multiple coding is indicated for any diagnoses. If a V code is reported in place of a case mix diagnosis, then optional item M0246 Payment Diagnoses (Columns 3 and 4) may be completed. A case mix diagnosis is a diagnosis that determines the Medicare PPS case mix group.

Code each row according to the following directions for each column:

Column 1: Enter the description of the diagnosis.

Column 2: Enter the ICD-9-CM code for the diagnosis described in Column 1;
Rate the severity of the condition listed in Column 1 using the following scale:
- 0 - Asymptomatic, no treatment needed at this time
- 1 - Symptoms well controlled with current therapy
- 2 - Symptoms controlled with difficulty, affecting daily functioning; patient needs ongoing monitoring
- 3 - Symptoms poorly controlled; patient needs frequent adjustment in treatment and dose monitoring
- 4 - Symptoms poorly controlled; history of re-hospitalizations

Column 3: (OPTIONAL) If a V code reported in any row in Column 2 is reported in place of a case mix diagnosis, list the appropriate case mix diagnosis (the description and the ICD-9-CM code) in the same row in Column 3. Otherwise, leave Column 3 blank in that row.

Column 4: (OPTIONAL) If a V code in Column 2 is reported in place of a case mix diagnosis that requires multiple diagnosis codes under ICD-9-CM coding guidelines, enter the diagnosis descriptions and the ICD-9-CM codes in the same row in Columns 3 and 4. For example, if the case mix diagnosis is a manifestation code, record the diagnosis description and ICD-9-CM code for the underlying condition in Column 3 of that row and the diagnosis description and ICD-9-CM code for the manifestation in Column 4 of that row. Otherwise, leave Column 4 blank in that row.

(M0230) Primary Diagnosis & (M0240) Other Diagnoses		(M0246) Case Mix Diagnoses (OPTIONAL)	
Column 1	Column 2	Column 3	Column 4
	ICD-9-CM and severity rating for each condition	Complete **only if** a V code in Column 2 is reported in place of a case mix diagnosis.	Complete **only if** the V code in Column 2 is reported in place of a case mix diagnosis that is a multiple coding situation (e.g., a manifestation code).
Description	ICD-9-CM / Severity Rating	Description/ ICD-9-CM	Description/ ICD-9-CM
(M0230) Primary Diagnosis	(V codes are allowed)	(V or E codes NOT allowed)	(V or E codes NOT allowed)
a. ______	a. (____.__) ☐0 ☐1 ☐2 ☐3 ☐4	a. ______ (____.__)	a. ______ (____.__)
(M0240) Other Diagnoses	(V or E codes are allowed)	(V or E codes NOT allowed)	(V or E codes NOT allowed)
b. ______	b. (____.__) ☐0 ☐1 ☐2 ☐3 ☐4	b. ______ (____.__)	b. ______ (____.__)
c. ______	c. (____.__) ☐0 ☐1 ☐2 ☐3 ☐4	c. ______ (____.__)	c. ______ (____.__)
d. ______	d. (____.__) ☐0 ☐1 ☐2 ☐3 ☐4	d. ______ (____.__)	d. ______ (____.__)
e. ______	e. (____.__) ☐0 ☐1 ☐2 ☐3 ☐4	e. ______ (____.__)	e. ______ (____.__)
f. ______	f. (____.__) ☐0 ☐1 ☐2 ☐3 ☐4	f. ______ (____.__)	f. ______ (____.__)

(M0250) Therapies the patient receives at home: **(Mark all that apply.)**

☐ 1 - Intravenous or infusion therapy (excludes TPN)
☐ 2 - Parenteral nutrition (TPN or lipids)
☐ 3 - Enteral nutrition (nasogastric, gastrostomy, jejunostomy, or any other artificial entry into the alimentary canal)
☐ 4 - None of the above

(M0275) Frailty Indicators: Which of the following signs or symptoms characterize this patient as at risk for major decline or hospitalization? **(Mark all that apply.)**

☐ 1 - Unstable vital signs
☐ 2 - Debilitating pain
☐ 3 - Recent change in mental status
☐ 4 - Recent functional decline
☐ 5 - Multiple hospitalizations (>1) in the past 12 months
☐ 6 - History of falls (2 or more falls - or any fall with an injury - in the past year)
☐ 7 - Other
☐ 8 - None of the above

(M0285) Stability Prognosis: Which description best fits the patient's overall status? [check one]

☐ 0 - The patient is stable with no heightened risk for serious complications and death (beyond those typical of the patient's age).
☐ 1 - The patient is temporarily facing high health risks but is likely to return to being stable without heightened risk for serious complications and death (beyond those typical of the patient's age).
☐ 2 - The patient is likely to remain in fragile health and have ongoing high risks of serious complications and death.
☐ 3 - The patient has serious progressive conditions that could lead to death within a year.
☐ UK - The patient's situation is unknown or unclear.

(M0291) Risk Factors characterizing this patient: **(Mark all that apply.)**

☐ 1 - Smoking
☐ 2 - Obesity
☐ 3 - Alcohol dependency
☐ 4 - Drug dependency
☐ 5 - None of the above
☐ UK - Unknown

(M1010) Urgent/Emergency Contact Information: Was the patient or caregiver provided patient-specific verbal and written instructions during the first visit regarding when and how to contact the HOME HEALTH AGENCY for urgent health-related problems during the day and after hours, and when to call 911 for a medical emergency?

☐ 0- No
☐ 1- Yes

(M1020) Influenza Vaccine: Has the patient received an influenza vaccination during this year's recommended time period?

☐ 0 - No
☐ 1 - Yes
☐ NA - Does not apply. SOC/ROC date is not within time period.
☐ UK - Unknown

(M1021) Influenza Vaccine: Did the patient receive the influenza vaccine from your agency during this year's recommended time period?

☐ 0 - No **(Complete M1025)**
☐ 1 - Yes **(Skip M1025)**
☐ NA - Does not apply because entire care episode is outside this year's recommended time period. **(Skip M1025)**

E

(M1025) Reason Influenza Vaccine not received: If the patient did not receive the influenza vaccine from your agency, state reason:

- ☐ 1 - Received from another health care provider (e.g., physician)
- ☐ 2 - Not eligible / Not indicated
- ☐ 3 - Offered and declined
- ☐ 4 - Not offered
- ☐ 5 - Inability to obtain vaccine due to declared shortage
- ☐ 6 - None of the above

(M1030) Pneumococcal Vaccine: Is the patient's pneumococcal polysaccharide vaccine (PPV) status up to date?

- ☐ 0 - No (skip pattern removed)
- ☐ 1 - Yes (skip pattern removed)
- ☐ UK - Unknown

(M1031) Pneumococcal Vaccine: Is the patient's pneumococcal polysaccharide vaccine (PPV) status up to date?

- ☐ 0 - No **(Complete M1035)**
- ☐ 1 - Yes **(Skip M1035)**

(M1035) If Pneumococcal Vaccine is not up to date, state reason:

- ☐ 1 - Not eligible / Not indicated
- ☐ 2 - Offered and declined
- ☐ 3 - Not offered

(M1040) Guidelines for Physician Notification: Have parameters (limits) related to the patient's health care problems been established (individually for this patient or using standard guidelines with patient-specific modifications as needed) for when to contact the physician for vital signs or other clinical findings?

- ☐ 0 - No
- ☐ 1 - Yes

LIVING ARRANGEMENTS

(M0345) Patient Living Situation: Which of the following best describes the patient's residential circumstance and availability of assistance? **(Check one box only)**.

	Availability of Assistance				
Living Arrangement	Around the clock	Day only	Night only	No assistance available	Unknown
a Patient lives alone	☐ 01	☐ 02	☐ 03	☐ 04	☐ 05
b Patient lives with other person(s)	☐ 06	☐ 07	☐ 08	☐ 09	☐ 10
c Patient lives in congregate situation (e.g., assisted living)	☐ 11	☐ 12	☐ 13	☐ 14	☐ 15

(M0382 and M0384 replaced by M0822 - M0824)

SENSORY STATUS

(M0390) Vision with corrective lenses if the patient usually wears them:

- ☐ 0 - Normal vision: sees adequately in most situations; can see medication labels, newsprint.
- ☐ 1 - Partially impaired: cannot see medication labels or newsprint, but can see obstacles in path, and the surrounding layout; can count fingers at arm's length.
- ☐ 2 - Severely impaired: cannot locate objects without hearing or touching them or patient nonresponsive.

(M0405) Ability to hear (with hearing aid or hearing appliance if normally used):

- ☐ 0 - Adequate: hears normal conversation without difficulty.
- ☐ 1 - Mildly to Moderately Impaired: difficulty hearing in some environments or speaker may need to increase volume or speak distinctly.
- ☐ 2 - Severely Impaired: absence of useful hearing.
- ☐ UK - Unable to assess hearing.

(M0406) **Understanding of Verbal Content** in patient's own language (with hearing aid or device if used):

- ☐ 0 - Understands: clear comprehension without cues or repetitions.
- ☐ 1 - Usually/Sometimes Understands: Comprehends only basic conversations or simple, direct phrases or requires cues to understand.
- ☐ 2 - Rarely/Never Understands
- ☐ UK - Unable to assess understanding.

(M0410) **Speech and Oral (Verbal) Expression of Language** (in patient's own language):

- ☐ 0 - Expresses complex ideas, feelings, and needs clearly, completely, and easily in all situations with no observable impairment.
- ☐ 1 - Minimal difficulty in expressing ideas and needs (may take extra time; makes occasional errors in word choice, grammar or speech intelligibility; needs minimal prompting or assistance).
- ☐ 2 - Expresses simple ideas or needs with moderate difficulty (needs prompting or assistance, errors in word choice, organization or speech intelligibility). Speaks in phrases or short sentences.
- ☐ 3 - Has severe difficulty expressing basic ideas or needs and requires maximal assistance or guessing by listener. Speech limited to single words or short phrases.
- ☐ 4 - Unable to express basic needs even with maximal prompting or assistance but is not comatose or unresponsive (e.g., speech is nonsensical or unintelligible).
- ☐ 5 - Patient nonresponsive or unable to speak.

(M0420) **Frequency of Pain** interfering with patient's activity or movement:

- ☐ 0 - Patient has no pain **(Go to M1070)**
- ☐ 1 - Patient has pain that does not interfere with activity or movement
- ☐ 2 - Less often than daily
- ☐ 3 - Daily, but not constantly
- ☐ 4 - All of the time

(M1050) Has this patient had a formal **Pain Assessment** using a standardized pain assessment tool (appropriate to the patient's ability to verbalize severity of pain)?

- ☐ 0 - Yes, and it does not indicate severe or persistent pain (skip pattern removed)
- ☐ 1 - Yes, and it indicates severe or persistent pain (skip pattern removed)
- ☐ 2 - No assessment conducted.

(M1060) **Pain Intervention:** Is intervention to monitor and mitigate pain severity included in the care plan for this home health episode of care?

- ☐ 0 - No
- ☐ 1 - Yes

Complete M1065 if M1050 = "1"or if M0420 is greater than "1".

(M1065) **Pain Intervention:** Have pain management steps been implemented to monitor and mitigate pain severity during this home health episode of care?

- ☐ 0 - No
- ☐ 1 - Yes

INTEGUMENTARY STATUS

(M1070) **Pressure Ulcer Assessment:** Was this patient assessed for the **Risk of Developing Pressure Ulcers**?

- ☐ 1 - No
- ☐ 2 - Yes, using a standardized tool
- ☐ 3 - Yes, using a clinical evaluation

(M0446) Does this patient have a high **Risk of Developing Pressure Ulcers**?

- ☐ 0 - No **(Skip M1072 at SOC/ROC; Skip M1073 at F/T/D)**
- ☐ 1 - Yes

(M1072) **Pressure Ulcer Prevention:** Is there a plan for relieving pressure (using a pressure-relieving or redistributing device such as an enhanced mattress or overlay, or instructing the patient/caregiver in other methods to reduce pressure)?

- ☐ 0 - No
- ☐ 1 - Yes

(M1073) Pressure Ulcer Prevention: Was there a plan for relieving pressure (using a pressure-relieving or redistributing device such as an enhanced mattress or overlay, or instructing the patient/caregiver in other methods to reduce pressure)?

☐ 0 - No
☐ 1 - Yes

(M0447) Current Number of Stage I Pressure Ulcers (Intact skin with non-blanchable redness of a localized area usually over a bony prominence. The area may be painful, firm, soft, warmer or cooler as compared to adjacent tissue.):

☐ 0 ☐ 1 ☐ 2 ☐ 3 ☐ 4 or more

(M0448) Does this patient have at least one unhealed (non-epithelialized) **Pressure Ulcer** at Stage II or higher or designated as "not stageable"?

☐ 0 - No **[If No, go to M0465]**
☐ 1 - Yes

(M0452) Current Number of Unhealed (non-epithelialized) Pressure Ulcers at Each Stage: (Circle one response for each line.)

Rows b.i, b.ii, c.i, and c.ii removed

Stage description – unhealed pressure ulcers	Number of unhealed pressure ulcers present						Number with onset during service by this agency **(Omit at SOC/ROC)**					
a. **Stage II:** Partial thickness skin loss – shallow open ulcer with red/pink wound bed without slough, or blister.												
i. Total currently present	0	1	2	3	4 or more		0	1	2	3	4 or more	
ii. Currently present and known to be present for at least 30 days	0	1	2	3	4 or more		0	1	2	3	4 or more	
b. **Stage III:** Full thickness skin loss--no exposure of bone, tendon, or muscle	0	1	2	3	4 or more	UK	0	1	2	3	4 or more	UK
c. **Stage IV:** Full thickness tissue loss with exposed bone, tendon or muscle.	0	1	2	3	4 or more	UK	0	1	2	3	4 or more	UK
d. Known or likely but not stageable due to non-removable dressing or cast	0	1	2	3	4 or more	UK	0	1	2	3	4 or more	UK
e. Known but not stageable due to coverage of wound bed by slough and/or eschar.	0	1	2	3	4 or more	UK	0	1	2	3	4 or more	UK
f. Suspected deep tissue injury in evolution.	☐ 0 – No ☐ 1 – Yes ☐ UK						☐ 0 – No ☐ 1 – Yes ☐ UK					

Directions for M0454 and M0456: If the patient has one or more unhealed (non-epithelialized) Stage III or IV pressure ulcers, identify the **pressure ulcer with the longest dimension** and record in centimeters:

(M0454) Pressure Ulcer Length: Longest length in any direction |___|___|.|___| (cm)

(M0456) Pressure Ulcer Width: Width of the same pressure ulcer, greatest width measured at right angles to length |___|___|.|___| (cm)

(M0461) Status of Most Problematic (Observable) Pressure Ulcer:

☐ 0 - Re-epithelialized or healed
☐ 1 - Fully granulating
☐ 2 - Early/partial granulation
☐ 3 - Not healing
☐ NA - No observable pressure ulcer

(M0465) [If patient has no pressure ulcers (M0447 = "0" and M0448 = "0", skip to M0469] **Stage of Most Problematic (Observable) Pressure Ulcer:**

☐ 1 - Stage I
☐ 2 - Stage II
☐ 3 - Stage III
☐ 4 - Stage IV
☐ NA - No observable pressure ulcer

Complete M1080 if patient has an open Stage II or higher pressure ulcer or a pressure ulcer that is designated as "not stageable", regardless of whether eschar is present.

(M1080) **Pressure Ulcer Intervention:** If the patient has an open Stage II or higher pressure ulcer or a pressure ulcer that is designated as "not stageable", are moisture retentive dressings specified on the plan of care?

- ☐ 0 - No
- ☐ 1 - Yes
- ☐ 2 - Moisture retentive dressings not indicated for this patient.

(M1085) **Pressure Ulcer Intervention:** If the patient had one or more open Stage II or higher pressure ulcers, were moisture retentive dressings used?

- ☐ 0 - No
- ☐ 1 - Yes
- ☐ 2 - Moisture retentive dressings not indicated for this patient

(M0469) Does this patient have a **Stasis Ulcer**?

- ☐ 0 - No **[If No, go to *M0483*]**
- ☐ 1 - Yes, patient has one or more (observable) stasis ulcers.
- ☐ 2 - Stasis ulcer known or likely but not observable due to non-removable dressing **[Go to *M0483*]**

(M0470) **Current Number of (Observable) Stasis Ulcer(s):**

- ☐ 0 - Zero
- ☐ 1 - One
- ☐ 2 - Two
- ☐ 3 - Three
- ☐ 4 - Four or more

(M0478) [At follow-up, skip to M0483 if patient has no stasis ulcers] **Status of Most Problematic (Observable) Stasis Ulcer:**

- ☐ 0 - Re-epithelialized or healed
- ☐ 1 - Fully granulating
- ☐ 2 - Early/partial granulation
- ☐ 3 - Not healing
- ☐ NA - No observable stasis ulcer

(M0483) Does this patient have a **Surgical Wound?**

- ☐ 0 - No **[If No, go to *M0489*]**
- ☐ 1 - Yes, patient has at least one (observable) surgical wound
- ☐ 2 - Surgical wound known or likely but not observable due to non-removable dressing. **[Go to *M0489*]**

(M0487) [At follow-up, skip to M0489 if patient has no surgical wounds] **Status of Most Problematic (Observable) Surgical Wound:**

- ☐ 0 - Re-epithelialized or healed
- ☐ 1 - Fully granulating
- ☐ 2 - Early/partial granulation
- ☐ 3 - Not healing
- ☐ NA - No observable surgical wound

(M0489) Does this patient have a **Skin Lesion** or **Open Wound,** excluding bowel ostomy, other than those described above that is receiving clinical intervention?

- ☐ 0 - No
- ☐ 1 - Yes

E

Complete M1090 or M1095 if patient has a diagnosis of diabetes.

(M1090) **Foot Care Education:** Does the care plan include patient education on both proper foot care and regular monitoring for the presence of skin lesions on the lower extremities?

- ☐ 0 - No
- ☐ 1 - Yes
- ☐ NA - Bilateral amputee

(M1095) **Foot Care Plan Follow-up:** Was the care plan regarding patient education and regular monitoring of foot care followed?

- ☐ 0 - No
- ☐ 1 - Yes
- ☐ NA - Bilateral amputee

RESPIRATORY STATUS

(M0490) When is the patient dyspneic or noticeably **Short of Breath**?

- ☐ 0 - Patient is not short of breath
- ☐ 1 - When walking more than 20 feet, climbing stairs
- ☐ 2 - With moderate exertion (e.g., while dressing, using commode or bedpan, walking distances less than 20 feet)
- ☐ 3 - With minimal exertion (e.g., while eating, talking, or performing other ADLs) or with agitation
- ☐ 4 - At rest (during day or night)

(M0500) **Respiratory Treatments** utilized at home: **(Mark all that apply.)**

- ☐ 1 - Oxygen (intermittent or continuous)
- ☐ 2 - Ventilator (continually or at night)
- ☐ 3 - Continuous positive airway pressure
- ☐ 4 - None of the above

CARDIAC STATUS

Complete M1102 (or M1105) & M1110 if patient has a diagnosis of heart failure .

(M1102) **Symptoms of Volume Overload:** Does the patient exhibit symptoms of volume overload indicated by clinical heart failure guidelines (including dyspnea, orthopnea, edema, or weight gain)?

- ☐ 0 - No **(Skip Item M1110)**
- ☐ 1 - Yes **(Complete Item M1110)**
- ☐ 2 - Not assessed. **(Skip Item M1110)**

(M1105) **Symptoms of Volume Overload:** Did the patient exhibit symptoms of volume overload indicated by clinical heart failure guidelines (including dyspnea, orthopnea, edema, or weight gain) at any point since the initial assessment?

- ☐ 0 - No **(Skip Item M1110)**
- ☐ 1 - Yes **(Complete Item M1110)**
- ☐ 2 - Not assessed. **(Skip Item M1110)**

(M1110) **Volume Overload Follow-up:** What action has been taken to respond to symptoms of volume overload?

- ☐ 0 - No action taken
- ☐ 1 - Patient's physician (or other primary care practitioner) contacted the same day, or patient advised to get emergency treatment (call 911 or go to emergency room)
- ☐ 2 - Other action taken

ELIMINATION STATUS

(M0510) Has this patient been treated for a **Urinary Tract Infection** in the past 14 days?

- ☐ 0 - No
- ☐ 1 - Yes
- ☐ NA - Patient on prophylactic treatment
- ☐ UK - Unknown

(M0520) Urinary Incontinence or Urinary Catheter Presence:

☐ 0 - No incontinence or catheter (includes anuria or ostomy for urinary drainage) **[If No, go to *M0540*]**
☐ 1 - Patient is incontinent
☐ 2 - Patient requires a urinary catheter (i.e., external, indwelling, intermittent, suprapubic) **[Go to *M0540*]**

(M0530) When does **Urinary Incontinence** occur?

☐ 0 - Timed-voiding defers incontinence
☐ 1 - During the night only
☐ 2 - During the day and night

(M0540) Bowel Incontinence Frequency:

☐ 0 - Very rarely or never has bowel incontinence
☐ 1 - Less than once weekly
☐ 2 - One to three times weekly
☐ 3 - Four to six times weekly
☐ 4 - On a daily basis
☐ 5 - More often than once daily
☐ NA - Patient has ostomy for bowel elimination
☐ UK - Unknown

(M0550) Ostomy for Bowel Elimination: Does this patient have an ostomy for bowel elimination that (within the last 14 days): a) was related to an inpatient facility stay, or b) necessitated a change in medical or treatment regimen?

☐ 0 - Patient does not have an ostomy for bowel elimination.
☐ 1 - Patient's ostomy was not related to an inpatient stay and did not necessitate change in medical or treatment regimen.
☐ 2 - The ostomy was related to an inpatient stay or did necessitate change in medical or treatment regimen.

NEURO/EMOTIONAL/BEHAVIORAL STATUS

(M0560) Cognitive Functioning: (Patient's current level of alertness, orientation, comprehension, concentration, and immediate memory for simple commands.)

☐ 0 - Alert/oriented, able to focus and shift attention, comprehends and recalls task directions independently.
☐ 1 - Requires prompting (cuing, repetition, reminders) only under stressful or unfamiliar conditions.
☐ 2 - Requires assistance and some direction in specific situations (e.g., on all tasks involving shifting of attention), or consistently requires low stimulus environment due to distractibility.
☐ 3 - Requires considerable assistance in routine situations. Is not alert and oriented or is unable to shift attention and recall directions more than half the time.
☐ 4 - Totally dependent due to disturbances such as constant disorientation, coma, persistent vegetative state, or delirium.

(M0570) When Confused (Reported or Observed):

☐ 0 - Never
☐ 1 - In new or complex situations only
☐ 2 - On awakening or at night only
☐ 3 - During the day and evening, but not constantly
☐ 4 - Constantly
☐ NA - Patient nonresponsive

(M0580) When Anxious (Reported or Observed):

☐ 0 - None of the time
☐ 1 - Less often than daily
☐ 2 - Daily, but not constantly
☐ 3 - All of the time
☐ NA - Patient nonresponsive

(Order revised--M1120 placed after M0590)

(M0590) Depressive Symptoms Reported or Observed in Patient: (Mark all that apply.)

- ☐ 1 - Depressed mood (e.g., feeling sad, tearful)
- ☐ 2 - Sense of failure or self reproach
- ☐ 3 - Hopelessness
- ☐ 4 - Recurrent thoughts of death
- ☐ 5 - Thoughts of suicide
- ☐ 6 - Other signs or symptoms
- ☐ 7 - None of the above feelings observed or reported **(Go to M0610)**

(M1120) Depression Screening: Has the patient been screened for depression, using a standardized depression screening tool?

- ☐ 0 - No
- ☐ 1 - Yes, and the patient displays no current symptoms of depression. **(Go to M0610)**
- ☐ 2 - Yes, and the patient displays some symptoms of depression.

(M1130) Depression Intervention/Referral: Is intervention for symptoms of depression or referral for other treatment or a monitoring plan for current treatment included in the care plan for this home health episode of care?

- ☐ 0 - No
- ☐ 1 - New intervention or referral initiated.
- ☐ 2 - Monitoring plan for patient already on treatment.

(M0610) Behaviors Demonstrated <u>at Least Once a Week</u> (Reported or Observed): (Mark all that apply.)

- ☐ 1 - Memory deficit: failure to recognize familiar persons/places, inability to recall events of past 24 hours, significant memory loss so that supervision is required
- ☐ 2 - Impaired decision-making: failure to perform usual ADLs or IADLs, inability to appropriately stop activities, jeopardizes safety through actions
- ☐ 3 - Verbal disruption: yelling, threatening, excessive profanity, sexual references, etc.
- ☐ 4 - Physical aggression: aggressive or combative to self and others (e.g., hits self, throws objects, punches, dangerous maneuvers with wheelchair or other objects)
- ☐ 5 - Disruptive, infantile, or socially inappropriate behavior (**excludes** verbal actions)
- ☐ 6 - Delusional, hallucinatory, or paranoid behavior
- ☐ 7 - None of the above behaviors demonstrated

(M0620) Frequency of Behavior Problems (Reported or Observed) (e.g., wandering episodes, self abuse, verbal disruption, physical aggression, etc.):

- ☐ 0 - Never
- ☐ 1 - Less than once a month
- ☐ 2 - Once a month
- ☐ 3 - Several times each month
- ☐ 4 - Several times a week
- ☐ 5 - At least daily

(M0630) Is this patient receiving **Psychiatric Nursing Services** at home provided by a qualified psychiatric nurse?

- ☐ 0 - No
- ☐ 1 - Yes

ADL/IADLs

(M0642) Grooming: Current ability to tend to personal hygiene needs (i.e., washing face and hands, hair care, shaving or make up, teeth or denture care, fingernail care).

- ☐ 0 - Able to groom self unaided, with or without the use of assistive devices or adapted methods.
- ☐ 1 - Grooming utensils must be placed within reach before able to complete grooming activities.
- ☐ 2 - Someone must assist the patient to groom self.
- ☐ 3 - Patient depends entirely upon someone else for grooming needs.

(M0652) Current **Ability to Dress <u>Upper</u> Body** (with or without dressing aids) including undergarments, pullovers, front-opening shirts and blouses, managing zippers, buttons, and snaps:

- ☐ 0 - Able to get clothes out of closets and drawers, put them on and remove them from the upper body without assistance.
- ☐ 1 - Able to dress upper body without assistance if clothing is laid out or handed to the patient.
- ☐ 2 - Someone must help the patient put on upper body clothing.
- ☐ 3 - Patient depends entirely upon another person to dress the upper body.

(M0662) Current **Ability to Dress <u>Lower</u> Body** (with or without dressing aids) including undergarments, slacks, socks or nylons, shoes:

- ☐ 0 - Able to obtain, put on, and remove clothing and shoes without assistance.
- ☐ 1 - Able to dress lower body without assistance if clothing and shoes are laid out or handed to the patient.
- ☐ 2 - Someone must help the patient put on undergarments, slacks, socks or nylons, and shoes.
- ☐ 3 - Patient depends entirely upon another person to dress lower body.

(M0672) Bathing: Current ability to wash entire body <u>SAFELY</u>. **<u>Excludes</u> grooming (washing face and hands only).**

- ☐ 0 - Able to bathe self in <u>shower or tub</u> independently, including getting in and out of tub/shower.
- ☐ 1 - With the use of devices, is able to bathe self in shower or tub independently, including getting in and out of the tub/shower.
- ☐ 2 - Able to bathe in shower or tub with the assistance of another person:
  - (a) for intermittent supervision or encouragement or reminders, <u>OR</u>
  - (b) to get in and out of the shower or tub, <u>OR</u>
  - (c) for washing difficult to reach areas.
- ☐ 3 - Able to participate in bathing self in shower or tub, <u>but</u> requires presence of another person throughout the bath for assistance or supervision.
- ☐ 4 - Able to bath self independently or with the use of devices in chair, or on commode, but unable to use the shower or tub.
- ☐ 5 - Able to participate in bathing self in bed, bedside chair, or on commode, but requires presence of another person throughout the bath for assistance or supervision and is unable to use the shower or tub.
- ☐ 6 - Unable to effectively participate in bathing and is totally bathed by another person.

(M0682) Toilet Transferring: Current ability to get to and from the toilet or bedside commode <u>SAFELY</u>, including transferring on and off toilet/commode.

- ☐ 0 - Able to get to and from the toilet and transfer independently with or without a device.
- ☐ 1 - When reminded, assisted, or supervised by another person, able to get to and from the toilet and transfer.
- ☐ 2 - <u>Unable</u> to get to and from the toilet but is able to use a bedside commode (with or without assistance).
- ☐ 3 - <u>Unable</u> to get to and from the toilet or bedside commode but is able to use a bedpan/urinal independently.
- ☐ 4 - Is totally dependent in toileting.

(M0684) Toileting Hygiene: Current ability to maintain perineal hygiene, adjust clothes before and after using toilet, commode, bedpan, urinal. If managing ostomy, include wiping opening but not managing equipment.

- ☐ 0 - Able to manage toileting hygiene without assistance.
- ☐ 1 - Able to manage toileting without assistance if hygiene supplies/implements are laid out for the patient.
- ☐ 2 - Someone must help the patient to maintain hygiene or adjust clothing.
- ☐ 3 - Patient depends entirely upon another person to maintain toileting hygiene.

(M0692) Transferring: Current ability to move SAFELY from bed to chair, or ability to turn and position self in bed if patient is bedfast.

- ☐ 0 - Able to independently transfer.
- ☐ 1 - Able to transfer with minimal human assistance or with use of an assistive device.
- ☐ 2 - Unable to transfer self but is able to bear weight and pivot during the transfer process.
- ☐ 3 - Unable to transfer self and is unable to bear weight or pivot when transferred by another person.
- ☐ 4 - Bedfast, unable to transfer but is able to turn and position self in bed.
- ☐ 5 - Bedfast, unable to transfer and is unable to turn and position self.

(M0702) Ambulation/Locomotion: Ability to SAFELY walk, once in a standing position, or use a wheelchair, once in a seated position, on a variety of surfaces.

- ☐ 0 - Able to independently walk on even and uneven surfaces and climb stairs with or without railings (i.e., needs no human assistance or assistive device).
- ☐ 1 - With the use of a cane, able to independently walk on even and uneven surfaces and climb stairs with or without railings.
- ☐ 2 - Requires use of a walker or crutches to walk alone on a level surface or requires human supervision or assistance to negotiate stairs or steps or uneven surfaces.
- ☐ 3 - Able to walk only with the supervision or assistance of another person at all times.
- ☐ 4 - Chairfast, unable to ambulate but is able to wheel self independently.
- ☐ 5 - Chairfast, unable to ambulate and is unable to wheel self.
- ☐ 6 - Bedfast, unable to ambulate or be up in a chair.

(M0712) Feeding or Eating: Current ability to feed self meals and snacks. Note: This refers only to the process of eating, chewing, and swallowing, not preparing the food to be eaten.

- ☐ 0 - Able to independently feed self.
- ☐ 1 - Able to feed self independently but requires:
  - (a) meal set-up; OR
  - (b) intermittent assistance or supervision from another person; OR
  - (c) a liquid, pureed or ground meat diet.
- ☐ 2 - Unable to feed self and must be assisted or supervised throughout the meal/snack.
- ☐ 3 - Able to take in nutrients orally and receives supplemental nutrients through a nasogastric tube or gastrostomy.
- ☐ 4 - Unable to take in nutrients orally and is fed nutrients through a nasogastric tube or gastrostomy.
- ☐ 5 - Unable to take in nutrients orally or by tube feeding.

(M0715) Change in Mobility: Is the patient's ability to transferring and/or ambulate more impaired better or worse than it was before the onset of the illness or injury that initiated this episode of care?

- ☐ 0 – Patient at least as able to transfer and ambulate now as s/he was before the onset of the illness or injury that initiated this episode of care.
- ☐ 1 – Patient is less able to transfer and ambulate now than before the onset of the illness or injury that initiated this episode of care.
- ☐ UK – Unknown

(M0717) Change in Self-care Ability: Is the patient's ability to perform self-care activities (grooming, dressing, and bathing) better or worse than it was before the onset of the illness or injury that initiated this episode of care?

- ☐ 0 – Patient is at least as able to perform self-care activities now as s/he was before the onset of the illness or injury that initiated this episode of care.
- ☐ 1 – Patient is less able to perform self-care activities now than before the onset of the illness or injury that initiated this episode of care.
- ☐ UK – Unknown

(M0722) Current **Planning and Preparing Light Meals** (e.g., cereal, sandwich) or reheat delivered meals:

- ☐ 0 - (a) Able to independently plan and prepare all light meals for self or reheat delivered meals; OR
  (b) Is physically, cognitively, and mentally able to prepare light meals on a regular basis but has not routinely performed light meal preparation in the past (i.e., prior to this home care admission).
- ☐ 1 - Unable to prepare light meals on a regular basis due to physical, cognitive, or mental limitations.
- ☐ 2 - Unable to prepare any light meals or reheat any delivered meals.

(M0732 eliminated)

(M0742) Laundry: Current ability to do own laundry -- to carry laundry to and from washing machine, to use washer and dryer, to wash small items by hand.

- ☐ 0 - (a) Able to independently take care of all laundry tasks; OR
  (b) Physically, cognitively, and mentally able to do laundry and access facilities, but has not routinely performed laundry tasks in the past (i.e., prior to this home care admission).
- ☐ 1 - Able to do only light laundry, such as minor hand wash or light washer loads. Due to physical, cognitive, or mental limitations, needs assistance with heavy laundry such as carrying large loads of laundry.
- ☐ 2 - Unable to do any laundry due to physical limitation or needs continual supervision and assistance due to cognitive or mental limitation.

(M0752) Housekeeping: Current ability to safely and effectively perform light housekeeping and heavier cleaning tasks.

- ☐ 0 - (a) Able to independently perform all housekeeping tasks; OR
  (b) Physically, cognitively, and mentally able to perform all housekeeping tasks but has not routinely participated in housekeeping tasks in the past (i.e., prior to this home care admission).
- ☐ 1 - Able to perform only light housekeeping (e.g., dusting, wiping kitchen counters) tasks independently.
- ☐ 2 - Able to perform housekeeping tasks with intermittent assistance or supervision from another person.
- ☐ 3 - Unable to consistently perform any housekeeping tasks unless assisted by another person throughout the process.
- ☐ 4 - Unable to effectively participate in any housekeeping tasks.

(M0762) Shopping: Ability to plan for, select, and purchase items in a store and to carry them home or arrange delivery.

- ☐ 0 - (a) Able to plan for shopping needs and independently perform shopping tasks, including carrying packages; OR
  (b) Physically, cognitively, and mentally able to take care of shopping, but has not done shopping in the past (i.e., prior to this home care admission).
- ☐ 1 - Able to go shopping, but needs some assistance:
  (a) By self is able to do only light shopping and carry small packages, but needs someone to do occasional major shopping; OR
  (b) Unable to go shopping alone, but can go with someone to assist.
- ☐ 2 - Unable to go shopping, but is able to identify items needed, place orders, and arrange home delivery.
- ☐ 3 - Needs someone to do all shopping and errands.

(M0772) Ability to Use Telephone: Current ability to answer the phone, dial numbers, and effectively use the telephone to communicate.

- ☐ 0 - Able to dial numbers and answer calls appropriately and as desired.
- ☐ 1 - Able to use a specially adapted telephone (i.e., large numbers on the dial, teletype phone for the deaf) and call essential numbers.
- ☐ 2 - Able to answer the telephone and carry on a normal conversation but has difficulty with placing calls.
- ☐ 3 - Able to answer the telephone only some of the time or is able to carry on only a limited conversation.
- ☐ 4 - Unable to answer the telephone at all but can listen if assisted with equipment.
- ☐ 5 - Totally unable to use the telephone.
- ☐ NA - Patient does not have a telephone.

(M0775) Change in Ability to Perform Routine Household Tasks: Is the patient's ability to perform routine household tasks (light housekeeping, light meal preparation, laundry) better or worse now than it was before the onset of the illness or injury that initiated this episode of care?

- ☐ 0 – Patient is at least as able to perform routine household tasks now as s/he was before the onset of the illness or injury that initiated this episode of care.
- ☐ 1 – Patient is less able to perform routine household tasks now than before the onset of the illness or injury that initiated this episode of care.
- ☐ UK – Unknown

(M1140) Has this patient had a multi-factor **Fall Risk Assessment** (such as falls history, use of multiple medications, mental impairment, toileting frequency, general mobility/transferring impairment, environmental hazards)?

- ☐ 0 - Yes, and it does not indicate a moderate or high risk for falls. **(Skip Item M1150)**
- ☐ 1 - Yes, and it indicates a moderate or high risk for falls. **(Complete Item M1150)**
- ☐ 2 - No multi-factor falls risk assessment conducted. **(Skip Item M1150)**

(M1150) **Falls Risk Intervention:** Is intervention to mitigate the risk of falls included in the care plan for this home health episode of care?

- ☐ 0 - No
- ☐ 1 - Yes

Complete M1155 if previous falls risk assessment indicates the presence or significant risk factors for falls.

(M1155) **Falls Risk Intervention:** Have fall prevention steps been implemented for this home health episode of care?

- ☐ 0 - No
- ☐ 1 - Yes

MEDICATIONS

(M1160) **Potential Adverse Effects/Reaction:** Does a complete drug regimen review indicate potential clinically significant adverse effects or drug reactions, including ineffective drug therapy, side effects, drug interactions, duplicate therapy, omissions, dosage errors, or noncompliance?

- ☐ 0 - No **(Skip Item M1170)**
- ☐ 1 - Yes **(Complete Item M1170)**
- ☐ 2 - Not assessed **(Skip Item M1170)**

(M1170) **Medication Follow-up:** Was the patient's physician (or other primary care practitioner) contacted within one calendar day to resolve clinically significant medication issues?

- ☐ 0 - No
- ☐ 1 - Yes

(M1180) **Patient/Caregiver Drug Education:** Has the patient/caregiver been instructed to monitor the effectiveness of drug therapy and potential adverse effects, and how and when to report problems that may occur?

- ☐ 0 - No
- ☐ 1 - Yes

(M0782) **Management of Oral Medications:** Patient's current ability to prepare and take all prescribed oral medications reliably and safely, including administration of the correct dosage at the appropriate times/intervals. **Excludes injectable and IV medications. (NOTE: This refers to ability, not compliance or willingness.)**

- ☐ 0 - Able to independently take the correct oral medication(s) and proper dosage(s) at the correct times.
- ☐ 1 - Able to take medication(s) at the correct times if:
  - (a) individual dosages are prepared in advance by another person; OR
  - (b) given daily reminders; OR
  - (c) someone develops a drug diary or chart.
- ☐ 2 - Unable to take medication unless administered by someone else.
- ☐ NA - No oral medications prescribed.

(M0792) **Management of Inhalant/Mist Medications:** Patient's current ability to prepare and take all prescribed inhalant/mist medications (nebulizers, metered dose devices, oxygen) reliably and safely, including administration of the correct dosage at the appropriate times/intervals. **Excludes all other forms of medication (oral tablets, injectable and IV medications).**

- ☐ 0 - Able to independently take the correct medication and proper dosage at the correct times.
- ☐ 1 - Able to take medication at the correct times if:
  - (a) individual dosages are prepared in advance by another person, OR
  - (b) given daily reminders.
- ☐ 2 - Unable to take medication unless administered by someone else.
- ☐ NA - No inhalant/mist medications prescribed.

(M0802) Management of Injectable Medications: Patient's current ability to prepare and take all prescribed injectable medications reliably and safely, including administration of correct dosage at the appropriate times/intervals. **Excludes IV medications.**

- ☐ 0 - Able to independently take the correct medication and proper dosage at the correct times.
- ☐ 1 - Able to take injectable medication at correct times if:
  - (a) individual syringes are prepared in advance by another person, OR
  - (b) given daily reminders.
- ☐ 2 - Unable to take injectable medications unless administered by someone else.
- ☐ NA - No injectable medications prescribed.

(M0805) Change in Ability to Manage Oral, Inhalant, or Injectable Medications: Is the patient's ability to prepare and take all prescribed medications (oral and, if applicable, inhalant or injectable medications) reliably and safely (including administration of the correct dosage at the appropriate times/intervals.) better or worse than before the onset of the illness or injury that initiated this episode of care?

- ☐ 0 – Patient is at least as able to prepare and take all prescribed medications now than before the onset of the illness or injury that initiated this episode of care
- ☐ 1 – Patient is less able to prepare and take all prescribed medications now than before the onset of the illness or injury that initiated this episode of care
- ☐ UK – Unknown

EQUIPMENT MANAGEMENT

(M0810) Patient Management of Equipment (includes ONLY oxygen, IV/infusion therapy, enteral/parenteral nutrition equipment or supplies, ventilator therapy equipment or supplies): Patient's ability to set up, monitor and change equipment reliably and safely, add appropriate fluids or medication, clean/store/dispose of equipment or supplies using proper technique. **(NOTE: This refers to ability, not compliance or willingness.)**

- ☐ 0 - Patient manages all tasks related to equipment completely independently.
- ☐ 1 - If someone else sets up equipment (i.e., fills portable oxygen tank, provides patient with prepared solutions), patient is able to manage all other aspects of equipment.
- ☐ 2 - Patient requires considerable assistance from another person to manage equipment, but independently completes portions of the task.
- ☐ 3 - Patient is only able to monitor equipment (e.g., liter flow, fluid in bag) and must call someone else to manage the equipment.
- ☐ 4 - Patient is completely dependent on someone else to manage all equipment.
- ☐ NA - No equipment of this type used in care (skip deleted)

M0820 deleted; incorporated into M0822

(M0822) Type of Assistance needed Patient needs assistance with (check all that apply)		(M0823) Caregiver Assistance (If patient needs assistance, check one on each row)				
		Caregiver(s) provides	Caregiver(s) will need training and/or other supportive services	Caregiver(s) not likely to provide	Unclear if Caregiver(s) will provide	No Caregiver available
a. ☐	a. ADL assistance (e.g., transfer/ambulation, bathing, dressing, toileting, eating/feeding)	a1. ☐	a2. ☐	a3. ☐	a4. ☐	a5. ☐
b. ☐	b. IADL assistance (e.g., meals, housekeeping, laundry, telephone, shopping, finances)	b1. ☐	b2. ☐	b3. ☐	b4. ☐	b5. ☐
c. ☐	c. Medication administration (e.g., oral, inhaled or injectable)	c1. ☐	c2. ☐	c3. ☐	c4. ☐	c5. ☐
d. ☐	d. Medical procedures/ treatments (e.g., changing wound dressing)	d1. ☐	d2. ☐	d3. ☐	d4. ☐	d5. ☐
e. ☐	e. Management of Equipment (includes oxygen, IV/infusion equipment, enteral/parenteral nutrition, ventilator therapy equipment or supplies)	e1. ☐	e2. ☐	e3. ☐	e4. ☐	e5. ☐
f. ☐	f. Supervision and safety	f1. ☐	f2. ☐	f3. ☐	f4. ☐	f5. ☐
g. ☐	g. Advocacy or facilitation of patient's participation in appropriate medical care (includes transportation to or from appointments)	g1. ☐	g2. ☐	g3. ☐	g4. ☐	g5. ☐
h. ☐	h. None of the above					

(M0824) How Often does the patient receive **ADL or IADL assistance** from any caregiver(s) (other than home health agency staff)?

☐ 1 - At least daily
☐ 2 - Two or more times per week
☐ 3 - One to two times per week
☐ 4 - Less often than weekly
☐ UK - Unknown*

* at discharge, omit unknown response.

THERAPY NEED

(M0826) Therapy Need: In the home health plan of care for the Medicare payment episode for which this assessment will define a case mix group, what is the indicated need for therapy visits (total of reasonable and necessary physical, occupational, and speech-language pathology visits combined)? **(Enter zero ["000"] if no therapy visits indicated.)**

(_ _ _) Number of therapy visits indicated (total of physical, occupational and speech-language pathology combined).

☐ NA - Not Applicable: No case mix group defined by this assessment.

EMERGENT CARE

(M0831) Emergent Care: Since the last time OASIS data were collected, has the patient utilized a hospital emergency department (includes holding/observation with or without hospital admission)?

- ☐ 0 - No **[Go to *M0855*]**
- ☐ 1 - Yes
- ☐ UK - Unknown **[Go to *M0855*]**

(M0845) Reason for Emergent Care: For what reason(s) did the patient receive emergent care (with or without hospitalization)? **(Mark all that apply.)**

Options 19 and 20 eliminated and list renumbered

- ☐ 1 - Improper medication administration, medication side effects, toxicity, anaphylaxis
- ☐ 2 - Injury caused by fall or accident at home
- ☐ 3 - Respiratory infection (e.g. pneumonia, bronchitis)
- ☐ 3 - Other respiratory problem
- ☐ 5 - Heart failure (e.g., fluid overload)
- ☐ 6 - Cardiac dysrhythmia (irregular heartbeat)
- ☐ 7 - Myocardial infarction or chest pain
- ☐ 8 - Other heart disease
- ☐ 9 - Stroke (CVA) or TIA
- ☐ 10 - Hypo/Hyperglycemia, diabetes out of control
- ☐ 11 - Upper GI obstruction, constipation, impaction
- ☐ 12 - Dehydration, malnutrition
- ☐ 13 - Urinary tract infection
- ☐ 14 - IV catheter-related infection
- ☐ 15 - Wound infection or deterioration
- ☐ 16 - Uncontrolled pain
- ☐ 17 - Acute mental/behavioral health problem
- ☐ 18 - Deep vein thrombosis, pulmonary embolus
- ☐ 19 - Other than above reasons
- ☐ UK - Reason unknown

DATA ITEMS COLLECTED AT INPATIENT FACILITY ADMISSION OR AGENCY DISCHARGE ONLY

(M0855) To which **Inpatient Facility** has the patient been admitted?

- ☐ 1 - Hospital **[Go to *M0896*]**
- ☐ 2 - Rehabilitation facility **[Go to *M0903*]**
- ☐ 3 - Nursing home **[Go to *M0900*]**
- ☐ 4 - Hospice **[Go to *M0903*]**
- ☐ NA - No inpatient facility admission

(M0870) Discharge Disposition: Where is the patient after discharge from your agency? **(Choose only one answer.)**

- ☐ 1 - Patient remained in the community (not in hospital, nursing home, or rehab facility)
- ☐ 2 - Patient transferred to a non-institutional hospice (skip removed)
- ☐ 3 - Unknown because patient moved to a geographic location not served by this agency (skip removed)
- ☐ UK - Other unknown (skip removed)

[Go to *M0903*]

(M0890) If the patient was admitted to an acute care **Hospital**, for what **Reason** was he/she admitted?

- ☐ 1 - Hospitalization for <u>emergent</u> (unscheduled) care
- ☐ 2 - Hospitalization for <u>urgent</u> (scheduled within 24 hours of admission) care
- ☐ 3 - Hospitalization for <u>elective</u> (scheduled more than 24 hours before admission) care
- ☐ UK - Unknown

(M0896) **Reason for Hospitalization**: For what reason(s) did the patient require hospitalization? **(Mark all that apply.)**

Options 19 and 20 eliminated and list renumbered

- ☐ 1 - Improper medication administration, medication side effects, toxicity, anaphylaxis
- ☐ 2 - Injury caused by fall or accident at home
- ☐ 3 - Respiratory infection (e.g. pneumonia, bronchitis)
- ☐ 3 - Other respiratory problem
- ☐ 5 - Heart failure (e.g., fluid overload)
- ☐ 6 - Cardiac dysrhythmia (irregular heartbeat)
- ☐ 7 - Myocardial infarction or chest pain
- ☐ 8 - Other heart disease
- ☐ 9 - Stroke (CVA) or TIA
- ☐ 10 - Hypo/Hyperglycemia, diabetes out of control
- ☐ 11 - Upper GI obstruction, constipation, impaction
- ☐ 12 - Dehydration, malnutrition
- ☐ 13 - Urinary tract infection
- ☐ 14 - IV catheter-related infection
- ☐ 15 - Wound infection or deterioration
- ☐ 16 - Uncontrolled pain
- ☐ 17 - Acute mental/behavioral health problem
- ☐ 18 - Deep vein thrombosis, pulmonary embolus
- ☐ 19 - Scheduled treatment or procedure
- ☐ 20 - Other than above reasons
- ☐ UK - Reason unknown

Go to *M0903*

(M0900) For what **Reason(s)** was the patient **Admitted** to a **Nursing Home**? **(Mark all that apply.)**

- ☐ 1 - Therapy services
- ☐ 2 - Respite care
- ☐ 3 - Hospice care
- ☐ 4 - Permanent placement
- ☐ 5 - Unsafe for care at home
- ☐ 6 - Other
- ☐ UK - Unknown

(M0903) **Date of Last (Most Recent) Home Visit:**

__ __/__ __/__ __ __ __
month / day / year

(M0906) **Discharge/Transfer/Death Date:** Enter the date of the discharge, transfer, or death (at home) of the patient.

__ __/__ __/__ __ __ __
month / day / year

INDEX

Note: Entries followed by "b" indicate boxes; "f" figures; "t" tables.